The Economics of Health and Medical Care

Fifth Edition

Philip Jacobs, PhD
Professor
Department of Public Health Sciences
University of Alberta
Edmonton, Alberta, Canada

John Rapoport, PhD
Professor
Department of Economics
Mount Holyoke College
South Hadley, Massachusetts

JONES AND BARTLETT PUBLISHERS
Sudbury, Massachusetts
BOSTON   TORONTO   LONDON   SINGAPORE

World Headquarters

Jones and Bartlett Publishers
40 Tall Pine Drive
Sudbury, MA 01776
978-443-5000
info@jbpub.com
www.jbpub.com

Jones and Bartlett Publishers
Canada
6339 Ormindale Way
Mississauga, ON L5V 1J2
CANADA

Jones and Bartlett Publishers
International
Barb House, Barb Mews
London W6 7PA
UK

Jones and Bartlett's books and products are available through most bookstores and online booksellers. To contact Jones and Bartlett Publishers directly, call 800-832-0034, fax 978-443-8000, or visit our website at www.jbpub.com.

Substantial discounts on bulk quantities of Jones and Bartlett's publications are available to corporations, professional associations, and other qualified organizations. For details and specific discount information, contact the special sales department at Jones and Bartlett via the above contact information or send an email to special-sales@jbpub.com.

This publication is designed to provide accurate and authoritative information in regard to the Subject Matter covered. It is sold with the understanding that the publisher is not engaged in rendering legal, accounting, or other professional service. If legal advice or other expert assistance is required, the service of a competent professional person should be sought.

Production Credits
Chief Executive Officer: Clayton Jones
Chief Operating Officer: Don W. Jones, Jr.
Executive V.P. & Publisher: Robert W. Holland, Jr.
V.P., Sales and Marketing: William J. Kane
V.P., Design and Production: Anne Spencer
V.P., Manufacturing and Inventory Control: Therese Bräuer
Publisher—Aspen: Michael Brown
Associate Editor: Chambers Moore
Production Assistant: Carolyn F. Rogers
Production Specialist: Anda Aquino-Eisenberg
Manufacturing and Inventory Coordinator: Amy Bacus
Printing and Binding: Port City Press

ISBN-13: 978-0-7637-2595-2
ISBN-10: 0-7637-2595-1

6048

Printed in the United States of America
11 10 09 08 07   10 9 8 7 6 5 4 3 2

Table of Contents

Introduction **1**
    Three Major Tasks of Economics 2
    Tools Used In Economic Analysis. 3
    Outline of Contents 10
    How To Use This Book 12

PART I—DESCRIPTIVE ECONOMICS **15**

Chapter 1 — Output of the Health Care Sector **17**
    1.1 Introduction 17
    1.2 Medical Care 18
    1.3 Risk Shifting and Health Insurance 21
    1.4 Health Status. 23
    1.5 Consumption and Investment Output 30

Chapter 2 — Economic Dimensions of the Health Care System **35**
    2.1 Introduction 35
    2.2 Economic Units and Economic Flows 36
    2.3 Cost of Activities 44

PART II—EXPLANATORY ECONOMICS **53**

Chapter 3 — Demand for Medical Care: A Simple Model **55**
    3.1 The Concept of Demand 55
    3.2 Individual Demand: The Price-Quantity Relation 56
    3.3 Deriving the Demand Relationship 60
    3.4 Market Demand 64
    3.5 Measuring Quantity Responsiveness To Price Changes 64
    3.6 Insurance, Out-of-Pocket Price, and Quantity Demanded 69
    3.7 Elasticity of Demand Estimates 73

**Chapter 4 — Additional Topics in the Demand for Health and
    Medical Care** **80**
    4.1 Introduction 80

4.2   Implications of Health Care for Life and Health 81
4.3   External and Social Demand for Medical Care 82
4.4   Influence of Quality on the Demand for Medical Care 83
4.5   Time and Money Costs 84
4.6   The Demand for Health 85
4.7   Agency Theory and Supplier-Induced Demand 86

Chapter 5 — Health Care Production and Costs **96**
5.1   Introduction 96
5.2   Production: The Input-Output Relation 97
5.3   Short-Run Cost-Output Relations 103
5.4   Cost Curve Position 108
5.5   Economies of Scope 110
5.6   Long-Run Cost Curves 112
5.7   Empirical Estimation of Cost Curves 113

Chapter 6 — Behavior of Supply **126**
6.1   Introduction 126
6.2   A Model of Supply Behavior: An Individual For-Profit
      Company 127
6.3   Market Supply 134
6.4   Supply Behavior of Nonprofit Agencies: The Output
      Maximization Hypothesis 135
6.5   Supply Decisions Involving Quality 138
6.6   Supply Behavior of Nonprofit Agencies: The
      Administrator as Agent Model 140

Chapter 7 — Provider Payment **147**
7.1   Introduction 147
7.2   Principal-Agent Relationships Among Payers and Providers . . . 148
7.3   Physician Reimbursement 148
7.4   Hospital Reimbursement 153
7.5   Diagnosis-Related Groups 157
7.6   Long-Term Care Facility Reimbursement 160
7.7   Health Maintenance Organizations 161
7.8   Provider Supply under Managed Care 163

Chapter 8 — Competitive Markets **174**
8.1   Introduction 174
8.2   The Competitive Model: Assumptions 175
8.3   The Competitive Model: Predictions 176
8.4   Evidence for and against the Competitive Model 185
8.5   Competitive Bidding 188
8.6   Supplier-Induced Demand 190

Chapter 9 — Market Power in Health Care **202**
9.1   Introduction 202
9.2   Monopolistic Markets 203
9.3   Monopsony—Buyers' Market Power 210

   9.4 Market Structure and Its Determinants 212
   9.5 Nonprice Competition and Market Power 217

Chapter 10—Health Insurance **228**
   10.1 Introduction 228
   10.2 Demand for Health Insurance 229
   10.3 Supply of Health Insurance 239
   10.4 Adverse Selection in Health Insurance Markets 242

Chapter 11—The Labor Market **248**
   11.1 Introduction 248
   11.2 Demand for Labor 249
   11.3 Labor Supply 252
   11.4 The Competitive Labor Market 256
   11.5 Market Power in Labor Markets 259

PART III—EVALUATIVE ECONOMICS **267**

Chapter 12—Value Judgments and Economic Evaluation **269**
   12.1 Introduction 269
   12.2 Values and Standards in Economic Evaluation 270
   12.3 Efficient Output Levels 271
   12.4 Optimal Health Insurance 280
   12.5 Extra-Welfarism 281
   12.6 Concepts of Equity 283
   12.7 Goals of Health Policy 285

Chapter 13—Financing Health Care **291**
   13.1 Introduction 291
   13.2 Financing Means and Burdens in the United States 292
   13.3 Economic Analysis of Alternative Payment Sources 293
   13.4 The Incidence of Alternative Types of Health
        Care Financing 301
   13.5 The Administrative Cost of Alternative Types of
        Health Care Financing 304

Chapter 14—Public Health Insurance **307**
   14.1 Introduction 307
   14.2 Public Health Insurance 307
   14.3 Uncovered Care 313
   14.4 Some Trends in Public Health Insurance 314
   14.5 Goals of Medicare 317
   14.6 Policy Alternatives for Medicare 318
   14.7 Policy Alternatives for Medicaid 322

Chapter 15—Reform of the Health Care Market **330**
   15.1 Introduction 330
   15.2 Insurance Market Reform 331

15.3 Managed Care 338
15.4 Information and Consumer Choice 344

Chapter 16—Regulation and Antitrust Policy in Health Care **350**
Ronald P. Wilder
16.1 Introduction 350
16.2 Regulation of Health Care 352
16.3 Antitrust Policy 357

Chapter 17—Economic Evaluation of Health Services **374**
17.1 Introduction 374
17.2 The Purposes of Economic Evaluation 375
17.3 Selecting the Right Type of Analysis 375
17.4 Guidelines for Conducting a Cost-Effectiveness Analysis 376
17.5 Cost-Benefit Analysis 386

Appendix A—Glossary of Health Economics Terms **395**

Appendix B—Answers to Odd-Numbered Questions **415**

Index **425**

Introduction

This book is an introduction to the economic approach to understanding health care problems. Our approach is based on the identification of scarcity as a major cause of many of today's health care problems. Scarcity can be defined as a deficiency in the quantity or quality of available goods and services as compared with the amounts that people desire. Perhaps the most glaring deficiency in the United States today is the lack of health insurance coverage on the part of roughly 40 million people, many of whom consequently have difficulty obtaining adequate care, especially primary care. Although there are others as well who have inadequate access to care, the size of the uninsured population has become a bellwether of the access problems in the U.S. health care system.

Yet the fundamental difficulty is not merely that there is "not enough" to go around. Side by side with problems of scarcity are problems of "too much." In 1998 total expenditures on health care in the United States reached over $1.1 trillion, over 13.5 percent of the gross national product (GNP), the dollar sum of all final goods and services produced. In 1965, health care expenditures were only 5.6 percent of the GNP. Included in these expenditures are high-cost services whose impact on health has been questioned, including large-volume "little ticket" items, such as radiographs and lab tests, which make up about a quarter of all hospital costs (Angell 1985); high-cost procedures, such as coronary artery bypass grafting and transplants, costly intensive care services, and new drugs, whose effectiveness is often still undocumented; and some hospital services for the terminally ill, which consume a disproportionate share of the health care dollar (Zook and Moore 1980; Long et al. 1984). A number of commentators have asserted that a considerable amount of "flat of the curve" medicine, that is, medical care that produces little or no improvement in health, is being practiced (Enthoven 1980). Accusations of "too much," when uttered side by side with cries of "not enough," point to the importance of studying the entire resource allocation process in health care.

Economics is the science that deals with the consequences of resource scarcity, and health economics deals with the consequences of resource scarcity in the health care industry. Because of its very broad scope, economics does not provide a body of rigid doctrines about scarce resources. Rather, economics offers an overall viewpoint intended to help in understanding the many problems related to various types of scarcity.

This book focuses on how to *do* economics; that is, how to think about economic problems in a systematic way. It divides the discipline into three separate areas, which can be regarded as the three main tasks of economics: description, explanation, and evaluation. The exposition of these tasks in a health context is the objective of this book; the performance of these tasks should be regarded as the objective of the reader.

Accomplishing the tasks involves asking specific questions and searching for answers to them. It should be stressed that searching for relevant questions is as critical a part of the process of analyzing economic problems as searching for answers. By formulating a problem in the context of scarcity, a deeper understanding of it can be obtained, and discovery of a solution or a means of accommodation might be the end result.

THREE MAJOR TASKS OF ECONOMICS

The three major tasks of economics covered in this book—description, explanation, and evaluation—will usually not be performed in isolation from one another. Rather, descriptive economics will be used to complement explanations and evaluations of events. But even though these tasks may be intermingled in economic analysis, the specific task being performed should be kept clearly in mind.

Descriptive Economics

Description involves the identification, definition, and measurement of phenomena. By performing this task, we obtain some notion of the existing facts. It should be pointed out that this task basically amounts to fact-finding. There is, at this stage, no explanation of why the facts are what they are and no evaluative pronouncement or judgment. Of course, the selection of which phenomena to describe is usually motivated by an ultimate explanatory or evaluative purpose.

The statement that, for example, in 1992 Americans 65 years and older visited physicians' offices on the average of 5.5 times per year while those in the 15- to 44-year-old age group paid 2.5 visits per year (U.S. Department of Health and Human Services, 1995, 173) falls within the realm of description.

Explanatory Economics

The second task of economics is explaining and predicting certain phenomena. This task involves conducting a cause-and-effect analysis. In undertaking such a task, we are moving one step beyond description; we are now identifying the causes of certain events that have occurred. This task is performed with the aid of models that classify various causal factors (assuming there is more than one) in a systematic framework. Based on this framework, hypotheses are developed about the net effect of each causal factor on the phenomena we want to explain. We do not do any further analysis at this stage. That is, we do not pass judgment on whether the phenomena we have observed are present in the desired amounts.

As an example of an explanation, suppose we want to determine why those in the 65-year-old and above age group utilized more medical care than those in the 15- to 44-year-old age group. First, we would develop a framework that incorporates the major causal factors relevant to this phenomenon. Let us say that our framework contains two essential causal factors: (1) the health status of each group and (2) the price paid by the members of each group for their medical care. Using these causal factors, we might then hypothesize that quantity of medical care demanded will increase when health status is lowered and when consumers pay less for their medical care. These causal factors relate to our example because (1) the health status of the older group is lower and (2) government-sponsored health insurance for the elderly reduces the amount the older group pays for medical care. Assuming these facts to be true, our hypothesis would predict that the older group will demand medical care in greater quantities. Should these increased quantities also be available, then the older group will utilize more medical care.

Evaluative Economics

The third task of economics is evaluation. This task involves judging or ranking alternative phenomena according to some standard. An acceptable standard is first chosen, then used to rank alternative ways of distributing scarce resources. In choosing the standard, one major criterion is acceptability. Standards are easy to come by; however, many are controversial, and the standard chosen should have some degree of acceptability.

Using the standard, alternative quantities of economic variables—that is, alternative uses of scarce resources—can be evaluated. For example, if we choose a standard that says that the more medical care one has the better off one is, then, according to this standard, the older group in our example is better off than the younger group. Furthermore, any measure that raises the utilization of the younger group (by lowering the price paid by this group and by increasing the resources available for use by this group) would, according to our standard, improve the well-being of the younger group (Hemenway 1982).

TOOLS USED IN ECONOMIC ANALYSIS

Several tools are used in economic analysis. One general tool is graphic analysis. The purpose of graphic analysis is to illustrate relations between economic variables. Also helpful are models that allow us to draw inferences about the relations we might expect to occur when specific underlying conditions are present. Such tools help us to be explicit about the underlying factors that are present in the workings of the resource-allocation process.

Economic Variables

An economic variable is an economically relevant phenomenon whose value or magnitude may vary. Examples of economic variables include prices, costs, incomes, and quantities of commodities. An economic variable can be measured along a scale once appropriate units of measurement have been chosen. For example, price can be measured in cents or dollars per unit, and quantities can be expressed in terms of number of visits, number of hospital days, number of hospital beds, and so on. Two examples of units of measurement are shown in Figure I–1. Along the vertical axis, values of the price of medical care are shown. The price per visit to a physician, which is the economic variable being examined, is expressed in terms of cents. Along this axis, the price can be 0, 100, 200, 300, and so on. Along

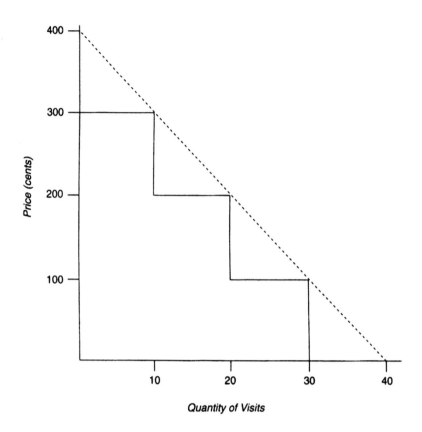

Figure I-1 Relation between price and quantity of visits. The dashed line shows continuous values, and the solid line shows discrete values.

the horizontal axis are alternative values of the quantity of visits to a physician's office. These are measured in terms of number of visits.

Relations between Economic Variables

The next step after the identification and measurement of economic variables is to determine the relations between these variables. The relations show how one variable changes with respect to another variable.

These relations can be causal or noncausal. For example, we can state that one variable (total health care costs) has increased while another variable (time) has also increased. This is an example of a noncausal relation, because it is not time itself that has caused the costs to increase. As time has passed, other influencing variables have changed, and these have caused the health care costs to increase.

In a causal relation, when the value of one economic variable changes, the value of a second economic variable also changes as a result. For example, if the price falls for a visit to the doctor, the lower price causes more visits to be demanded. Causal relations are usually expressed in the form of hypothetical statements (e.g., "If price falls, then the quantity demanded will increase").

Graphic Representation of Relations

Let us start with a simple relation between price and quantity of visits: When the price is 400 cents, the quantity of visits is 0; when the price is 300, the quantity of visits is 10; when the price is 200, the quantity of visits is 20; and when the price is 100, the quantity of visits is 30. Associated with each price is a specific quantity: 0 visits with 400 cents, 10 visits with 300 cents, and so on. Each of the associations can be represented by a point, as shown in Figure I–1. All these points together form the relation. If we knew only these values, we could draw this relation diagrammatically as the solid line in Figure I–1. This solid line is known as a step function and relates only to the values specified. However, we could go further and generalize about the nature of our function by saying that the values between 0 and 100 cents (or 100 and 200 cents) and between 0 and 10 visits (or 10 and 20 visits) could also be specified as part of the relation. We could draw a continuous curve joining all the points specified in the relation in order to represent the values not explicitly expressed, such as 155 cents, 5 visits, and so on (consider the dashed line in Figure I–1). Once we have drawn a continuous curve, we have a more complete specification of the relation between price and quantity. Any value of price, within our specified ranges, has an associated quantity of visits.

The Direction of Relations

We can now be more specific about the nature of the relation between the two variables. The first characteristic to be examined is the direction of the relation. A relation can have four possible directions, as shown in Figure I–2. First, the relation may be positive, as shown by curve *B*. Here higher values of price are associated with higher values of quantity of visits. If there was a causal relation between them, and if the direction of causation ran from price to quantity, we would hypothesize that, as price increases, so does quantity. The opposite type of relation is shown by curve *D*. The relation is a negative: the greater the price, the smaller the quantity. Thus higher values of price are associated with lower values of quantity of visits. The remaining cases show where variables are unrelated. For curve *C*, whatever the quantity of visits, the price stays the same (i.e., 200 cents). Curve *A* shows that, whatever the price may be, the quantity of visits will remain the same (i.e., 30 visits).

The Slope of Relations

The slope of a geometric relation shows how much of a change in one variable is associated with a given change in a related variable. In causal terms, slope can be expressed as the magnitude of response. Several examples are shown in Figure I–3.

Curve *F* touches the price axis where the price equals 200 cents. This price is associated with a quantity of visits of 0. If we raise the price by 50 cents to a level of 250 cents, the associated new quantity of visits, as shown by *F*, is 10. A 50-cent increase in the price is associated with a 10-visit increase in quantity. The slope of *F* is thus 50/10 with regard to the quantity axis (or 10/50 with regard to the price axis). Because *F* is a straight line, the slope remains constant at every point on the line. (Some nonlinear relations are presented later.)

Relation *E* also has a positive slope. As can be seen in Figure I–3, *E* shows a greater change in price associated with a given change in quantity than does *F*. From the

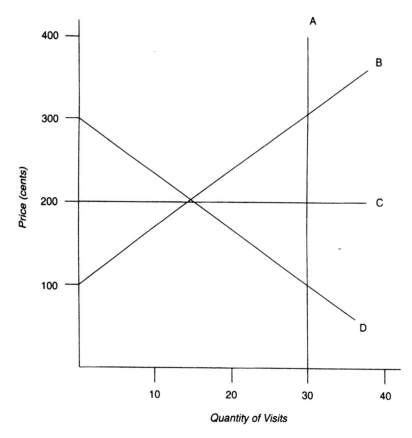

Figure I–2 Direction of relations: curve *A*, constant quantity of visits for all prices; curve *B*, price and quantity positively related; curve *C*, constant price; and curve *D*, price and quantity negatively related.

initial price of 200 cents and 0 visits, a quantity change of 10 visits is associated with a price change from 200 to 300 cents. The slope is thus 100/10 with regard to the quantity axis (or 10/100 with regard to the price axis). Comparing *E* and *F*, we can say that for the same quantity change, the price change in *E* must be double that in *F*.

Relations *G* and *H* can be regarded in a similar manner, but now the direction of these relations is such that a higher price is associated with a lower quantity. In relation *G*, a fall in price of 50 cents is associated with an increase in quantity of 10 visits. The slope is thus the same as the slope of *F* but in the opposite direction. Relation *H* shows a change in price of 100 associated with a quantity change of 10—the same as relation *E*, except the slope is in the opposite direction. Where the two variables change in the same direction (as occurs in curves *E* and *F*), the slope is considered to be positive; where the change is in the opposite direction (as occurs in curves *G* and *H*), the slope is considered to be negative.

The Position of Relations

The next characteristic of a relation is its position. In Figure I–4, two relations, *J* and *K*, are shown with similar slopes but different positions. Each relation exhibits

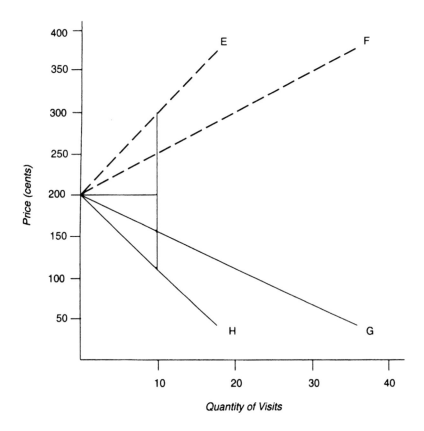

Figure I–3 Slope of relations. In relation *E*, the price increases more than in relation *F* for a given increase in quantity. In relation *H*, the price decreases more than in relation *G* for a given increase in quantity.

a 100-cent change in price associated with a change of 10 visits. Relation *J* shows no visits at a price of 300 cents, 10 visits at a price of 200, and so on. By comparison, *K* shows 10 visits at a price of 300 cents, 20 visits at a price of 200, and so on. The essential point of this figure is to show how the two relations are positioned with respect to each other. Relation *K* is higher than *J* in the sense that, at any specific price, the related quantity of visits for *K* is greater than the related quantity for *J*.

The Shape of Relations

The examples so far have involved only linear relations, in which the change in one variable with regard to a given change in another variable is fixed. This is not the only type of relation, however. Sometimes we also encounter nonlinear relations. For this type of relation, the magnitude of the response will vary along the curve. Relations *L* and *M* in Figure I–5 are both nonlinear relations.

M indicates the correspondence between the total cost of production of lab tests and the number of tests produced. At a quantity of 0, the total cost is $10; at a

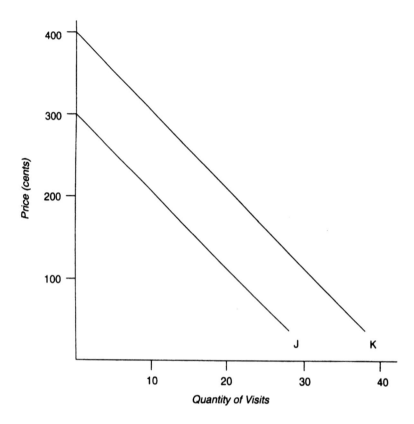

Figure I–4 Position of relations. *K* shows a greater quantity of visits than *J* for any given price.

quantity of 1, it is $11; at a quantity of 2, it is $14; and at a quantity of 3, it is $19. The slope of the relation changes as more lab tests are produced. For the first test, the slope is such that a $1 change in cost is associated with a change of one lab test. The next change of one lab test is associated with a $3 change in cost, and the next with a $5 change in cost. The slope with reference to the lab test axis increases as the number of lab tests increases. *M* is a smoothed-out version of this relation.

Relation *L* shows declining slopes with increasing production. A total cost of 0 is associated with a 0 level of output. An output level of 1 is associated with a cost of $5, an output level of 2 is associated with a cost of $8, and an output level of 3 is associated with a cost of $9. The slope of the relation between 0 and 1 units of production, with regard to the production axis, is 5/1; for the next unit of production, it is 3/1; and for the next it is 1/1.

The Nature of Economic Propositions

Many statements in this book regarding the resource allocation process in the health care field are basically attempts to spell out the consequences of certain conditions. The propositions are hypothetical statements of the form "if . . . then . . . "

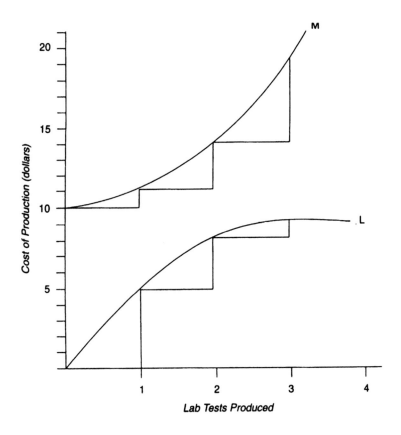

Figure I-5 Shape of relations. *M* shows higher additional costs at successively higher levels of lab tests produced. *L* shows lower additional costs at successively higher levels of tests.

For example, we might claim that if certain conditions *x*, *y*, and *z* hold, then, as a consequence, phenomenon *q* will occur. In making this statement, we essentially make a prediction of what will cause the phenomenon we want to explain. The "if" portions of these statements are called *conditions* or *assumptions;* the "then" portions are *conclusions, implications,* or *predictions.*

As an example, let us form a model to explain how much medical care an individual will demand. Our model contains initial assumptions. The first, A1, is that the price of medical care charged to an individual is $5 per visit; this $5 includes all services provided by the doctor, including transfusions, intravenous feedings (should they be needed), and so on. The second assumption, A2, states that the individual has a weekly income of $100 that can be spent on any of a number of commodities. This assumption brings the example within the realm of economics, since scarcity is now introduced. The third assumption, A3, is about the behavior of the individual; the individual has as an objective the consumption of medical care only; he does not want to consume any other commodity. We also assume that this is entirely feasible. If the individual does not consume food, for example, he would begin to starve and have to visit a physician, where, for a fee of $5, he could receive nutrition intravenously.

What are the implications of these assumptions? The main implication is that the individual will consume 20 physician's office visits. Given his economic situation, this is all he can afford to consume, and given that he wants only medical care and can survive by consuming this commodity, then he will not consume less than 20 visits. This implication is a prediction of our model; the prediction is based on the initial conditions or assumptions of the model. Predictions are derivatives of the assumptions and can be regarded as the consequences that would result if the assumptions were to hold.

Let us now replace one of our initial assumptions, A1, with the assumption that the price of medical care is $1 per visit. Now our model implies that the quantity of visits will be 100. With a fall in price, the quantity demanded will increase. This is a prediction of our model when we consider all the assumptions and do a comparative analysis.

We can also predict the consequences that would result if the individual's income increases. Suppose we replace assumption A2 with the assumption that the individual's weekly income is $110. This new assumption, coupled with the original assumptions A1 and A3, yields the conclusion that the quantity of visits demanded will increase. By performing a comparative analysis of the original conditions and the new conditions, we can conclude that an increase in income will lead to an increase in the quantity of medical care demanded.

The mere predicting or deriving conclusions about the resource allocation process is not the end of our task, however. Our conclusions are implications about what would result if the assumptions we have posited in the model are adequate approximations of the conditions that exist in reality. In explanatory economics, implications are tested against actual data to see if what we predicted actually does occur. The true test of an explanatory model is how well it explains or predicts actual phenomena. In evaluative economics, our task is somewhat different: we compare actual against ideal sets of events. Nevertheless, whether we are deriving explanatory or evaluative principles, we put our propositions into a logical form that allows us to incorporate a number of variables into our analysis simultaneously.

OUTLINE OF CONTENTS

This book introduces the analysis of health care economics in the context of the three tasks mentioned above: description, explanation, and evaluation. Part I, which consists of Chapters 1 and 2, describes the economic dimensions of the health care field. Part II, consisting of Chapters 3–11, presents explanatory analyses of a number of health-related issues. Part III, which consists of Chapters 12–17, develops evaluative analyses of several important aspects of health care resource use. The analyses in the book focus on three distinct markets: the medical care market, the health insurance market, and the labor market. Throughout the book, tools are developed to analyze the economic behavior of all three markets.

Chapter 1 contains a discussion of the output of the health care sector. Three types of output are identified: (1) health care, which consists of activities designed to improve health; (2) health itself; and (3) health insurance coverage. (Types of input, such as the hiring of health care personnel, are also discussed.) Measurements of each type of output are presented. In Chapter 2, economic dimensions of the health care sector are identified and some measures of these dimensions are presented. In particular, economic flows of the various components of the health care system are described, and the concept of cost is analyzed.

Chapter 3, the first explanatory chapter, develops a model to explain the demand for medical care by consumers. A number of separate factors are identified as influences on the demand for medical care. These are incorporated into a single model that allows us to predict the effects of each factor when all other relevant factors are held constant. In this chapter, the demand for medical care is presented as if medical care were an ordinary commodity in the consumer's budget.

However, medical care has characteristics that combine to warrant special treatment. These include the importance of medical care in influencing health status, uncertainty when illness occurs, people's concern about others' health status and health care consumption, and the asymmetry in the medical knowledge possessed by providers and consumers. In Chapter 4, a number of these characteristics are introduced and analyzed in light of the standard model developed in Chapter 3.

Chapters 5–7 focus on the behavior of health care providers, such as physicians, hospitals, and laboratories. Chapter 5 discusses the relationships between resource use and output, quality of care and output, and cost of care and output. All these relationships are examined with regard to each individual provider. Chapter 6 presents an analysis of the supply behavior of individual providers and of groups of providers (i.e., market supply). The behavior of for-profit providers and the behavior of nonprofit providers are treated separately, since nonprofit and government providers play such an important role in the health care field. The chapter also considers a model of the supply behavior of health insurers as well as a model of the demand for labor (which is based on the supply model). Chapter 7 deals with one important aspect of supply analysis—provider reimbursement. In health care there are many examples of providers being paid by a third party (an insurer or the government). The important economic concept of the principal-agent relationship is introduced and is used to analyze alternative payment schemes for physicians, hospitals, long-term care providers, and health maintenance organizations.

Chapter 8 examines a standard textbook explanation of how the market resource allocation process works. This is the competitive market model, which has drawn a good deal of attention recently. Included in this chapter is an exposition of a phenomenon that has received considerable attention in health economics: supplier-induced demand. Not all market behavior is competitive. Chapter 9 looks at the concept of market power: how it is acquired by suppliers and demanders and how its acquisition affects market phenomena (e.g., prices and quantity and quality of output).

Chapters 10 and 11 consider two types of markets whose functioning is closely tied to health care. Chapter 10 describes the market for health insurance, and Chapter 11 presents an analysis of the labor market and of several variants of this market that are associated with health care.

The third part of the book focuses on evaluation and health policy issues. Chapter 12 introduces the topic of evaluation by identifying several alternative standards that have been used in evaluating resource use in the health care field. These standards include efficiency and equity. Two frameworks used to evaluate efficiency are presented: the narrower efficiency framework and the broader "extra-welfarist" framework. A set of specific goals for the health care system are derived from these welfare analyses.

Chapter 13 discusses alternative types of health care finance: out-of-pocket reimbursement, health insurance, and taxation. It uses economic models to identify the burden of each type.

Chapter 14 discusses two major public insurance programs, Medicare and Medicaid. It presents specific policy problems and, using the explanatory economic models developed in Chapters 3–11, evaluates the effects of policy measures in light of specific policy goals.

Chapter 15 focuses on methods to reform health insurance and health care markets. It discusses various proposals for restructuring the health insurance market so that the preferred risk selection of the health insurers might discriminate less against high-risk individuals, thereby increasing the equity of these markets. Chapter 15 also introduces the emerging concept of "consumerism."

The role of government policy in influencing the performance of the health care market is the topic of Chapter 16. Two views of regulation are presented there. According to the first, the public-interest approach, the government establishes regulations to ensure that providers act in the public interest. Evidence of the effectiveness of this approach has not been very convincing. The second view of regulation is based on a wider picture of the market. According to this view, the government is a participant in a marketplace that encompasses both the suppliers and demanders of the traded product as well as politicians and regulators. In this marketplace, various regulations and laws that have an impact on the supply-demand situation are "traded." The market outcome is thus influenced by regulation. Faced with discontent over the results of traditional market regulation, some observers have proposed that the medical market should be reshaped in the competitive mold. Also included in Chapter 16 is an analysis of anti-trust regulation, a topic of considerable policy interest in recent years.

There is a great deal of controversy over whether health care markets can ensure that health care is delivered efficiently to consumers. One way to study this issue is to gauge whether specific interventions improve health status in an efficient way. Cost-benefit and cost-effectiveness analyses are two techniques by which we can judge the economic impact of various interventions and policies on health status. Chapter 17 offers an introduction to these tools.

HOW TO USE THIS BOOK

There is a considerable amount of material in this book, much more than would be included in a typical introductory course in health care economics. As a rough guide, a typical student without any prior economics background should be able to cover a chapter a week. In a 14-week course, perhaps 13 chapters could be covered comfortably. Although more advanced students could handle more, instructors will probably want to be selective in covering the subjects.

The book could be used as the main text for a basic health care economics course for public health students and for a similar course in which the emphasis is more on health policy and finance. Our suggestions for coverage in each kind of course are listed below.

At the end of each chapter we have provided a set of questions and problems. The student is encouraged to work through these problems, as it is easier to learn and retain the material by doing actual problems and testing yourself. At the end of the book we provide the answers to every second problem. The answers to the other problems are contained in the instructor's manual.

Orientation	Chapters
Public health	1–6, 8, 9, 11–14, 17
Health finance and policy	1–10, 12, 13, 15, 16

BIBLIOGRAPHY

Aaron, H.J., and W.B. Schwartz. 1984. *The painful prescription*. Washington, DC: Brookings Institution.

———. 1990. Rationing health care. *Science* 247:418–422.

Angell, M. 1985. Cost containment and the physician. *JAMA* 253:1203–1207.

Arrow, K.H. 1972. Problems of resource allocation in United States medical care. In *The challenge of life*, ed. R.M. Kunz and H. Fehr. Basel: Birkhauser-Verlag.

Culyer, A.J., and J.P. Newhouse. 2000. *Handbook of health economics*. Vol. 1a and 1b. Amsterdam: Elsevier Publishers.

Earl-Slater, A. 1999. *Dictionary of health economics*. Abingdon, England: Radcliffe Medical Press.

Enthoven, A.C. 1980. *Health plan*. Reading, MA: Addison-Wesley.

Evans, R.G. 1984. *Strained mercy*. Toronto: Butterworths.

Feldstein, P.J. 1999. *Health economics*. 5th ed. Albany: Delmar Publishers.

Folland, S., et al. 2000. *Economics of health and health care*. New York: Prentice Hall.

Fuchs, V. 1974. *Who shall live?* New York: Basic Books.

Getzen, T.E. 1997. *Health economics*. New York: John Wiley.

Hemenway, D. 1982. The optimal location of doctors. *New England Journal of Medicine* 306:397–401.

Jack, W.P. 1999. *Principles of health economics for developing countries*. Washington, DC: World Bank.

Littenberg, B., and D. Newhauser. 1981. To hell with economics? *American Journal of Public Health* 71:363–365.

Long, S.H., et al. 1984. Medical expenditures of terminal cancer patients during the last year of life. *Inquiry* 21:315–327.

Mooney, G.H. 1994. *Key issues in health economics*. New York: Harvester Wheatsheaf.

Mooney, G.H., et al.1986. *Choices for care*. 2nd ed. London: MacMillan Press.

Reinhardt, U. 1985. Future trends in the economics of medical practice and care. *American Journal of Cardiology* 56:50C–58C.

———. 1987. Resource allocation in health care. *Milbank Quarterly* 65:153–176.

Senterre, R.E., and S.P. Neun. 2000. *Health economics*. Orlando, FL: Dryden Press.

U.S. Department of Health and Human Services. 1995. *Health United States, 1994*. Hyattsville, MD: U.S. Department of Health and Human Services, Public Health Service.

Weisbrod, B. 1975. Research in health economics: A survey. *International Journal of Health Services* 5:643–661.

———. 1991. The health care quadrilemma: An essay on technological change, insurance, quality of care, and cost containment. *Journal of Economic Literature* 29:523–552.

Zook, C., and F.D. Moore.1980. High cost users of medical care. *New England Journal of Medicine* 302:996–1002.

Part I

Descriptive Economics

Chapter 1

Output of the
Health Care Sector

1. Describe the product *medical care* and its components.
2. Define the concepts of *risk* and *risk shifting* and show why they are relevant to medical care.
3. Describe health care and its components.
4. Describe the concept of *health outcome*.
5. Explain the theoretical relationship between health and medical care and demonstrate the meaning of the term *flat-of-the-curve medicine*.

1.1 INTRODUCTION

In this chapter we introduce the descriptive elements in the study of the health care system. This involves identifying the phenomena with which we are concerned, defining them so we can know their nature precisely, and measuring them so we can obtain an understanding of their magnitude. At this stage, we only wish to discover what phenomena exist, not what causes them (explanation) or in what quantities they should exist (evaluation).

The processes generated within the health care system can be looked at in two ways. The first approach is to directly examine factors that influence health. These health-influencing factors can be classified as lifestyle elements, such as diet, sleep, and other individual behaviors; environmental factors, such as air and water purification; genetic factors; and medical care, such as examinations and treatments. Section 1.2 focuses on the definition and measurement of medical care. It identifies and defines the phenomena associated with medical care and discusses measures that indicate how much medical care is provided. Section 1.3 describes another aspect of the health care system: risk shifting. Because most medical expenditures do not occur with certainty, individuals will place a value on buying insurance to cover possible losses. Risk shifting provides benefits to consumers and is an important output of the health care sector.

The second approach stems from the assertion that the true end of the health care sector is not the care itself but rather the health that results from this care. When measuring the output of health care, according to this approach, we should be measuring how much health is being produced. If we feel that the volume of medical care provided is not necessarily a good indicator of the benefits provided, a more fundamental approach would be to measure what medical care is ideally supposed to produce, that is, health. Section 1.4 examines issues of definition and measurement associated with health.

Section 1.5 focuses on the output of the health care system derived from the education of health care personnel. The health care system includes the training of the professionals who work within the system, and these individuals will produce output (health care) during their training and after it is completed. In economic terms, the output of the production process is called "human capital."

1.2 MEDICAL CARE

Medical care is a process in which certain inputs or factors of production (e.g., health care provider services, medical instrument and equipment services, and pharmaceuticals) are combined in varying quantities, usually under a physician's supervision, to yield an output. An individual visiting a physician's office receives an examination involving the services of the physician or a nurse practitioner, nurse, or medical technician and the use of some equipment. The inputs vary from one visit to another. One patient may receive more friendly treatment than another, and health care providers vary in their thoroughness, knowledge, and technique. Thus the quality of one visit may differ considerably from the quality of another.

Much of the difficulty in measuring the medical care process stems from the issue of quality. If we measure physician care by the number of patient visits to a physician's office, two cursory examinations count as two visits. But one cursory examination followed by a thorough examination involving a battery of tests also counts as two visits, even though more medical care was provided.

It should be stressed that *quality* is a very broad term and its meaning is elusive (Donabedian 1988). For example, organizations providing medical care can have substantially different characteristics. To begin with, they can differ in terms of structure, that is, the amount and type of training of the care providers and the type of medical equipment used. Further, differences in structure are associated with the use of different techniques in the provision of care. For example, a computerized axial tomography (CAT) scan machine that takes cross-sectional radiographs is generally considered to provide a higher-quality product than a standard radiology machine (Sisk et al. 1990). A second aspect of the quality of care involves the process of providing care, in particular, the amount of personal attention providers devote to consumers. Examples of quality-of-care measures that reflect the degree of personal attention given to consumers include the volume of services performed per individual and patient evaluations of physician performance.

Another set of characteristics is associated with outcomes, that is, with the accuracy of diagnoses and the effectiveness of treatments in producing health. Examples of measures reflecting this set of characteristics include hospital mortality rates adjusted for patient condition and the rates of other adverse events in hospitals, such as postsurgical infections.

All the above characteristics, as well as others, have been identified as aspects of quality. The challenge of measuring quality, then, derives from the fact that there are many ways of viewing quality—many different ideas as to what constitutes quality. For this reason, the raw measure "visits" should be only guardedly used as a measure of physician care.

The measurement of hospital care requires the same caution. Hospital output has frequently been measured by bed days or by the number of cases admitted to the hospital. Over time, however, the typical admitted patient receives a greater intensity of services as a result of advances in technology. To count an admission in 1965 as having the same output as an admission in 1996 (given the type of case) would be to neglect the greater intensity of services likely to be provided at the later date.

Despite these objections, physician visits as a measure of the output of medical care and hospital admissions or bed days as a measure of the output of hospital care have frequently been used because of their immediate availability. Recently, efforts have been made to develop additional measures that incorporate the changing quality of inputs per admission or per bed day.

Output measurements are usually conducted to make comparisons, either against other output measures or against some standard. There are two types of output comparisons: time series and cross-sectional comparisons. A time series comparison measures the output of the same commodity at different times. A cross-sectional comparison measures the output of the commodity among different groups at the same time (e.g., the medical care provided to consumers in different age groups, ethnic groups, or geographic areas or with different diagnoses).

Medical care output can be measured at three sources:

1. The providers can be surveyed to determine how much medical care they have produced.
2. The payers for medical care can be surveyed to determine how much medical care they have paid for.
3. The consumers can be surveyed to determine the quantity of consumption.

With perfect measurement, all three sources will yield the same results; however, because of measurement difficulties, considerable differences will arise. A continuing source of data on medical care received by consumers is the National Health Interview Survey, an annual nationwide sample survey of households on health-related matters compiled for the U.S. Public Health Service. Much of the information from this survey is summarized in the Public Health Service's annual compendium of health-related data, *Health United States*.

The National Health Interview Survey is also the major source of data on medical care administered by physicians outside the hospital; this care is measured by the number of visits to physicians (the numbers of visits are often adjusted for the size of the relevant populations to yield utilization rates), with utilization defined as the amount of services consumed. As an illustration of the use of time series data, comparisons were made of physician's office visits per year for individuals in the 65 and over age group. For this group, visits per person were 4.5 in 1975, also 4.5 in 1985, and 5.3 in 1995. These numbers indicate that there was no increase in the output of physician office care for this group between 1975 and 1985 but that a marked increase did occur in the following decade (see U.S. Department of Health and Human Services, *Health United States*, 1994 and 1999). Also, one visit in 1975 was counted as the equivalent of one visit in 1995 because quality-difference adjustments were not made. It is very likely that quality did increase in this period because of new technology, better equipment, and better training. Unfortunately, this aspect of output is usually neglected in data collection efforts (Freiman 1985).

An alternative way of measuring physician output is to focus on procedures or services. Procedures (e.g., an appendectomy) can be measured in a number of dimensions (e.g., average time of performance, complexity, overhead expenses), and based on these dimensions comparable weights can be developed for each procedure (Hsiao and Stason 1979; Hsiao et al. 1992). This approach better captures the differences between various physician tasks.

There are several different measures of hospital output. One way of measuring output is to examine the number of admissions on a per population basis. In 1964 there were 190 admissions per 1,000 population, while in 1996 there were 268 admissions. However, the length per admission has changed radically in this time period, from 12 days per admission to 6.7 days. As a result, total days in hospital per 1,000 population fell from 2,292 to 1,818. Days is a better measure of resources used than admissions, but even days does not tell the whole picture, as it leaves out the consideration of quality. (U.S. Department of Health and Human Services, *Health United States*, 1999).

Because of the vast differences in types of illnesses, in disease severity, and in medical treatment patterns (including quality of care), hospital output is difficult to characterize from an economic viewpoint. One method of doing so that captures a mixture of illness types and severities as well as treatment patterns is the diagnosis-related group (DRG) classification system. The DRG system has many variants. In the 1998 version of the DRG system, which was used by the Health Care Financing Administration to reimburse hospitals, hospital inpatient output was divided into 511 different groups based on the major reason for hospitalization, whether the case was medical or surgical, patient age, and the presence of significant complications and comorbidities (conditions in addition the the primary). In a nationwide study of hospital costs conducted at the Agency for Health Care Policy and Research (AHCPR), average annual charges for specific DRGs were as follows: normal delivery, $3,094; craniotomy without complications, $32,594; liver transplant, $204,000 (Agency for Healthcare Research and Quality 1997). Despite the fact that the DRG system develops average costs among groups, the range of costs within as well as between DRGs is very considerable.

DRGs do not measure "quality of care." To gather a picture of hospital product quality, we must look at data collected from hospitals. Hospital output data are available from *Vital and Health Statistics* (Series 13), published by the Public Health Service; *Hospital Statistics,* the annual compendium of the American Hospital Association (AHA), and various issues of *Hospitals: Journal of the American Hospital Association.*

The AHA formerly published a series of indexes that extensively covered the concept of measuring quality changes in hospital care over time (Phillip 1977). This index attempted to measure the quality change of a day of care by changes in service intensity, which was defined as the quantity of real services that go into one typical day of hospitalization. The AHA's Hospital Intensity Index (HII) incorporated 46 services, including the number of dialysis treatments, obstetric unit worker hours, and pharmacy worker hours. A weighted average of these 46 services was calculated annually for data from a sample of hospitals to derive an average number of services per patient day offered during the year. With the calculation for 1969 as a baseline (the value for that year equals 100), the annual averages formed an index that measured changes in the service intensity component of output over time. Although these data are no longer published, they provide an excellent illustration of how important service intensity is as a component of medical care output.

In Table 1–1, national data are shown for three components of hospital care: services per day, average length of hospital stay, and number of admissions during the time period when the HII was compiled. Services per day are presented in the form of an index (the HII, with 1969 = 100). Average length of stay is presented in average days per stay and as an index (1969 = 100) in parentheses beside the average-length figure. Admissions are shown in millions and also as an index (1969 = 100). As can be seen from the three indexes, service intensity was by far the largest growth component of hospital output, increasing by 68 percent in seven years. Admissions rose by 18 percent, while the length of stay fell slightly. This indicates the importance of intensity of output in medical care. However, although we often equate intensity with quality, this presupposition has been questioned because additional intensity of services may not always result in additional health.

1.3 RISK SHIFTING AND HEALTH INSURANCE

Another type of health care sector output is risk shifting through the purchase of health insurance. Illnesses are often unexpected and are often accompanied by monetary losses. These losses can be in the form of medical expenses, lost earnings from work, and other expenses. Individuals can be said to face a *risk* of losing some of their wealth, which means that the existence of the loss and its amount are uncertain. This risk creates concern on the part of the consumers, and they are usually willing to pay something to avoid the risk.

One way of dealing with the risk is to shift it to someone else. Insurers are organizations that specialize in accepting risk. When an insurer accepts a large amount of risk, the average loss to the insurer becomes predictable. Of course, there are costs of operating such a risk-sharing organization. These include the administrative expenses associated with determining probabilities, setting prices, selling policies, and adjudicating claims. The owners also expect a return on their investment (profits). These expenses and profits are included in the fee (called a *premium*)

Table 1–1 Components of Output in Short-Term Hospital Care in the United States

Year	Index of Services per Day (1969=100)[a]	Average Length of Stay and as an Index (1969=100)[b]	Total Admissions in Millions and as an Index (1969=100)[b]
1969	100	8.2 (100)	20.3 (100)
1970	108.7	8.2 (100)	20.9 (102)
1971	115.5	8.1 (98)	21.5 (106)
1972	119.5	8.0 (97)	21.8 (107)
1973	125.4	7.9 (96)	22.4 (110)
1974	136.9	7.9 (96)	23.3 (114)
1975	153.5	7.8 (95)	23.7 (116)
1976	168.6	7.9 (96)	24.1 (118)

[a]Data compiled from the Hospital Intensity Index, American Hospital Association.
[b]Data compiled from *Hospital Statistics: 1978 Edition*, American Hospital Association.

that each individual must pay to obtain insurance. The essential point here is that, in its own right, risk shifting is an additional output that is distinct from the output called *medical care*. Someone can obtain medical care without risk shifting (by paying for it when the product is received). Such an individual is still faced with the risk of incurring losses but has done nothing to shift the risk. It is the *additional* activity of shifting the risk in advance—taking action to reduce the loss should illness occur—that is the output.

There are a variety of ways in which risk can be shifted. It can be done privately, by the purchase of insurance. Insurance organizations such as Blue Cross, Blue Shield, Prudential, and Aetna sell health insurance policies either directly to individuals (individual policies) or through groups such as employers and professional associations (group policies). In addition, health maintenance organizations (HMOs) act as both insurers and providers of care. The government also acts as a payer of health care bills for large numbers of individuals, although strictly speaking it is not an insurer: Most of its revenues are in the form of taxes, not premiums, and often the covered individuals are not the ones who pay these taxes. Thus the government does not manage its health care–related expenditures on an insurance (risk assessment) basis. Government-style risk sharing is referred to as *risk pooling*.

Health insurance can cover all an individual's expenses. Full insurance has become quite costly, and so insurers have come to resort to "cost-sharing" provisions according to which insured persons pay a portion of their health care bills and the insurer covers the rest. These provisions allow the insurers to limit expected payouts and charge the insured persons lower premium rates. In cost-sharing arrangements, the risk shifting is not complete.

Cost sharing can be done in several ways. The insurance policy can require the individual to cover the first dollars of expenses, and the insurer then pays all, or a portion, of the rest. For example, the individual might be required to pay a deductible of $100 before the insurer begins to kick in. The insurer can also specify a limit above which payments will cease. For example, it might cover expenses up to a lifetime limit of $100,000. Beyond that, the individual would again bear the risk. So-called catastrophic insurance can be obtained to cover very large losses.

The amount and type of insurance coverage is inextricably tied to the workings of the medical care market. Thus, although insurance and medical care should be thought of as separate products, they do affect one another. In the case of insurance coverage, distribution issues have arisen as a cause for concern. In the United States in 1998, roughly 44.3 million people under age 65, 16.3 percent of the population, were uninsured (U.S. Census Bureau, 1999). Among those lacking insurance were a large number of children (15.4 percent of those under 15), a fact that has generated a considerable amount of concern. Additionally, many employed individuals have no insurance. Since employment is the traditional source of health insurance in the United States, the lack of insurance among workers is viewed as a worrisome development (Monheit and Short 1989).

The mere possession of some sort of coverage does not guarantee adequate risk protection. Medicare is a government plan that covers hospital expenses and (optionally) medical expenses for individuals over 65. Because of the cost-sharing arrangements incorporated into the program, many of those who are covered under Medicare still face a substantial financial risk should they become ill. Indeed, 60 percent of those who are over 65 now purchase private "Medigap" coverage to cover the risk resulting from the cost-sharing elements (Health Care Financing Administration, 1998).

At the same time, it also should be pointed out that a complete absence of risk on the part of insured individuals (the shifting of the entire risk onto insurers) has its problems as well. A totally riskless policy may be very expensive, since individuals are more prone to demand care when it has a zero price (as under full insurance coverage). The costs of such care must still be covered by the insurer, and so premiums must increase to cover these costs.

1.4 HEALTH STATUS

1.4.1 Concepts

The concept of health seems so familiar to us that we can almost reach out and touch it. It seems easy to distinguish the 97-pound weakling from the bodybuilder who kicks sand in his face at the beach or to recognize a radiant complexion when we see one in a facial soap commercial on television. More precise measures, however, are hard to obtain. The categories "healthy" and "unhealthy" are not exact. The main reason for this is that we have not defined health precisely. Lacking such a definition, two observers can have different opinions as to whether one person is healthier than another. An essential task of the scientific method is to obtain widespread agreement about the nature of a phenomenon. If we lack an operational definition, we can hardly expect two independent observers to reach agreement about the status of the phenomenon. A definition is useful if it helps pinpoint the characteristics of the phenomenon we are trying to describe and eventually measure.

Health is not an easy concept to define with any degree of precision. As the English epidemiologist Sir Richard Doll remarked concerning the concept of health, "Positive health seems to be as elusive to measure as love, beauty, and happiness" (Doll 1974). Yet in an effort to give some hold on the concept, the World Health Organization has defined health as "a complete state of physical, mental and social well-being, and not merely the absence of illness or disease." This is a very broad definition, and the characteristics of health suggested by it are not easy to pinpoint and measure. The definition stresses that there are three components of health, and even if a person is physically healthy, he or she can still be lacking in the other categories.

1.4.2 Measures of Individual Health

For many years health was identified by the presence of disease (morbidity) or by death (mortality). Individual measures, such as the diagnosis rates for certain conditions or rates of hospitalization, were used as indicators for morbidity. Mortality was usually adjusted for population factors such as age and sex. More recently, mortality has been addressed in terms of premature mortality, with the difference between expected age of death and the actual age of death being forwarded as a measure of life-years lost prematurely. Thus if the expected age of death for a male aged 20 is 75, a 20-year-old man who dies in a car accident is considered to have lost 55 years of life.

Researchers have been looking for other measures of health with a more positive focus. Attempts at identifying and measuring health have focused on certain characteristics we would expect in a healthy person. These characteristics include the physical functioning of the individual's body in relation to some norm, the physical capability of the individual to perform certain acts (e.g., getting up or dressing), the social capabilities of the individual (i.e., how well he or she interacts with others), and how the individual feels. These characteristics are by no means distinct from one another, a fact that has led to much disagreement among researchers who have tried to invent a unique measurement of health status. Different research efforts have focused on clinical characteristics; on individual capabilities (Boyle and Torrance 1984; Culyer 1976); on the physical functioning of people's bodies in relation to some norm (Kass 1975; Williamson 1971); and on a mixture of physical, mental, and social characteristics (Breslow 1972).

Despite the considerable difficulties in arriving at widely acceptable indexes of health status, the importance of the topic ensures that researchers will keep trying. One widely used measure is the 15-D (for 15 health dimensions), which categorized health status into 15 groups, as shown in Table 1–2. These groups include breathing, hearing, moving, and so on. Subjects rate each dimension on a 5-point scale. For the breathing dimension, for example, a "1" would indicate normal breathing and a "5" would indicate that the individual experiences breathing difficulties almost always. Within each dimension, each point on the scale is assigned a value, which scores the functioning level. For example, normal breathing is scored as 1.0000, and level 1 breathing is scored as 0.093. The 15-D investigators have assigned a second set of weights to each of the 15 dimensions. These weights were obtained from community surveys and reflect the importance of each dimension. Example weights are shown in Table 1–2. For example, breathing has an importance weight of 0.0805. The 15 importance weights sum to 1.0000.

Investigators can use instruments such as the 15-D to provide measures of an individual's quality of life. Further, a time dimension can be added to provide a

Table 1–2 Health Dimensions in the 15-D Health-Related Quality of Life Index

Dimension	Importance Weight
Breathing	.075
Mental functioning	.044
Speech	.065
Vision	.075
Mobility	.046
Usual activities	.057
Vitality	.074
Hearing	.104
Eating	.040
Eliminating	.033
Sleeping	.090
Distress	.079
Discomfort/symptoms	.072
Sexual activity	.084
Depression	.062
Total	1.000

Source: Based on H. Sintonen, The 15D Instrument of Health-related Quality of Life: Properties and Applications, *Annals of Medicine*, Vol. 33, pp. 328–335, © 2001.

measure of quality adjusted life years, or QALYs. Investigators often standardize these measures, with a score of 1.0000 being the highest level of health, and 0.0000 being the lowest (or perhaps even death). Thus, for example, a group of patients with asthma had an average overall 15-D score of 0.89 (out of a maximum possible score of 1.00) (Kaupinnen et al. 1998). If the condition persisted for 1 year, then the average patient's quality of life index would be 0.89 QALYs for the period. The individual would have lost 0.11 QALYs due to his asthmatic condition. The figure 0.11 represents the loss of full health over the year. If the condition persisted over 2 years, then the individual would have experienced 1.78 QALYs during that period.

The translation of health-related quality of life (HRQOL) measures into QALYs has one very convenient benefit. By evaluating death as 0.0000, one can compare interventions some of which result in death. For example, if one person lived for 5 years at a QALY value of 0.5 rather than being dead (QALY value is 0.0000), then the difference in QALYs would be 2.5000–0.0000, or 2.5 QALYs. Of course, there are conceptual problems with placing a 0.0000 value on death; death is beyond the conscious experience of people, and so they may have great difficulty comparing different levels of health with death.

The 15-D weights can be used both to assess the HRQOL of an individual over time or to compare different individuals or groups. For example, women with breast cancer can take different forms of chemotherapy. The 15-D can measure differences in health-related quality of life between the interventions. There are several general HRQOL measures in use (Bowling, 1997); those used mostly by economists include the Euroquol 5D (Kind, 1996) and the Health Utilities Index (Feeny et al. 1996). In addition, there are a large number of HRQOL measures for specific diseases (Bowling, 1995).

1.4.3 Population Health Measures

The most commonly used population health measures have been mortality rates and morbidity (usually hospitalization) rates. Mortality or death rates are standardized by age and sometimes gender and can be expressed for the entire population or for subgroups, such as whites and blacks. In Figure 1–1 we show the trends in death rates for the total population and for whites and blacks from 1950 to 1997 in the United States. All rates have been falling, but the death rate for blacks is substantially above that for whites. Death rates are also used for subgroups; for example, the neonatal mortality rate, which expresses deaths up to the first 28 days of life as a percentage of total live births, was 5.7 in 1998. For the white and black populations the respective rates were 4.7 and 11.1 (U.S. Department of Health and Human Services, 1999).

Increasingly, analysts have been focusing on survival time as an indicator of health status. They choose survival-time indicators because these place emphasis on the duration component of health status; a person's well-being is a function of the time spent in each health state, not merely the health state at a given moment in time. Measures that look at survival time adopt this important dimension of health. One such measure is that of potential years of life lost (PYLL) before a target age. The analyst selects a target age below which most individuals are expected to live. Deaths that occur at an age earlier than the target age are considered to be premature. The measure of premature deaths is considered to be one of the best population-level indicators of health. This indicator for whites and blacks in the

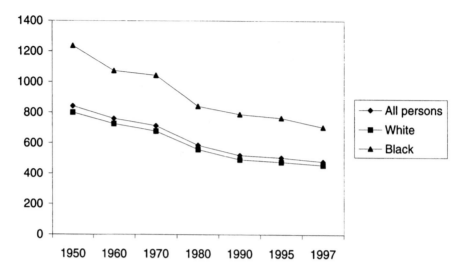

Figure 1–1 Age-adjusted death rates by group, United States, 1950–1997 (deaths per 100,000 residents). *Source:* Reprinted from National Center for Health Statistics, Health, United States, Table 30, 1999, U.S. Department of Health and Human Services.

United States is shown in Table 1–3. The PYLL for white males, expressed in terms of 100,000 persons, is over 11,000 life years, a figure that is half that for black males and twice that for white females. White and black females maintain about the same relative magnitudes as do males.

Of course, mortality rates do not take quality of life into account. In an effort to incorporate both mortality and quality of life into a single index, analysts at the World Health Organization have developed an index called *disability adjusted life expectancy* (DALE) (Mathers et al. 2000). To estimate DALE, the investigators determined the prevalence of nonfatal conditions in each country and adjusted life years in light of disability rates. The results for selected countries are displayed in Table 1–4. This table shows the life expectancy for females in six countries, including the United States, both adjusted and unadjusted for disability, for 1998. For the United States, the life expectancy at birth was 79.6 years before adjusting for disability. After making disability adjustments, this figure was reduced to 72.6 years. The difference, 7 disability-adjusted years, is the reduction in quality of life of those who survived. The greater the gap between the two figures, the poorer is the measure

Table 1–3 Years of Potential Life Lost before Age 75, per 100,000 population under 75 years of age, United States, Selected Years

Year	White Males	White Females	Black Males	Black Females
1980	11,877	6,185	22,338	11,863
1990	10,614	5,255	21,250	10,662
1995	9,546	4,005	20,278	10,179
1997	8,533	4,821	17,373	9,475

Source: Reprinted from National Center for Health Statistics, Health, United States, Table 31, 1999, U.S. Department of Health and Human Services.

Table 1–4 Life Expectancy at Birth, Unadjusted and Adjusted for Disability
(Selected Countries, 1999)

Country	Life Expectancy at Birth, Females	Disability-Adjusted Life Expectancy at Birth, Females	Expected Years Lost to Disability at Birth
Japan	84.3	77.2	7.1
Australia	81.9	74	7.9
United Kingdom	79.9	73.7	6.0
United States	79.6	72.6	7.0
New Zealand	79.4	71.2	8.2
Argentina	77.8	69.6	8.2

Source: Reprinted with permission from S.D. Mathers, et al., *Estimates of DALE for 191 Countries: Methods and Results*, Global Programme on Evidence for Health Policy Work, Paper No. 16, © 2000, World Health Organization

of health of the surviving population. For those countries shown in the table, the gap is between 6 and 8 disability years.

1.4.4 Outcome

The final output of the health care sector is health. If there is a close relationship between health and medical care, then indicators of *medical care* output can be used as indicators of the true output of the health care sector. It has been contended that there is not necessarily such a correspondence and that the quantity of medical care utilized is therefore not a good indicator of output.

The true output of the health care sector is measured by the net change in health produced by the medical care provided. That is, output is measured, not by the level of the health index (e.g., by the infant mortality rate), but rather by the *change* in the index due to the medical care—in other words, the effects of the care. For example, if the infant mortality rate fell from 12 to 10 deaths per 1,000 births subsequent to the program to introduce a new drug, the output of the program would be that proportion of the reduction in infant mortality that was due to the program. It may be that other factors, such as the mothers' diets, also contributed to the change in infant mortality. The presence of such confounding factors creates difficulties in finding an accurate measure of output; medical care is seldom the only factor contributing to changes in health status. Other factors may be difficult to identify (e.g., changes in personal behaviors) and equally difficult to measure.

In addition to the identification of confounding factors, there is the problem of measuring changes in health status. We have seen how many difficulties are posed in trying to measure levels of health status. The measurement of changes in health status merely adds to these problems. For example, assume that an individual with a gastrointestinal disorder will have a quality-of-life index of 0.5 for a seven-week period in the absence of any treatment. She can be treated using one of two different drugs. The less effective drug we will call Treatment A. With Treatment A, the individual will have a quality-of-life index of 0.7 for two weeks, of 0.8 for an additional two weeks, and 1.0 for the fifth to seventh weeks (see Figure 1–2). With Treatment B, the individual will have a quality of life of 0.8 for two weeks and will be completely cured after that. Over the entire seven week period, the individual would have a total quality-of-life measure of 3.5 quality-adjusted weeks with no

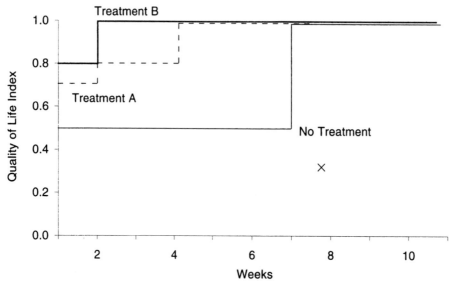

Figure 1–2 Quality of life indexes under three alternative treatment options. With no treatment (see thin solid line), the individual has a quality of life index of 0.5 over 7 weeks and then recovers fully (quality of life level 1.0). Under Treatment A (broken line), the quality of life index is 0.7 for 2 weeks, 0.8 for the next two weeks, and 1.0 thereafter. Under Treatment B (darker solid line), the quality of life index is 0.8 for 2 weeks and full recovery (1.0) there after.

treatment, 6 quality-adjusted weeks ([2 × 0.7] + [2 × 0.8] + [3 × 1.0]) with Treatment A, and 6.6 weeks with Treatment B.

The outcome measure will depend on what the alternative is. If the alternative is no care, then the outcome for Treatment A is 2.1 quality-adjusted weeks, and for Treatment B it is 3.1 quality-adjusted weeks. That is, the outcome is the difference in the value of the index between the two treatments (Williams, 1994).

It has been contended that, in general, there is a limit to how much good medical care can do; as more medical care is provided (to the same individuals), the additional output becomes less. This is illustrated in Figure 1–3, where health is shown on the vertical axis and the quantity of medical care on the horizontal axis. The medical care "outcome" curve showing the relation between health and medical care is drawn so as to indicate that there would be some level of health without any medical care (H_o) and that additional levels of medical care make some contribution to health. However, the additional contribution declines as the quantity of medical care increases. Such an output curve assumes all other factors (environmental, genetic, personal) are held constant and only medical care varies. The additional output is expressed as $\Delta H/\Delta M$, where ΔM is the additional medical care and ΔH is the additional health. Note that, because of the way the curve is drawn, $\Delta H/\Delta M$ declines in value as more medical care (M) is provided. This eventual flattening of the output curve has given rise to the expression "flat-of-the-curve medicine" (Enthoven 1980). Drawing the curve in this way illustrates geometrically that, as medical care provision is increased, the additional effectiveness of medical care declines.

Researchers have attempted to establish the relation between medical care and health in different ways. Several early studies attempted to identify statistically a relation between mortality rates and various measures of medical input per capita using state data (Auster et al. 1969) and national data (Stewart 1971). Both studies

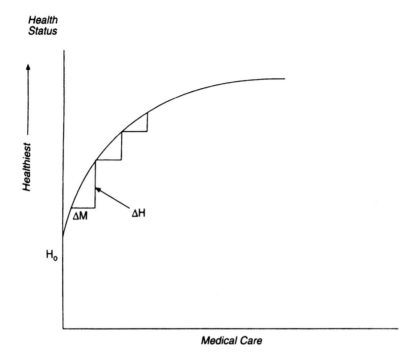

Figure 1–3 Hypothesized relationship between health and medical care. In this representation, additional doses of medical care have a diminishing impact on health; eventually, a situation of low medical productivity, termed "flat-of-the-curve medicine," is reached.

---

found a small relationship or none at all. One explanation given was that we may have reached the leveling-out point on the curve. Furthermore, it was estimated that the self-care components of health care (e.g., quitting smoking, eating right, getting exercise) may indeed be more important than the medical care components (Newhouse and Freidlander 1979). However, subsequent statistical research that examined specific groups such as infants did find significant evidence of the impact of medical care (Hadley 1982).

Because such studies are so broadly focused, their results are often difficult to interpret, and it may be that health output is more reasonably measured only by experimental means. Setting up clinical trials in which one group receives a certain treatment and another group with similar characteristics (a control group) does not is an experimental method of establishing output. The difference in cure rates, if any, between the two groups could be taken as a measure of the output produced by the resources (Cochrane 1972). In a number of instances, less aggregated studies have sometimes failed to turn up evidence that certain medical practices impact health (e.g., no relationship was found between appendicitis death rates and appendectomies performed) (see Enthoven 1980, chap. 2). However, such findings should not automatically be generalized (Angell 1985). Although it may have some analytic appeal, a broad-brush approach may pass over many situations where we are not on the "flat of the curve."

1.5 CONSUMPTION AND INVESTMENT OUTPUT

The production of any output requires the use of inputs, including services and supplies. These inputs themselves have to be produced. Many of them are capital inputs, which means that they are durable and last for fairly long periods of time. The totality of resources at any point in time is called a *stock*. In contrast, the amount of activity that occurs during a given time period is called a *flow*.

An output is measured over a given period of time, such as a year. Outputs fall into two classes: those that serve current wants, such as the treatment of patients, and those that serve future wants, such as the production of capital inputs. The use of output for current wants is called *consumption* activity. In health care, much of the output is used up as soon as it is produced. Curing a common cold using drugs is a consumption activity because the treatment is brief. The production of capital resources is called *investment* activity; the effects themselves are designed to last for several years or more.

Capital inputs can be of the physical variety (radiological equipment) or the human variety (trained radiologists and radiology technicians). Physical capital is the stock of physical means of production. Examples include equipment and buildings. Human capital is the stock of talents, skills, and knowledge embodied in individuals. An example of investment in physical capital is the production of radiology machines. Undergraduate and postgraduate medical education is an example of investment in human capital.

One feature of the health care sector is that much of the human capital investment activity is a byproduct of medical care consumption activity. Much undergraduate medical education and most postgraduate medical education occurs in hospitals and clinics. In many cases, education and patient care activities are inseparable, physically and financially. For many years teaching hospitals have relied on labor from medical interns and residents for patient care. Because the supply of physicians, including the ratio of specialists to primary care physicians, has become such an important issue in the United States, much attention is being paid to the process by which physicians and specialists are produced.

There is a distinct relationship between capital and production activities. Imagine a given stock of capital at the beginning of 1995 (e.g., magnetic resonance imaging [MRI] machines). Net new investment is the additional stock added during the year (new machines produced minus any machines retired). The stock at the beginning of 1996 is the original capital stock plus the net new investment in MRIs. Important related concepts include the capacity of the capital equipment, actual production, and the percent utilization (or occupancy) rate. If there are 1,000 MRIs in existence, and it takes one hour to produce one image, then the daily capacity is 24,000 images and the yearly capacity is 8.76 million images. If, in any year, 2 million images were produced, the utilization rate would be 23 percent.

Measures of capacity have a particular importance in the health care field. Some analysts believe that the supply of resources directly influences the demand. Commonly used terms and sayings such as "supplier-induced demand" and "an available bed is a filled bed" reflect this view. One of its implications is that, in order to control consumption activity, the investment of capital inputs must be controlled.

EXERCISES

1. Distinguish between three different views of the quality of medical care and provide examples of types of care that would be considered indicators of quality by each view.
2. What is risk and how can people reduce it? Is it costless to do so?
3. What is the difference between morbidity and utilization? Identify an indicator that has been used to measure both and state a reason why it is not an ideal measure of morbidity.
4. What is the World Health Organization definition of health? How does this differ from the concept of utilization? Why is it important to distinguish between these two concepts?
5. What is a health-related quality of life index? What is the difference between "social importance" weights and "level values" in constructing such indexes?
6. What is a quality-adjusted life year? How can it be used to compare differences in health status between someone who is healthy and someone who is not? Can it be used to compare health outcomes of someone who is ill with someone who has died?
7. What is the weakness of using an unadjusted mortality rate as an indicator of population health status?
8. Which issues in the measurement of population health do potential years of life lost (PYLL) and disability adjusted life expectancy (DALE) address?
9. Specify a hypothesized relationship between medical care and health. How does flat-of-the-curve medicine fit in with this concept?
10. Indicate at which point flat-of-the-curve medicine is experienced in the following example (imagine that antibiotics have been prescribed for a given population of 1,000 elderly persons).

Number of Prescriptions	Hospitalizations for Community Acquired Pneumonia
0	60
100	50
200	40
300	32
400	28
500	28

BIBLIOGRAPHY

Measurement of Medical Care

Agency for Healthcare Research and Quality. 1997. *Statistics from the Nationwide Inpatient Sample for 1994 Hospital Inpatient Stays*. AHCPR pub. no. 97-0056. http://www.ahcpr.gov/data/hcup/1991) (September 1997). Accessed 7 April 2001.

Bailey, R. 1970. Philosophy, faith, fact and fiction in the production of medical services. *Inquiry* 7:37–53.

Berry, R.E. 1973. On grouping hospitals for economic analysis. *Inquiry* 10:5–12.

Center for Disease Control. 1986. Premature mortality in the United States: Public health issues in the use of years of potential life lost. *MMWR Supplements* 35 (2S): 1s–11s.

Freiman, M.P. 1985. The rate of adoption of new procedures among physicians. *Medical Care* 23:939–945.

Hornbrook, M. 1982. Hospital case mix: Its definition, measurement, and use. Parts 1, 2. *Medical Care Review* 39:1–43, 73–123.

Hsiao, W.C., and W.B. Stason. 1979. Toward developing a relative value scale for medical and surgical services. *Health Care Financing Review* 1:23–39.

Hsiao, W.C., et al. 1992. An overview of the development and refinement of the resource-based relative value scale. *Medical Care* 30 (suppl.): NS1.

Lave, J.R., and L.B. Lave. 1971. The extent of role differentiation among hospitals. *Health Services Research* 5:15–38.

Phillip, P.J. 1977. HCI/HII: Two new AHA indexes measure cost, intensity. *Hospital Financial Management*, April, 20–26.

Reder, M.W. 1967. Some problems in the measurement of productivity in the medical care industry. In *Production and productivity in the service industries*, ed. V.R. Fuchs. New York: Columbia University Press.

Russell, L.B. 1976. The diffusion of new hospital technologies in the United States. *International Journal of Health Services* 6:557–580.

Sisk, J.E., et al. 1990. Assessing information for consumers on the quality of medical care. *Inquiry* 27:263–272.

U.S. Department of Health and Human Services. 1999. *Health, United States, 1999.* Hyattsville, MD: National Center for Health Statistics.

Measurement of Health

Ahlburg, D. 1998. Intergenerational transmission of health. *American Economic Review* 88:265–270.

Bowling, A. 1995. *Measuring disease.* Buckingham, England: Open University Press.

———. 1997. *Measuring health.* 2nd ed. Buckingham, England: Open University Press.

Boyle, M.H., and G.W. Torrance. 1984. Developing multiattribute health indexes. *Medical Care* 22:1045–1057.

Breslow, L. 1972. A quantitative approach to the World Health Organization definition of health: Physical, mental, and social well-being. *International Journal of Epidemiology* 1:347–355.

Culyer, A.J. 1972. Appraising government expenditure on health services: The problems of "need" and "output." *Public Finance* 27:205–211.

———. 1976. *Need and the national health service.* London: Martin Robertson Co.

Cutler, D.M., and E. Richardson. 1998. The value of health, 1970–1990. *American Economic Review* 88:97–100.

Donaldson, C., et al. 1988. Should QALYs be programme-specific? *Journal of Health Economics* 7:239–257.

Feeny, D., et al. 1996. Health utilities index. In *Quality of life and pharmacoeconomics in clinical trials,* ed. B. Spilker. Philadelphia: Lippincott-Raven.

Goldsmith, S.B. 1973. A re-evaluation of health status indicators. *Health Services Reports* 88:937–941.

Gonnella, J.S., et al. 1984. Staging of disease. *JAMA* 251:637–644.

Hellinger, F.J. 1989. Expected utility theory and risky choices with health outcomes. *Medical Care* 27:273–279.

Hornbrook, M.C. 1983. Allocative medicine. *Annals: American Association of Political and Social Science* 468:12–29.

Israel, S., and G. Teeling-Smith. 1967. The submerged iceberg of sickness in society. *Social Policy and Administration* 1:43–57.

Kass, L.R. 1975. The pursuit of health. *Public Interest* 40:11–42.

Kauppinen, R., et al.1998. One-year economic evaluation of intensive versus conventional patient education and supervision for self-management of new asthmatic patients. *Respiratory Medicine* 92:300–307.

Kind, P. 1996. The EUROQUOL instrument: An index of health related quality of life. In *Quality of life and pharmacoeconomics in clinical trials,* ed. B. Spilker. Philadelphia: Lippincott-Raven.

Mathers, S.D., et al. 2000. *Estimates of DALE for 191 countries: Methods and results.* Global Programme on Evidence for Health Policy Work Paper No. 16. Geneva: World Health Organization.

Sintonen, H. 1981. An approach to measuring and valuing health states. *Social Science and Medicine* 15C:55–65.

————. 1995. *The 15D-measure of health-related quality of life. II. Feasibility, reliability, and validity of its valuation system.* West Heidelberg, Australia: National Centre for Health Program Evaluation.

Sintonen, H., and M. Pekurinen. 1992. A fifteen-dimensional measure of health-related quality of life and its applications. In *Quality of life assessment,* ed. S.R. Walker and R.M. Rosser. Dordrecht, Netherlands: Kluwer Academic.

Smith, G.T. 1988. *Measuring health: A practical approach.* Chichester, England: Wiley.

Sullivan, D.F. 1966. *Conceptual problems in developing an index of health.* Vital and Health Statistics, series 2, no. 17, pub. no. HRA 74-1017. Washington, DC: U.S. Department of Health, Education and Welfare.

U.S. Congress, Office of Technology Assessment. 1988. *The quality of medical care.* Pub. no. OTA-H-386. Washington, DC: U.S. Government Printing Office.

U.S. General Accounting Office. 1996. *Public health: A health status indicator for targeting federal aid to states.* Washington, DC: U.S. General Accounting Office.

Williams, A. 1985. The nature, meaning, and measurement of health and illness. *Social Science and Medicine* 20:1023–1027.

————. 1988. The importance of quality of life in policy decisions. In *Quality of life: Assessment and application,* ed. S.R. Walker and R.M. Rossier. Lancaster, England: MTP Press Limited.

————. 1999. Calculating the global burden of disease: Time for a strategic appraisal? *Health Economics* 6:1–8.

Williamson, J.W. Evaluating quality of patient care. *JAMA* 218:564–569.

World Bank. 1993. *World development report: Investing in health.* Washington, DC: World Bank.

————. 2000. *World development indicators.* Washington, DC: World Bank.

World Health Organization. 2000. *The world health report 2000.* Geneva: World Health Organization.

The Health–Medical Care Relationship

Angell, M. 1985. Cost containment and the physician. *JAMA* 254:1203–1207.

Auster, R., et al. 1969. The production of health. *Journal of Human Resources* 4:412–436.

Cochrane, A. 1972. *Effectiveness and efficiency*. New York: Oxford University Press.

Doessel, D.P., and J.V. Marshall. 1985. A rehabilitation of health outcome in quality assessment. *Social Science and Medicine* 21:1319–1328.

Doll, R. 1974. Surveillance and monitoring. *International Journal of Epidemiology* 3:305–314.

Donabedian, A. 1988. The quality of care. *JAMA* 260:1743–1748.

Enthoven, A.C. 1980. *Health plan*. Reading, MA: Addison-Wesley.

Erickson, P., et al. 1989. Using composite health status measures to assess the nation's health. *Medical Care* 27:S66–S76.

Hadley, J. 1982. *More medical care, better health?* Washington, DC: Urban Institute.

Newhouse, J.P., and L.J. Friedlander. 1979. The relationship between medical resources and measures of health. *Journal of Human Resources* 15:200–218.

Russell, L.B. 1986. *Is prevention better than cure?* Washington, DC: Brookings Institution.

Scheffler, R.M., et al. 1982. Severity of illness and the relationship between intensive care and survival. *American Journal of Public Health* 72:449–454.

Stewart, C.T. 1971. Allocation of resources to health. *Journal of Human Resources* 6:103–122.

Williams, A. 1974. Measuring the effectiveness of the health care system. *British Journal of the Preventive Medicine Society* 28:196–202.

Health Insurance

Cafferata, G.C. 1984. *Private health insurance coverage of the Medicare population*. National Health Care Expenditures Study, data preview, 18 September 1984. Rockville, MD: National Center for Health Services Research.

Health Care Financing Administration. 1998. *A profile of Medicare*. Chartbook. Baltimore, MD: Health Care Financing Administration.

Monheit, A.C., and P.F. Short. 1989. Mandating health coverage for working Americans. *Health Affairs* 8 (winter): 22–38.

Short, P.F., et al. 1988. *Uninsured Americans: A 1987 profile*. Rockville, MD: National Center for Health Services Research.

U.S. Census Bureau. 1999. *Health insurance coverage 1998*. Washington, DC: U.S. Census Bureau.

Data Sources

American Hospital Association. *Hospital statistics*. Chicago: American Hospital Association. Various years.

U.S. Department of Health and Human Services. *Health, United States*. Rockville, MD: National Center for Health Statistics.

U.S. Department of Health and Human Services. *Morbidity and Mortality Weekly Report*. Atlanta, GA: Centers for Disease Control and Prevention.

U.S. Department of Health and Human Services. *NCHS Monthly Vital Statistics Report*.

U.S. Department of Health and Human Services. *Vital and Health Statistics*. Rockville, MD: National Center for Health Statistics.

Economic Dimensions
of the Health Care System

2.1 INTRODUCTION

The purpose of this chapter is twofold: to introduce readers to some basic concepts used in describing health care activity and to provide a description of some of the key elements of health care in the United States. To achieve its purpose, it focuses on three aspects of economic activity. First, it will examine the basic economic units that participate in the health care economy. Second, it explains how simple flow analysis can be used to describe the economic relationships between the various units. Finally, it presents the concept of economic cost, which is used in measuring the amount of economic activity performed to produce economic output as well as the potential impact of illness.

It should be pointed out that this chapter describes what happens over time as a result of activity in the health care economy. It identifies the economic units and their characteristics and describes the flows of money and services that occur.

Section 2.2 identifies the main "actors" in our analysis—the economic units of the health care sector—and describes some of their central characteristics. It also identifies the concepts economists use to study how these units are organized. Finally, using flow diagrams, it shows how transactions between the various economic units can be understood.

Of considerable importance is the measurement of the magnitude of economic activity. Section 2.3 elucidates the concept of "economic cost," which is a measure of economic activity in terms of money. This concept is used to measure various aspects of health care activity, including the total expenditures on health care services, the total economic costs of illness, and the burden of economic costs on various groups.

2.2 ECONOMIC UNITS AND ECONOMIC FLOWS

2.2.1 Economic Units

Units observed for economic analysis include individuals and organizations. In examining the activity of consuming health care, one can take the economic unit to be an individual or a household. Both alternatives are commonly employed by economists in describing and explaining economic activity. One reason the household is so frequently used is that more consistent data can be collected at this level. For example, if one examined housewives' consumption of health care in relation to their *personal* incomes, a biased picture of the relationship might emerge, because their consumption of health care is more closely related to the income of their households. The roles of individuals include those of demanders of health care and health insurance, employees, and taxpayers. Employers are also economic units in the health care system, primarily in their role as demanders of health care insurance for their employees.

Insurers are firms that have the function of taking on the health care expenditure risk of their customers. They collect premiums from their customers and reimburse the providers for the care they provide for their customers. Providers of health care can include physicians, nurse practitioners, nurses, hospitals, long-term care facilities, and providers of various forms of ambulatory care.

There has been a trend in recent years toward the integration of units. "Horizontal integration" is a term that refers to joining together of providers (and sometimes consumers) of the same type. Physicians have joined group practices. Hospitals and long-term care facilities have joined chains. And there have been some instances of small business joining together to form group purchasing cooperatives for health insurance. There has also been a considerable movement towards "vertical integration," which is the amalgamation of purchasers and sellers. Insurers and providers have joined together to create health maintenance organizations (HMOs).

2.2.2 Flows between Units

Economic flows can involve both money and services. Generally, a flow will summarize a transaction in which a service or commodity is exchanged for money. Such transactions occur in simple markets, with the degree of concentration influencing the terms of the exchange. The market for lettuce is a simple market in which vendors provide lettuce to consumers in exchange for money. The exchange is at a price, which is determined, in part, by how concentrated the vendor market is. In this section, we are concerned with describing which flows take place, not with the terms of the transactions. Further, as we shall see presently, the flows in typical health care markets are much more complex than those in markets for lettuce, since they often contain two sets of flows—one for insurance and one for health care services.

2.2.2.1 Flows in a "Generic" Health Care Market

The flows in a simple, or "generic," health care market are shown in Figure 2–1. In this market, consumers purchase health insurance from insurers. The cash payments by the consumers and employers are called *premiums*. When a consumer uses services that are covered by the insurer, the insurer *reimburses* the provider for the services.

The contract between the insurer and the consumer can have another very important dimension. The consumer can purchase varying degrees of insurance coverage. If the consumer is partially covered, the insurer reimburses the provider for only a portion of the bill; the consumer must pay the remainder. The consumer's portion is called a *copayment* (or an *out-of-pocket payment*). If the consumer is fully insured, there is no out-of-pocket payment. The reimbursement provided by the insurer is payment in full for the services.

The economic importance of out-of-pocket payments is that they are borne by the consumer. It is this cost that governs the consumer's decision as to how much of the service he or she demands. Among the types of direct consumer payments are deductibles, which are fixed upfront payments, and copayments, which are payments related to quantity used. For example, an insurance policy might have a deductible of $200 and a copayment of 10 percent. This means that the consumer pays the first $200 for services rendered before insurance coverage begins. After the deductible is used up, the consumer pays 10 percent of the bill and the insurer reimburses the other 90 percent. Typically, hospital care has the highest coverage,

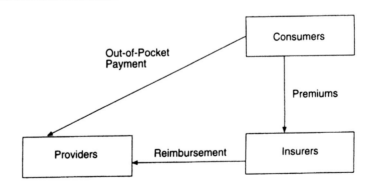

Figure 2–1 Diagrammatic representation of the flow of funds in a typical health care market. Consumers purchase insurance from third-party insurers, who reimburse providers for services. Providers include physicians, hospitals, nursing homes, and other health care organizations.

with 90 percent of expenses being covered; physician care has a lower degree of coverage (75 percent on average), and nursing home care has less still (50 percent).

With regard to insurer payments, there are numerous bases on which providers can be reimbursed. Hospitals can be reimbursed on the basis of a given budget or on a unit basis—per patient day, per case, or per service. In the past decade there has been a movement on the part of some insurers toward reimbursing hospitals on a per case basis, recognizing differences in resource use among different case types. In this instance, hospital cases are categorized into *diagnosis-related groups* (DRGs), and a separate reimbursement rate is set for each DRG. Each time a patient is admitted to the hospital, the hospital is paid a rate corresponding to the patient's particular DRG. Physicians are largely reimbursed on a fee-for-service basis, and long-term care facilities on a per diem basis.

2.2.2.2 Introducing the Employer

Almost three-quarters of all health insurance is provided through employers (Health Insurance Association of America 1989). A basic set of flow relationships for employer-provided health insurance is shown in Figure 2–2. In these circumstances both the employer and the employee pay a share of the premiums. Typically, the employer pays about two-thirds of the premium, though the percentage will vary depending on the plan (Levit et al. 1989).

Note that the employer's share of the premiums is not a "free" benefit given to the employee. It is, rather, a form of compensation received by the employee. Total compensation takes the form of money benefits (wages) and nonmonetary benefits, such as health insurance coverage. From a financial standpoint, the employer is affected the same by either form of compensation: a dollar in wages costs the same to the employer as a dollar in noncash benefits. But the employee will have a preference because of income tax regulations.

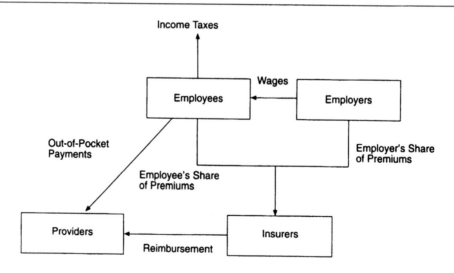

Figure 2–2 Representation of health care services and insurance markets with employer-provided health insurance. Employers and employees typically share premiums. Health insurance premiums are a tax-free benefit to the employee.

Unlike wages, many noncash benefits are not subject to income tax. Thus noncash benefits, such as health insurance, are cheaper to obtain if they are "purchased" through an employer rather than paid for out of after-tax income. As an example, assume that a family's tax rate is 20 percent and that the family wants to buy $100 of health insurance. If the employee takes compensation in the form of wages, the employee must earn $125 in order to have $100 after paying the 20-percent tax (20 percent of $125 is $25). The employee need earn only $100 if compensation is taken in the form of benefits. Or put another way, $100 of compensation in the form of nontaxable benefits will buy more health insurance than the employee could with $100 in wages. The economic importance of this is that present taxation arrangements make health insurance cheaper and encourage more of it to be bought.

It was mentioned above that when economic units are bigger or have a larger share of the market, they may be able to obtain better terms when selling or purchasing services. One type of arrangement that has been increasing in importance is the employer coalition. Employer coalitions are formed by businesses in local markets. Coalition members share information on provider prices, utilization trends, and so on, and they also cooperate with each other in developing benefit designs (e.g., common copayment arrangements). The original purpose of forming coalitions was to develop a sort of countervailing power in the market so that the buyers—the employers—would be able to exert some degree of market influence over price (McLauchlin et al. 1989). Another type of arrangement is the health insurance purchasing coalition (HIPC), which is a coalition of purchasers of insurance designed to garner the benefits associated with group purchasing (Reinhardt 1993). HIPCs have been set up in some states to improve the access of smaller purchasers to health insurance.

2.2.2.3 Medicare

Many individuals are insured by government programs. Medicare is a program of the federal government that covers individuals 65 years old and over, certain disabled groups, and individuals with certain kidney diseases. The essential flows in Medicare are shown in Figure 2–3. Medicare has two parts, an institutional portion and a noninstitutional portion. The institutional portion, called *Part A* (or *hospitalization insurance*), covers hospital care, home care, and a small amount of long-term care (limited to short-term skilled nursing facility care). As shown in Figure 2–3, there is no Part A premium. Part A is largely financed by a federal payroll tax paid by both employers and employees. In 2000 this tax amounted to 1.45 percent of taxable earnings of each employee and employer. The proceeds from this tax go into the Hospital Insurance Trust Fund and form the bulk of the fund's revenues. Hospital expenditures, which form most of the trust fund's payments, have greatly outpaced the fund's receipts (from the payroll tax). As the fund is set up, it cannot be supplemented to any great extent by other forms of receipts, such as general taxes (which could be allocated by the legislature), without major changes in legislation. Indeed, projections made in the early 1980s indicated significant deficits in the fund would occur during the 1990s. These gloomy forecasts, which were predicated on projections of rapidly rising hospital costs, led to significant changes in the method by which Medicare reimbursed hospitals.

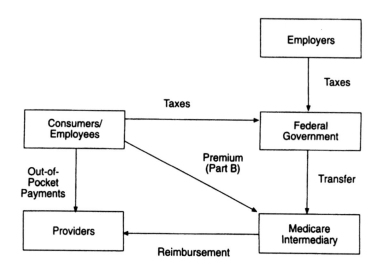

Figure 2–3 Representation of Medicare Parts A and B flows. Consumer and employer taxes include the payroll tax, which is paid into the Hospital Insurance Trust Fund (part of the federal government). Medicare enrollee premiums are only for Part B.

Although Part A Medicare has no premiums, the level of copayments is high. In 2000 there was a deductible of $776, which covered the first 60 days of care, and for anyone needing 61 to 90 days of hospitalization, there was a coinsurance payment of $194 for each day. If someone exceeded 90 days of care during a year, they could draw upon a lifetime reserve totaling 90 days. For many enrollees, the out-of-pocket payments have been considerable, and many individuals have purchased a private form of insurance called *Medigap*, which covers Medicare direct expenses.

Part B coverage is for noninstitutional care, such as physician care, lab and radiology services, and physiotherapy. Enrollment in Part B, called *supplemental medical insurance*, is voluntary and can be purchased with a premium payment ($45.50 monthly in 2000). This premium entitles the holder to partial coverage—there is an annual deductible of $100 of provider charges (billings) and a copayment of 20 percent after that. These direct payments can be insured against by purchasing a Medigap policy from a private insurer.

Unlike Part A, whose revenues come primarily from a single source, Part B revenues come from several sources. The main sources are enrollee premiums and allocations from general taxation. Although Part B expenses have increased considerably, there has been more flexibility in financing them through additional allocations. Nevertheless, there has been substantial growth in Part B expenditures as well as in the Medicare program's share and the out-of-pocket burden of enrollees.

2.2.2.4 Medicaid

Medicaid (Figure 2–4) is a joint federal-state program introduced in 1966 to cover poor individuals. Federal guidelines set basic minimum criteria for eligibility.

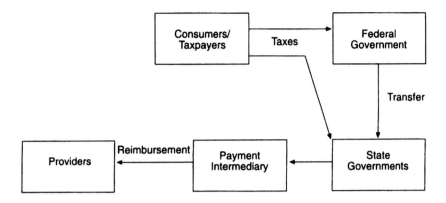

Figure 2–4 Flow of funds for Medicaid program. Federal transfers to state governments are for federal share of the combined state-federal program. Beneficiaries pay no premiums, and direct consumer payments are minimal.

Medicaid covers families who receive payments from Aid to Families with Dependent Children (AFDC), a program whose purpose is to provide financial aid where one parent is absent or the prime income earner is unemployed or cannot work. Medicaid also covers the aged poor and the blind. Eligibility for Medicaid above the basic, federally mandated coverage is determined by state governments, and there is a wide variation. Recently Medicaid coverage has been expanded to include recipients of cash assistance, poor children under the age of 5, and low-income pregnant women. The mandated services covered by the program include inpatient hospital and outpatient care, laboratory and radiology services, physiotherapy, and skilled nursing facility care. States have the option of covering drugs and intermediate care. Generally Medicaid-covered services do not have a copayment or deductible, though for some services direct prices can be charged.

The sharing of Medicaid expenses between state and federal governments is determined by a formula. States receive a proportion equal to 45 percent of the ratio of state to federal per capita income. However, the state's share can be no less than half of Medicaid expenditures and no more than 83 percent.

2.2.2.5 Health Maintenance Organizations

Managed care refers to forms of insurance coverage in which enrollee utilization patterns and provider service patterns are monitored by the insurer or an intermediary with the aim of containing costs. An HMO is one type of managed care organization.

Payment of HMO premiums are on a "capitation" basis. That is, there is a set fee for each enrollee, and the HMO receives a single annual amount for each enrollee whether it provides much or little care. This form of payment puts the HMO at risk for all expenses incurred when serving enrollees, which incidentally means that the HMO serves as an insurer as well as a provider.

Traditionally, an HMO had one of two forms: either it was a self-contained unit that functioned as insurer and provider or it was an amalgamation of private practice physicians (called an independent practice association) who were separately reimbursed by the HMO on a fee-for-service basis. Recently, there have sprung up many new forms of HMOs, many owned by traditional insurance companies such as Blue Cross or commercial companies. These new types receive the capitation fee and contract out for services with providers that the HMO enrollees use.

One of the salient features of any HMO is the restriction of access to providers. Whereas under traditional coverage individuals can go to any provider, enrollees in an HMO must use a group of designated providers. This closed panel arrangement allows the HMO to monitor the providers and possibly have some impact on provider behavior. The providers on the panel may be employees of the HMO or contractors; in either case, monitoring providers is more likely to be feasible than if the enrollees have an unrestricted choice of providers. Such monitoring can potentially encourage providers to practice in a more conservative, less costly manner.

Since the beginning of the 1980s, HMO enrollment has expanded rapidly. In 1997, an estimated 67 million individuals had HMO-type coverage. HMO coverage is offered to enrollees of Medicare and Medicaid as well as those who are traditionally covered. A simple flow diagram for HMO coverage is presented in Figure 2–5. HMO receipts would typically include employer contributions as well. It should be noted that, unlike in the case of traditional insurance coverage, there is typically no pass through from insurer to provider; the insurer is, in essence, the provider. However, there are some types of HMOs that do contract with independent providers.

2.2.2.6 Preferred Provider Organizations

A major drawback of HMO coverage is that enrollees can only choose from a limited panel of providers. In many cases, an enrollee may be attached to or prefer a specific physician. If the physician is not on the provider panel, the enrollee must

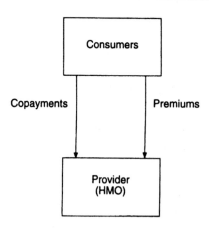

Figure 2–5 Flow of funds for an HMO. Consumers pay premium to the HMO, which is also the provider. Copayment levels vary among plans, and some plans do not require any copayment.

pay the provider's full price. Preferred provider organizations (PPOs) were designed to expand consumer choice while maintaining many of the monitoring benefits of managed care.

A PPO will contract with certain providers ("preferred providers") who agree to charge low prices and submit to utilization monitoring in exchange for being designated as a preferred provider (see Figure 2–6). The PPO will then contract on behalf of these providers with insurance companies to gain their business. The insurers offer their enrollees a dual pricing system—one price for those who use the preferred providers and a higher price for those who use nonpreferred providers. This price differential might take the form of varying copayment rates, for example, a low (or zero) copayment rate for those who use the preferred group and a higher direct payment for those who use nonpreferred providers. This creates an economic incentive for the consumers to use the preferred group, but it allows partial coverage when a consumer chooses a nonpreferred provider.

Preferred providers gain from the fact that they will likely get a greater volume of business from the enrollees. Their agreeing to submit to some form of utilization monitoring will, if the monitoring is successful, translate into lower utilization patterns and lower premiums, which in turn translates into savings for the employer and employees.

A PPO can be a separate contractor that receives a fee from the insurer. It can be part of the insurance company itself. Or it can be owned by provider groups and used as a marketing mechanism. In fact, there are many types of PPOs. What distinguishes them from HMOs is their allowance of greater choice of provider. Recently, however, HMOs have been relaxing their closed panel restrictions in favor of coverage that is more akin to PPO coverage. An HMO that allows members to seek care from nonpanel providers for a differential fee is called a point-of-service plan.

PPOs have been growing in popularity in recent years. Between 1992 and 1995, the proportion of all insured persons who were enrolled in PPOs increased from 23 percent to 40 percent (Health Insurance Association of America 1999). In fact, their popularity has earned them a place in a popular health insurance package now

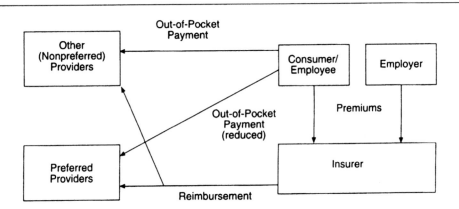

Figure 2–6 Outline of flows in a preferred provider arrangement. The preferred provider organization (PPO), not shown, arranges the preferred reimbursement rate from the preferred providers and conducts reviews of utilization. The PPO could be the preferred provider, the insurer, or an independent organization.

offered by many employers: the "triple option" package. With such a package, the employer offers each employee a choice among types of coverage: traditional coverage, HMO coverage, and PPO coverage. In order to make the three types roughly comparable, the employer can alter the out-of-pocket payments and employee premiums. For example, for traditional care, the least restrictive in terms of consumer choice, the employer might set higher copayments, and enrollees who choose the more restrictive managed care options might be offered lower copayments.

2.2.2.7 The Meaning of "Managed Care"

Managed care is most frequently associated with HMOs and PPOs, because these types of organizations were the first to try to control the utilization of care. In a traditional HMO, providers are typically employed by the HMO or are contractually tied to it and subject to some degree of regulation. More recently, indemnity insurers have begun to introduce regulatory controls over providers, such as second-opinion requirements for surgery and length-of-stay reviews. Providers transact with indemnity insurers at arm's length, and so indemnity insurers have had to develop such mechanisms to restrain utilization. Also, HMOs have been changing in form. In many cases, providers are more loosely tied to the HMO than has been true historically. In this type of arrangement, controlling utilization requires the establishment of contractual mechanisms. For example, providers who serve HMO members often have to obtain permission from the HMO before initiating expensive therapies.

The regulatory function of indemnity and contractual HMOs is shown in Figure 2–7. In this diagram, the financial flows are shown as before. The flow of services from the providers to the consumers is also shown. A dotted line from the insurer to the service flow line indicates the care-management function established by the insurer. Under managed care, the service flow is regulated.

In order to set standards for providers, HMOs engage in profiling, which involves collecting comparative data on the treatment patterns of providers. Using this information, the insurers can set benchmarks that can be used to regulate the utilization of care. In addition to specific controls on services, managed care organizations can also affect utilization through choosing providers to employ or with whom to contract. A cost-efficient practice style may be one characteristic such an organization is seeking when recruiting new providers.

2.3 COST OF ACTIVITIES

Having identified productive activities as efforts involving resource inputs whose aim is to create commodities, we now need to find some common measure. The concept of *cost* is often used. In the context of a flow, cost is taken to be the magnitude of the resources devoted to an activity during a given period of time. Several different meanings can be attached to this concept. One definition of cost is the money outlay or expenditure that has been paid to the providers for their services. For example, if an optometrist performs an eye pressure test, the money cost is simply what is paid for the optometrist's services. Money cost is a convenient way to measure the magnitude of an activity, but it is not always a complete measure. The same optometrist may do the same test for free; in this case the money

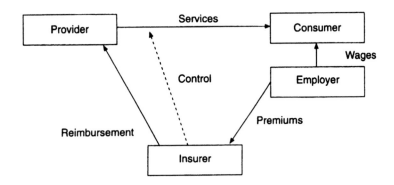

Figure 2–7 The flows of money and services shown in this diagram are consistent with any insurance arrangements. What is added is a control function by which the insurer establishes some form of control over the provider, thus regulating the flow of services from the provider to the consumer.

cost would be zero. Yet some activity has taken place, and this activity has used scarce resources.

In the health care sector, there are many examples of free (i.e., zero money cost) services. Clinical teachers in medical schools frequently donate their efforts. Volunteer collectors for such organizations as the American Heart Association, United Way, and March of Dimes donate their time. The notion of *opportunity cost*, defined as the value of the most valuable alternative course of action given up for the chosen course of action, is used as a measure that does not depend on whether providers are paid in money for their services. Opportunity cost is relevant when a resource has several alternative uses. If the resource is used in activity A, the opportunity cost is what that resource would have earned if it had been used in alternative activity B, where B is the highest valued alternative employment for that resource. Let us say that an optometrist who performs a refraction for free in a clinic could have obtained a fee of $20 had he or she performed it in the office. By valuing this service at $20, we make it comparable to services performed for a fee. Whenever a service is provided at a price below its alternative value, the money cost will not take into account the portion of cost that is, in effect, subsidized; opportunity cost is a better measure of the true size of the total resources committed to an activity.

Costs can be categorized, among other ways, as direct or indirect. *Direct costs* are money expenditures, while *indirect costs* (also called *lost-productivity costs*) are unpaid resource commitments. Though these are unpaid, they may still have significant opportunity costs.

Table 2–1 shows the estimated value of all direct national health expenditures for one year (1998) in the United States (Levit et al. 2000). These expenditures amount to $1,149 billion. The largest portion of funds went to hospital care (33.3 percent), followed by physician care (20 percent). The prescription drug portion has been growing considerably, and in 1998 it equaled 7.9 percent of the total. Twenty years earlier it had been only 4.8 percent of the total.

The growth in health expenditures, on a per capita basis, is shown in Figure 2–8. Since 1960, the growth has been steady. In 1989, health expenditures equaled $2,500 per person. By 1998, they had reached $4,200 per person.

Table 2–1 National Health Expenditures by Type of Service, United States, 1998

Expenditure Category	Amount (billions of dollars)	Percent of Total
Hospital care	382.8	33.3
Physician services	229.5	20.0
Dental services	53.8	4.6
Other professional services	66.6	5.8
Home health care	29.3	2.5
Prescription drugs	90.6	7.9
Vision products and other medical durables	15.5	1.3
Nursing home care	87.8	7.6
Other personal health care	32.1	2.8
Private insurance administration	57.7	5.0
Public health	36.6	3.2
Research and construction	35.3	3.1
Total national health expenditures	$1,149.1	100.0

Source: Reprinted from National Health Expenditure Tables, Health Care Financing Administration, www.hcfa.gov/stats/nhe/oact/tables/, 2000.

A frequently used benchmark for health spending is total health spending expressed as a ratio of the total of all final goods and services produced in the economy during a year (the gross domestic product [GDP]). The ratio in 1998 for the United States was 13.5 percent. That is, 13.5 percent of all final goods and services were health care services. The ratio of national health expenditures to the GDP is generally considered a critical indicator of resource use in the health care sector. In fact, as seen in Figure 2–9, this ratio had been growing steadily and significantly over the past several decades (Fuchs 1990), but since 1993 the ratio has been falling. The declining ratio may be partly due to reductions in government spending for health care services, but in general, as seen in Figure 2–8, per capita spending on

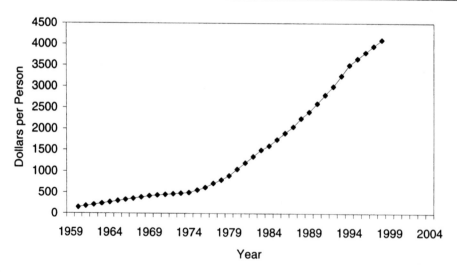

Figure 2–8 Per capita health expenditures, United States, 1960–1998. *Source:* Reprinted from National Health Expenditure Tables, Health Care Financing Administration, www.hcfa.gov/stats/nhe/oact/tables/, 2000.

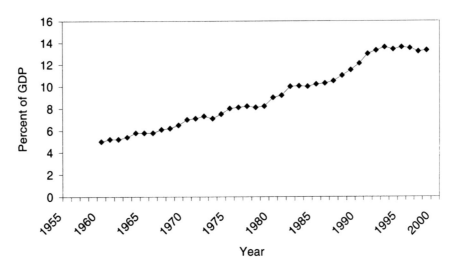

Figure 2–9 National health expenditures as a percent of gross domestic product (GDP), United States, 1960–1998. *Source:* Reprinted from National Health Expenditure Tables, Health Care Financing Administration, www.hcfa.gov/stats/nhe/oact/tables/, 2000.

health care was unabated after 1993. In fact, the national economy experienced tremendous growth during the 1990s, and this increase (which is the denominator in the ratio of health spending to GDP) helped reduce the ratio.

Despite the reduction in health spending relative to the GDP, when compared with other developed countries, the United States still has a very costly health care system. As can be seen in Figure 2–10, the health spending to GDP ratio is much lower for other countries (World Health Organization 2000; Organization for Economic Cooperation and Development 2000). In Germany, for example, the ratio was 10.8 percent, in Japan it was 7.1 percent, and in the United Kingdom it was 5.8 percent. Investigators have focused on this statistic as an important indicator of the economic performance of the health care system (Anderson 1997).

The above data provide us some idea of the direct costs of services provided. They do not, however, provide an indication of the total "burden" of costs—direct and indirect—that falls on all members of society as a result of illness. This total measure comprises what are called the *social costs*.

Ideally, a cost-of-illness study will include all of the relevant resources that are influenced by the illness. The economic effects of illness can be experienced for years, and they can have a very broad impact in terms of the types of resources that are affected.

An illness can be diagnosed years after it was acquired. For example, a person can be affected with the hepatitis C virus for many years before finally being diagnosed. It is only when he or she has been diagnosed that one can measure the economic impact of the illness. Further, the illness can generate economic costs for years after it has been diagnosed, even after the person has died. Chronic diseases last for years, and resources can be used as long as an illness lasts. If the person with the disease dies prematurely because of the disease, earnings that would have been experienced but were not are an indirect cost and part of the economic picture.

The following resource components might be affected by the illness: health care resources used in diagnosis and treatment (also called *direct care costs*); direct nonhealth resources such as transportation, special diets, and household goods;

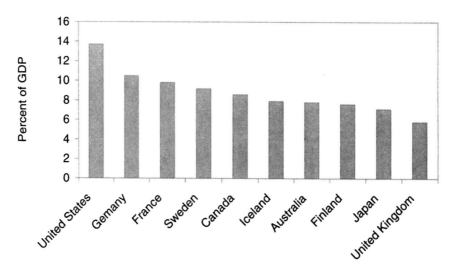

Figure 2–10 Health expenditures as a percentage of GDP, selected countries, 1997. *Source:* Reprinted from National Health Expenditure Tables, Health Care Financing Administration, www.hcfa.gov/stats/nhe/oact/tables/, 2000.

---

patient loss of work time due to illness and injury (also called *indirect care costs*); and other related indirect costs, such as work time lost by unpaid caregivers. The collection of all of these data is expensive, and so most studies will not include all the components.

Cost-of-illness studies can be conducted on a prevalence or incidence basis. With a prevalence basis, the annual costs of all existing cases during a year (including newly and previously diagnosed) are included. The future mortality–related costs for all persons with the disease who died during the year are also included (Rice 1990). In contrast, an incidence-based analysis includes all present and future costs *only for cases newly diagnosed during the year.* In theory, one can also conduct an incidence-based analysis for cases that were contracted during the year, although this is seldom done for chronic diseases because of a lack of data. The cost of a premature death would include the lost work time from future deaths.

The prevalence approach is useful for budgeting purposes. For many purposes, the incidence approach is preferred, although it is much easier to obtain prevalence data than incidence data. If we are conducting a study on the economic effects of preventing or detecting illness, we should obtain data on the costs of all down-stream events of the illness. The incidence approach would provide that information. If we used the prevalence approach, we would be obtaining the cost of many of the cases in midstream.

Data on the cost of several of the more economically important illnesses are shown in Figure 2–11. The costliest condition is injuries, with direct costs of $89 billion and indirect costs of $248 billion. The disease with the highest direct medical costs is heart disease, with annual costs of $101.8 billion. However, persons who suffer from injuries are younger than those who suffer from heart disease, and so their indirect costs are higher. Diabetes and cancer have roughly the same total cost of illness, but diabetes occurs in older persons, and so the ratio of direct to indirect costs is greater for diabetes. Arthritis has low direct costs because the cost of treatment is much lower than for the other illnesses shown in the graph.

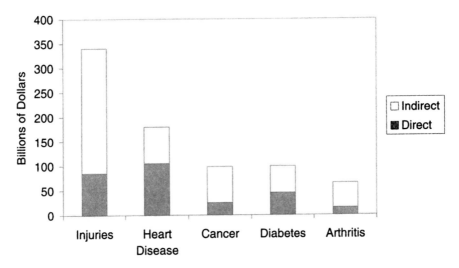

Figure 2–11 Cost of illness, selected diseases, United States, c. 1995. *Source:* Reprinted from *Disease Specific Estimates of Direct and Indirect Costs of Illnesss and NIH Support*, 1997, National Institutes of Health.

Cost-of-illness studies can provide valuable information that can be used in budgeting decisions and in cost-effectiveness studies. Cost-of-illness studies focus on the economic component of trends in disease and consequently are useful for policy makers. It is important for policy makers to have a notion of the impact of disease changes on expenditures. Much debate and misunderstanding has surrounded this topic. It should be understood that cost-of-illness studies are descriptive studies. One should not use the results of these studies by themselves to make policy recommendations. For these studies to be useful for evaluation purposes, the investigator must add additional information. Put another way, cost-of-illness studies describe what has happened. This can be most useful. But decision making requires more information: we must know why costs are what they are and what our objectives are.

EXERCISES

1. What is the difference between an insurance premium and a deductible?
2. Through what mechanism do most people in the United States purchase private health insurance?
3. What population does the Medicare program cover? What is Part A Medicare? Is there a premium, deductible, or copayment for Part A Medicare?
4. What is Part B Medicare insurance? Is there a premium, deductible, or copayment for Part B?
5. What populations does Medicaid cover? In general, is there a deductible or copayment for Medicaid? Why is there no premium?
6. On what basis is an HMO reimbursed? What is the relationship between the insurer and the provider in the HMO?

7. What distinguishes a preferred provider organization from a traditional health maintenance organization?
8. What is "managed" in managed care?
9. When would it be preferable to use opportunity costs rather than money costs?
10. What are direct and indirect costs?
11. What is a cost-of-illness study? What is the difference between measuring the cost of illness using the prevalence and incidence approaches?

BIBLIOGRAPHY

Overall Dimensions

Angell, M. 1985. Cost containment and the physician. *JAMA* 253:1203–1207.

Bauerschmidt, A.D. 1969. Sources and uses of healthcare funds in South Carolina. *Business and Economics Review of the University of South Carolina* 3:2–7.

Health Insurance Association of America. 1989. *Source book of health insurance data.* Washington, D.C.: Health Insurance Association of America.

Letsch, S.W., et al. 1988. National Health Expenditures, 1987. *Health Care Financing Review* 10 (winter): 109–122.

Levit, K.R., et al. 1989. Health spending and the ability to pay. *Health Care Financing Review* 10 (spring): 1–12.

Mullner, R., and J. Hadley. 1984. Interstate variations on the growth of chain-owned proprietary hospitals. *Inquiry* 21:144–151.

Rice, D.P., and J.J. Feldman. 1983. Living longer in the United States. *Milbank Quarterly* 61:362–396.

Sutcliffe, E.M. 1972. The Social Accounting of Health. In *The Economics of Medical Care*, ed. M.M. Hauser. London: George Allen and Unwin.

Costs, Prices, and Expenditures

Anderson, G., and J.R. Knickman. 1984. Patterns of expenditure among high utilizers of medical services. *Medical Care* 22:143–149.

Burner, S.T., and D.R. Waldo. 1995. National health expenditure projections, 1994–2005. *Health Care Financing Review* 16:221–242.

Cromwell, J., and D. Pushkin. 1989. Hospital productivity and intensity trends. *Inquiry* 26:366–380.

Freeland, M.S., et al. 1979. National hospital input price index. *Health Care Financing Review* 1 (summer):37–61.

Fuchs, V.R. 1990. The health sector's share of the gross national product. *Science* 247:534–538.

Ginsburg, D.H. 1978. Medical care services in the consumer price index. *Monthly Labor Review* 101:35–40.

Hellinger, F.J. 1990. Updated forecasts of the costs of medical care for persons with AIDS. *Public Health Reports* 105 (January): 1–12.

———. 1993. The lifetime cost of treating a person with AIDS. *JAMA* 270:474–478.

Kelly, J.V., et al. 1989. Duration and cost of AIDS hospitalizations in New York. *Medical Care* 27:1085–1098.

Klarman, H.E. 1972. Increases in the cost of physician and hospital services. *Inquiry* 7:22–36.

Long, S.H., et al. 1984. Medical expenditures for terminal cancer patients during the last year of life. *Inquiry* 22:315–327.

McCall, N. 1984. Utilization and costs of Medicare services by beneficiaries in their last year of life. *Medical Care* 22:329–342.

Pope, G. 1990. Physician inputs, outputs, and productivity; 1976–1986. *Inquiry* 27:151–160.

Rice, D.P., et al. 1985. The economic cost of illness. *Health Care Financing Review* 7 (fall): 61–80.

Scitovsky, A.A. 1984. The high cost of dying. *Milbank Quarterly* 62:591–608.

Scitovsky, A.A., and N. McCall. 1977. *Changes in the cost of treatment of selected illness.* Publication no. HRA 77–3161. Hyattsville, MD: National Center for Health Services Research.

Scitovsky, A.A., and D.P. Rice. 1987. Estimating the direct and indirect costs of acquired immunodeficiency syndrome in the United States, 1985, 1986, and 1991. *Public Health Reports* 102:5–17.

Sisk, J.E. 1987. The cost of AIDS: A review of the estimates. *Health Affairs* 6, no. 2:5–21.

Sloan, F.A., et al. 1985. The teaching hospital's growing surgical caseload. *JAMA* 254:376–382.

Zook, C.J., and E.D. Moore. 1980. High cost users of medical care. *New England Journal of Medicine* 302:996–1002.

New Institutions

de Lissovoy, G., et al. 1987. Preferred provider organizations one year later. *Inquiry* 24:127–135.

Gabel, J., et al. 1986. The emergence and future of preferred provider organizations. *Journal of Health Politics, Policy, and Law* 11:305–321.

Gruber, L.R., et al. 1988. From movement to industry: The growth of HMOs. *Health Affairs* 7, no 3:197–208.

McLauchlin, C.G., et al. 1989. Health care coalitions. *Inquiry* 26:72–83.

Health Insurance

DiCarlo, S., and J. Gabel. 1989. Conventional health insurance: A decade later. *Health Care Financing Review* 10 (spring): 77–89.

Gabel, J., et al. 1994. The health insurance picture in 1993. *Health Affairs* 13:325–336.

Reinhardt, U.E. 1993. Reorganizing the financial flows in American health care. *Health Affairs* 12:172–193.

Rotwein, S., et al. 1995. Medicaid and state health care reform. *Health Care Financing Review* 16 (spring): 105–120.

Rubin, R.M., et al. 1989. Private long-term care insurance. *Medical Care* 27:182–193.

Short, P.F. 1988. Trends in employee health insurance benefits. *Health Affairs* 7, no. 3:186–196.

Smeeding, T.M., and L. Straub. 1987. Health care financing among the elderly. *Journal of Health Politics, Policy, and Law* 12:35–52.

Data

Anderson, G.F. 1997. In search of value: An international comparison of cost, access, and outcomes. *Health Affairs* 16, no. 6:163–171.

Health Insurance Association of America.1999. *Source book of health insurance data 1999–2000.* Washington, DC: Health Insurance Association of America.

Levit, K., et al. 2000. Health spending in 1998: Signals of Change. *Health Affairs* 19, no. 1:124–132.

Organization for Economic Cooperation and Development. 2000. *OECD health data 2000.* Paris: Organization for Economic Cooperation and Development.

U.S. Department of Health and Human Services. 1999. *Health United States, 1999.* Hyattsville, MD: U.S. Department of Health and Human Services.

World Health Organization.2000. *World health report 2000.* Geneva: World Health Organization.

Cost of Illness

Cutler, D.M., et al. 1998. Are medical prices declining? Evidence from heart attack treatments. *Quarterly Journal of Economics* 63:991–1024.

Byford, S., et al. 2000. Cost of illness studies. *BMJ* 320:1335.

Frank, R.G., et al. 1998.Measuring prices and quantities of treatment for depression. *American Economic Review* 88:106–111.

Hodgson, T.A., and M.R. Meiners. 1982. Cost of illness methodology: A guide to current practices and procedures. *Milbank Quarterly* 60:429–462.

Hodgson, T.A., and A.J. Cohen. 1999. Medical care expenditures for selected circulatory diseases. *Medical Care* 37:994–1012.

———. 1999. Medical expenditures for major disease. *Health Care Financing Review* 21 (winter): 119–164.

Keeler, E.B., et al. 1989. The external costs of a sedentary lifestyle. *American Journal of Public Health* 79:975–981.

McClellan, M., and H. Noguchi. 1998. Technological change in heart-disease treatment. *American Economic Review* 88(2):90–96.

Moore, R., et al. 1997. *Economic burden of illness in Canada, 1993.* Ottawa: Health Canada.

Rice, D.P. 1990. Cost-of-illness studies: fact or fiction? *Lancet* 344:1519–1520.

Rice, D.P., et al. 1985. The economic cost of illness: A replication and update. *Health Care Financing Review* 7 (fall):61–80.

Rice, D.P., et al. 1990. *The economic costs of alcohol and drug abuse and mental illness: 1985.* San Francisco: University of California, Institute for Health and Aging.

Sheill, A., et al. 1987. Cost of illness studies: An aid to decision-making? *Health Policy* 8:317–323.

Ungar, W., and P. Coyte. 2000. Measuring productivity loss days in asthma patients. *Health Economics* 9:37–46.

Zook, C.J., et al. 1980. Repeated hospitalization for the same disease. *Milbank Quarterly* 58:454–471.

Part II

Explanatory Economics

Chapter 3

Demand for Medical Care: A Simple Model

1. Identify two hypotheses used to predict the behavior of quantity demanded for a health care service.
2. Explain the demand hypothesis and distinguish between the concepts of *demand* and *quantity demanded.*
3. Know the individual factors that influence demand and explain how each affects the demand curve.
4. Explain how we can derive an individual's demand curve for medical services from basic assumptions about the economic behavior of consumers.
5. Explain how to derive a market demand curve from data on individual demand curves.
6. Define the concept of elasticity of demand and explain how to measure the concept using data on prices and utilization.
7. Know the various types of health insurance arrangements and explain how each affects the out-of-pocket or direct price and the demand curve for medical services.

3.1 THE CONCEPT OF DEMAND

The purpose of explanatory economics is to predict economic behavior. When analyzing demand behavior, our attention focuses on the quantity demanded by consumers of a specific commodity or service. To perform the analysis, we use a demand model that serves two purposes: It provides a categorization of the separate factors that might cause demand or quantity demanded to increase or decrease, and it provides a specific hypothesis about how economic factors (e.g., price and income) influence demand or quantity demanded.

Models are the devices we use to obtain our results. A model is a representation of reality, not a complete description of it. The purpose of a model, however specified, is to present us with an "If . . . then . . ." type of explanation. In the case of the demand model, the reasoning is of this form: "If factor *x* increases, then demand or quantity demanded will increase (or decrease, depending on what factor *x* is)." A good model screens essential causal factors and incorporates them into a logical, coherent system.

Even though every model is conjectural, it should tell us something about movements in real phenomena (e.g., the quantity of medical care demanded). In assessing a model, it is therefore sufficient to examine whether its predictions concerning movements in selected phenomena are realized by comparing the predictions with actual movements in the phenomena as measured by data. In other words, accuracy of prediction is the test of an explanatory model.

This chapter introduces a simple model of the demand for a commodity. Section 3.2 sets forth the model, using an individual's demand for medical care as an example. Section 3.3 takes us behind the scenes and shows how the model of demand can be derived. Several key shortcomings of the simple model when applied to the medical care context are emphasized; these shortcomings are central to the extended analyses of Chapter 4. Section 3.4 examines the factors influencing the market demand for the commodity. Section 3.5 develops the concept of *elasticity*, a tool used to measure the magnitude of the hypothesized movements, and Section 3.6 presents the demand analysis when insurance is present. Finally, Section 3.7 presents some actual estimates of the demand relationship.

3.2 INDIVIDUAL DEMAND: THE PRICE-QUANTITY RELATION

3.2.1 Demand and Quantity Demanded

We begin our exposition of the price-quantity relation with a specification of the terms of reference and definitions of the variables used. The unit of analysis is the individual consumer. In the present context, we examine the economic behavior of a typical or representative consumer. This behavior involves attaining or attempting to attain commodities. Since our focus is on health care, the commodity *physician care* is used as the major example. Physician care is defined as examinations and treatments administered by physicians to their patients. Physician care is only one of many commodities in the health care sector. Thus, when following the analysis, keep in mind that the relations specified in this chapter can be applied to other health-related commodities as well, including hospital services, pharmaceuticals, dental care, home care, preventive measures, nutritional services, nursing care, and the services of other health professionals.

Having identified the commodity in our analysis, we must next find an appropriate unit of measurement. Here we encounter a problem that is pervasive in medical care organization analysis: defining and measuring quality differences among units of medical care. Examinations and treatments can vary in thoroughness, in the physician's technical competence, and in the physician's bedside manner, among other factors. Quality differences constitute differences in these characteristics. When analyzing physician care as a commodity, all these variations should be kept in mind. In this chapter, we will abstain from quality differences to avoid complicating our initial entrance into explanatory economics.

Our commodity, physician care, is measured by the number of visits to a physician by the typical consumer. Each visit is taken as identical with all others. Finally, we specify the time span as being one year. Given this time frame, our commodity measure becomes the number of physician visits per year.

With this background, the demand hypothesis used to predict the effect of a change in direct per unit price on the quantity demanded of a commodity can be presented. The hypothesis is that the lower the out-of-pocket price offered to consumers (all other factors held constant), the greater the number of units of that commodity they will demand. A number of conventions or interpretations are related to this hypothesis. By "quantity demanded" we mean the quantity demanded at any specific price, all other causal factors held constant. Quantity demanded is the amount that the consumer is willing and able to buy at the specified price. By "demand" we mean the set of quantities demanded at various prices, all other causal factors held constant. By "out-of-pocket price" we mean the price paid directly by consumers for a particular unit of the commodity. By "all other factors" we mean those variables other than price that influence consumer demand behavior. The economic approach to consumer behavior is to specify an initial relation between out-of-pocket price and quantity demanded and then to introduce other causal factors to see how they affect the basic demand relation.

One such demand relation, assuming all other factors remain unchanged, is illustrated diagrammatically as line d_1 in Figure 3–1. The specific relation shown by this line, or curve, entails that, at a price of $7 per visit, the consumer would be willing to visit the physician twice a year; at a price of $6 per visit, the consumer would be willing to make three visits; and so on. Assuming that the quantities demanded at all other prices trace out a straight-line relation, d_1 represents a particular demand curve at one specific level of demand. The lowercase letter d is used to indicate that we are representing the behavior of a single individual.

The downward slope of the demand curve is explained by the possibility of substitution. The economic approach implies that very few, if any, commodities are absolute musts. Substitutes exist for most commodities; some are almost identical and others are less similar. The longer the time span during which the consumer adapts his or her behavior to any substitutes, the more relevant they become. A sore throat, for example, can be treated by a physician or by resorting to drugs or home remedies. Furthermore, even if the malady is treated by a physician, alternative types of broad-spectrum antibiotics can be used. In recent years, use of outpatient treatment instead of hospitalization has been suggested for many types of ailments. In the long term, health foods and other preventive services are substitutes for medical care in maintaining desired health levels. In these as well as other instances, the hypothesized relation applies: the lower the price of any specific alternative, the more it will be demanded.

Other hypotheses than this demand relation might be put forward to explain consumer demand behavior. One alternative hypothesis that has received much attention in the medical care literature is that at higher prices individuals will still demand and pay for the same quantity of medical care. This alternative hypothesis would be represented by a vertical demand curve. Similar vertical demand curves have also been hypothesized for other items considered necessities, such as housing, basic foods, and even alcohol.

Having two alternative hypotheses, we are faced with the problem of determining which is the more useful for explaining actual behavior. Debating the issue by itself cannot resolve the controversy, however. The hypothesis chosen should be the one that most closely fits the actual data. The empirical testing of hypotheses is discussed in Section 3.7.

Before proceeding with qualifications to our hypothesis, we should emphasize that we are focusing solely on consumer behavior. Our hypothesis relates only to how much the consumer is willing to buy at any price. We are not inquiring at this stage about whether the amount demanded will be supplied or available.

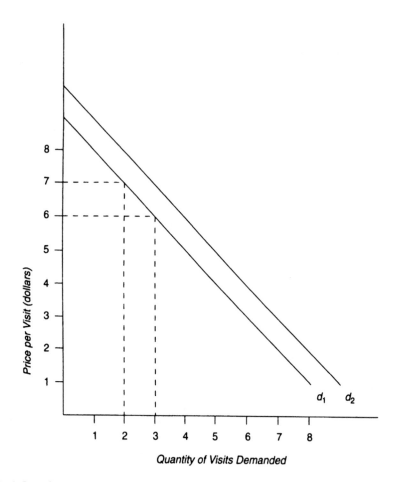

Figure 3–1 Graphic representation of the demand relation, the famous downward-sloping demand curve. Curves d_1 and d_2 show the quantity demanded increasing as the direct price decreases. Each curve represents a separate level of demand. With reference to curve d_1, curve d_2 represents an increase in demand.

3.2.2 Changes in Demand

The effects of factors other than the out-of-pocket price on the economic behavior of consumers are introduced by way of their influence on the basic price-quantity relation. These other factors can be placed into three broad categories: (1) income, (2) prices of other (related) commodities, and (3) tastes. Each category is considered in turn.

3.2.2.1 Income

The income of the consumer is generally assumed to be positively related to demand. That is, if income increases, the quantity demanded at each price will be greater. The basic relation between income and demand can be illustrated with the use of demand curves. In Figure 3–1, curve d_1 can now be interpreted as representing a level of demand at some initial level of income. Let us suppose that, from this initial level, income increases. The hypothesized effect on demand is such that at a price of $7 there will be three visits demanded instead of two, at a price of $6 there will be four visits demanded instead of three, and so on. The new demand level, corresponding to the higher income level, can be represented by the curve d_2. In the diagram, the relative position of the two curves summarizes the net influence of income on consumer behavior. A shift in demand from curve d_1 to curve d_2 is called an *increase* in demand.

The same reasoning can be applied in reverse to a fall in income. This decline causes the consumer to demand less of the commodity at each price. The change in the level of demand might, for example, be represented by a shift from d_2 to d_1. This is called a *decrease* in demand.

Income is frequently defined as an individual's earnings in a specific time period. It is a variable used to measure the ability of the individual to afford medical care, but it is only an approximate measure. Another measure of an individual's ability to purchase medical care is the individual's level of wealth, including bonds, bank deposits, real estate, and other assets, less any debt, such as bank loans and mortgages. A third measure is after-tax income. This measure is particularly important to take into account when considering changes in tax rates and their effects on purchasing power. Whatever measure is used should be a good approximation of the individual's ability to pay for medical care.

3.2.2.2 Prices of Related Commodities

The demand for a particular commodity is also influenced by the quantities of related commodities consumed. The quantities of these related commodities are, in turn, influenced by their prices. Two classes of commodity relations are of concern to us: complements and substitutes. A complementary commodity is one whose use is generally accompanied by the use of the commodity in question. Examples might include penicillin and syringes, the services of a surgeon and the hospital's surgical services, and the services of a radiologist and radiograph film. The hypothesis relating the demands of complementary commodities is as follows: a fall in the price of a commodity increases the quantity demanded of that commodity, and it also leads to an increase in the demand for commodities that are complements. Similar reasoning, in reverse, applies to an increase in the price of one commodity in a complementary set. As an example of this relation, we can hypothesize that a fall in the out-of-pocket price of the surgical services involved in tonsillectomies will lead to an increase in the quantity of services demanded; it will also increase the demand for hospital room services.

Complements play an important role in medical care demand. The close relation between radiology machines and radiologist services has frequently led to the assertion that much hospital demand is really determined by the quantity of physician services consumed.

The second type of commodity relation is that of substitution. A substitute is a commodity that can replace the original commodity. The hypothesis is that a fall in the price of a commodity increases the quantity demanded and leads to a reduced demand for substitute commodities. This relation can be illustrated using an example of two substitute services, postoperative recuperation time in the hospital versus home care. A rise in the price the patient pays for an additional day of hospital care decreases the quantity of hospital days demanded. At the same time, it increases the demand for home care.

Substitution was also the reason given for the downward slope of the demand curve for any commodity. For example, quantity of inpatient care demanded is negatively related to patient price because inpatient care can be substituted for home care when the price of inpatient care falls and vice versa. This assumes, of course, that the price of home care remains constant. When the price of home care rises, this leads to additional substitution, which is accounted for in our model by an outward shift in the inpatient care demand curve. The slope of the demand curve of any commodity, as well as how much it shifts when substitute prices change, depends on how similar the patient perceives the substitutes to be. Services such as inpatient and outpatient surgery (e.g., for hernia repair and tonsillectomies) are highly substitutable, as are nursing home care and home care in many instances.

3.2.2.3 Tastes

Consumer taste is a catchall category covering all other factors that might influence demand. Tastes have sometimes been called *wants*, a term connoting the intensity of desire for particular commodities. The elements that influence the intensity of an individual's desire for medical care include health status, educational background, sex, age, race, and upbringing. Any of these can explain differences among individuals in the intensity of desire for medical care. That is, with other factors (incomes, prices of other commodities, and so on) held constant, these differences can be used to explain why one individual's demand curve is d_1 (Figure 3–1) whereas another's is d_2. (The explanation might simply be that the health status of the first individual is lower than that of the second individual.)

Tastes are usually considered to be fixed from the standpoint of economic analysis, although some economic models recognize that advertising by firms can influence consumer tastes. Although tastes differ among individuals, they are hypothesized, for most commodities, to be stable over fairly short periods of time. If they are stable, once the factors that underlie tastes are accounted for, differences in demand can be attributed to differences in incomes, prices of other commodities, and factors influencing tastes. However, controversy exists over the stability of individual tastes for medical care. In addition to the dependence of tastes on health, which is itself transitory, physicians potentially can exert considerable influence over tastes for medical care. Changing tastes have played a large role in health economics. Because of this, it is necessary to go behind the scenes to discover the role of tastes in medical care demand.

3.3 DERIVING THE DEMAND RELATIONSHIP

In Section 3.2, the demand for medical care was analyzed as if medical care were an ordinary commodity like carrots or shoes. However, certain characteristics of medical care make it unlike many ordinary commodities. We must pay closer attention to these characteristics to determine if and when standard demand analysis is appropriate for medical care. To do this, we present a theoretical model focusing on the conditions that are required for the demand relation to hold; special attention is paid to whether these conditions are likely to be met in the case of medical care.

The factors influencing a consumer's behavior with regard to the demand for a commodity can be placed under the categories of income, prices, and tastes. Let us assume that a typical individual has a choice of purchasing only two commodities. These two commodities are carrots and physician care (as measured by physician's office visits). In what follows, we will specify the assumptions underlying our model for the demand for these two products.

3.3.1 Tastes

Tastes are essentially desires for products. These desires, or wants, are quantified using an index that we call *utility*. Although it is a hypothetical construct, the concept of utility is very valuable as an instructive device. It is often equated with the notion of satisfaction. The utility of carrots for a hypothetical individual is shown in Table 3–1. The numbers in this table were devised to show an increasing total amount of utility (total utility) as more carrots are consumed, but, more importantly, they were devised so that the increases gradually diminish. The concept used to represent the increases in utility from successive quantities of a commodity is called *marginal utility*. Marginal utility is the change in total utility resulting from a unit change in the consumption of the commodity. Thus the marginal utility for the first carrot is 6, it is 5 for the second, and so on. This decrease in the size of the utility of successive quantities of a commodity is called *diminishing marginal utility*. Note that, in general, total satisfaction will still increase. This is a key assumption of demand analysis.

The same assumption can be applied to medical care as well, but the circumstances in which the relationship of diminishing marginal utility will hold needs to be explored in greater detail. We therefore list the conditions that must occur.

3.3.1.1 Health Status

The initial health status of the individual (H) is given and known by the individual. That is, the individual knows what medical condition she has.

Table 3–1 Relationship between Quantity Consumed of Two Commodities and Utility of (Satisfaction Derived from) the Commodities

Quantity	Medical Care		Carrots	
	Total Utility	Marginal Utility	Total Utility	Marginal Utility
1	22	22	6	6
2	42	20	11	5
3	60	18	15	4
4	76	16	18	3
5	90	14	20	2
6	102	12	21	1

3.3.1.2 Consumer Information

The relationship between medical care (*MC*) and health status (*H*) is also known by the individual. That is, she knows how "productive" medical care will be in influencing her health.

3.3.1.3 Productivity of Medical Care

In general, we assume that the marginal productivity of medical care in influencing health is constant. As more units of medical care (visits) are consumed, equal additions to health status will result. Obviously, there must be a limit to how healthy an individual can become, and we will show what happens when this assumption is altered. For the moment, we will hold with the assumption of constant productivity.

3.3.1.4 Quality

The quality of medical care is constant. All visits are of the same quality.

3.3.1.5 Other Taste-Influencing Variables

It should be noted that the utility function is dependent on a host of other variables, each of which may influence the individual's intensity of desire for medical care. These variables include the individual's education, upbringing, marital status, and age, among others. For example, it is believed that increasing education increases an individual's desire for good health. Thus we should be aware that in back of any taste function lies a series of formative factors that cause the utility-quantity relation to be what it is. We will assume that there are no other sources of utility other than medical care and carrots.

Given these assumptions, we can hypothesize the type of relations between utility and medical care shown in Table 3–1, where each added visit results in a smaller increment of added utility. Unless the individual is a competitive bodybuilder, the hypothesis is a plausible one.

3.3.2 Income

The second variable in our demand model is the individual's income. We will assume that the individual's income is $10 for the time period and that the individual lacks any accumulated wealth usable for purchasing care.

3.3.3 Prices of Other Commodities

Other variables include the prices charged for medical care and carrots. We will initially set these at $1 per carrot and $4 per physician's office visit. The purpose of our analysis is to predict what happens when the price of medical care changes and, in the process, to make explicit what variables are initially being held constant in the analysis.

3.3.4 Behavioral Assumption: Utility Maximization

Finally, we come to our behavioral assumption, which is what sets the model in motion. Our assumption is that the individual is a utility maximizer (i.e., the individual desires to gain the most satisfaction or benefit from his or her income).

3.3.5 Predictions

The model's conclusion stems from these assumptions together with assumptions about price changes. Let us first determine what quantities of medical care and carrots are demanded at the initial prices. In doing this, we need to focus on the marginal utility per dollar of expenditure, or the ratio of marginal utility to price (*MU/P*). It is this variable that expresses the satisfaction per dollar of expense for each alternative use. At a price of $1 per carrot, buying a carrot will be the best bet for the first $1 of expenditure, since the first carrot yields 6 units of utility. The next item purchased will not be another carrot, because an additional expenditure here would yield 5 units of utility per $1, whereas a visit to the doctor would yield 5.5 units (22 units/$4). Therefore, the individual makes a visit to the doctor. The individual has now spent a total of $5 and has $5 left. The next items of expenditure will be a carrot and another visit to the doctor (indeed, both have an *MU/P* ratio of 5). At this point the individual will have used up all income and will have achieved an equal marginal utility per dollar for the last purchases of each commodity. The total utility (53) is the highest that can be attained with $10. This equality of *MU/P* in each use indicates that the individual's income cannot be reallocated to obtain more utility.

To show that the individual is maximizing utility, let us assume that, after the second carrot, the individual allocates the remaining $4 to the purchase of carrots instead of medical care. The marginal utility of the third, fourth, fifth, and sixth carrot would be 4, 3, 2, and 1, respectively. The individual would now be getting 1 unit of utility per $1 of expenditure instead of the 5 units obtainable by purchasing medical care. The total utility would be 43. That is, the individual would have been better off with two carrots and two visits than with this alternative set of purchases.

Having shown that there is a utility-maximizing "equilibrium" quantity for each commodity, let us now change the assumption about prices of other commodities and lower the price of medical care to $3. A carrot will still cost $1. This fall in the price of medical care results in an increase in the utility per dollar of medical care for all visits and makes medical care more valuable in dollar terms. Under this altered assumption, the individual will maximize utility by "consuming" three visits and only consume one carrot.

The essential implication of this analysis is that when the price of medical care falls, the quantity demanded increases (assuming all other variables, including other prices as well as incomes and tastes, remain the same). This is thus a derivation of the demand relationship. It should be noted that the model only holds when other variables are held constant. Changing them will shift the demand relationship in one direction or the other, depending on the variable and the degree of change. For example, a more educated person may perceive health as having a greater utility relative to carrots, thus causing a shift in tastes. This will shift the demand for medical care as well.

With regard to one particular loose end, our assumption about the productivity of medical care, let us consider the probable effect of a more realistic assumption. In particular, let us assume that medical care has diminishing marginal productivity with respect to health. If additional units of health diminished in size with successive visits, this would make the marginal utility of medical care fall more quickly and would reduce the relative desirability of additional units of medical care. There would still be a downward-sloping demand curve, but it would be shifted inward in comparison to the situation where the productivity of medical care was constant.

3.4 MARKET DEMAND

The model developed previously provided a means of analyzing an individual's demand for medical care. To generalize the model to explain market demand, we must make an additional assumption. (By "market" we mean the network of buyers and sellers of a commodity.) The assumption is that the more individuals there are who seek the product, the greater will be the market demand and the quantity demanded in the market at any price.

This is illustrated in Figure 3–2, which shows the demand curves of three individuals: d_b is Mr. B's demand curve, d_k is Ms. K's demand curve, and d_j is Mrs. J's demand curve. At a price of $20 per visit, Mr. B will demand 3 visits, Ms. K will demand 2, and Mrs. J will demand none. At $15 per visit, Mr. B., Ms. K., and Mrs. J will demand 5 visits, 4 visits, and 1 visit, respectively. At $10, the number of visits will be 7, 6, and 4. Using information on individual demand curves and on the number of individuals, we can derive a market demand curve.

Given the three individual demand curves, the market quantity demanded at a given price will be the sum of the quantities demanded by all three individuals at that price. At a price of $20, the quantity demanded in the market will be 5 visits; at $15, the quantity will be 10; and at $10, it will be 17. The market demand curve is shown in Figure 3–2 as D_m.

We can now divide the factors influencing market demand into two categories: (1) factors influencing individual demand only and (2) factors influencing market demand. The former includes prices, incomes, and tastes. If any of these change, individual demand or the quantities demanded will also change. If individual demand curves shift out, market curves, being based on individual curves, will shift out as well. In addition to responding to changes in individual curves, market demand is influenced by changes in the number of participants in the market. For example, an influx of people into an area will cause market demand to increase. It is also possible that people in the area who did not demand any medical care at higher prices will become consumers of care as the price falls.

3.5 MEASURING QUANTITY RESPONSIVENESS TO PRICE CHANGES

In the preceding sections, we developed a model that enabled us to predict how a particular factor will affect quantity demanded or demand. Thus, we can predict that, when the out-of-pocket price falls, the quantity demanded will rise. We can now ask, by how much will the quantity demanded rise? The answer to this question is likely to play an important role in setting policy.

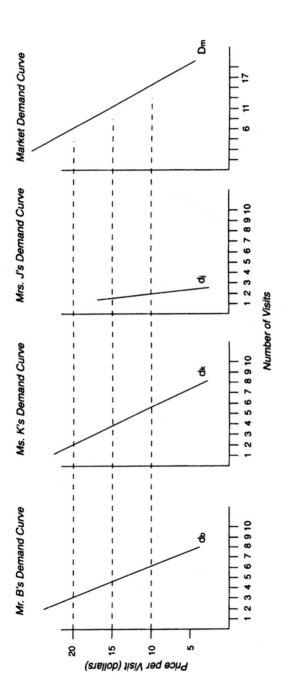

Figure 3–2 Derivation of the market demand curve from individual demand curves. The quantity demanded at each price by all consumers in the market is the sum of the individual demanded. The market demand curve is the horizontal sum of all individual demand curves.

The concept used to measure quantity responsiveness to out-of-pocket price changes is the concept of *price elasticity of demand.* Price elasticity is designed to measure the responsiveness of demand to a price change at a given point or between two given points on a single demand curve. That is, it attempts to measure responsiveness when the only factor undergoing change and thereby influencing the quantity demanded is price.

The elasticity of demand is designed to measure changes independent of the units of measurement. That is, the measure of elasticity is a measure of relative magnitudes and will not change if cents rather than dollars are used to measure price or units rather than thousands are used to measure quantity. Elasticity is thus a pure measure of the magnitude of change. The formula used for small changes in price is the percentage change in quantity demanded over the percentage change in price. In symbolic terms, this is written

$$E = \frac{\Delta Q / Q}{\Delta P / P}$$

where E is elasticity, Q is the original quantity, P is the original price, and ΔQ and ΔP are changes in Q and P. This formula is known as a *point elasticity formula.* The point elasticity formula is appropriate for very small changes along the demand curve. If the change in price is at all appreciable, an average elasticity measure over the range of the demand curve covered by the change is more appropriate. This measure, known as the *arc elasticity of demand,* is written as

$$E = \frac{(Q_2 - Q_1) / Q_2 + Q_1)}{(P_2 - P_1) / (P_2 + P_1)}$$

where Q_1 and P_1 refer to one price and quantity set and Q_2 and P_2 refer to a second set at another point on the same demand curve. In fact, both the price and quantity changes are expressed as ratios to average price and quantity levels, that is, as $(P_1 + P_2)/2$ and $(Q_1 + Q_2)/2$. The 2s would cancel out, leaving us with the formula as presented.

An example will help to illustrate the use of this formula. Assume that the Richland County Health Department charges \$3.00 per syphilis test and that in May it performed 1,200 tests. In June the County Council decided to raise the charges to \$3.25 per test. Only 1,150 people requested tests in June. What is the elasticity of demand?

The elasticity measure of a price change is supposed to be a measure of responsiveness along a demand curve, that is, when all factors other than price remain constant. If other factors have indeed remained constant, we can use the elasticity formula as an approximation of the responsiveness of quantity demanded to price changes. If other factors have changed, we must make some adjustment to take into account the extent to which these other factors influenced the quantity demanded. Assume in our example that these other factors remained constant and that only price influenced quantity. In this case, we can use the elasticity formula directly:

$$E = \frac{(1,150 - 1,200)/(1,150 + 1,200)}{(3.25 - 3)/(3.25 + 3)} = -0.53$$

The elasticity of demand at that point is –0.53. (The minus sign is frequently dropped from discussions, so one will often see the price elasticity quoted as the absolute value, e.g., 0.53. The reader should remember that, in the case of price elasticity, the negative sign, if dropped, is taken for granted.) We thus have a figure indicating the responsiveness of quantity to price.

Price elasticity is related to how total consumer expenditures respond to a change in the out-of-pocket price. For any elasticity measure whose absolute value is less than 1, total out-of-pocket expenditures will increase with a decrease in price; at such points on the demand curve, demand is said to be inelastic. In our example, total expenditures ($P \times Q$) were $3,600.00 before the price change and $3,737.50 after. Receipts from this source rose by $137.50 because of the nature of the responsiveness at that point on the demand curve. An elasticity measure of –0.53 is thought of as relatively unresponsive; that is, a small relative price rise or fall will generate a smaller relative quantity change. If price increases by 1 percent, the quantity will decrease by only about 0.5 percent, and the total amount spent on syphilis tests will increase. With an elasticity of –0.53, a reduction in price will lower total expenditures (i.e., total consumer expenditures in terms of dollars) because the relative increase in quantity purchased will not be sufficient to overcome the relatively greater price decrease. Thus, if the Richland County Health Department wants more revenue and does not care about how many tests are performed, it should raise its price to $3.25.

Demand curves can also have unitary elastic and elastic portions. Where the elasticity measures –1, demand responsiveness is said to be *unitary elastic*. In the case of a small change in price, total expenditures will remain constant. When the demand responsiveness is elastic (i.e., greater than 1 in absolute value), it means that the relative change in quantity consumed exceeds the relative change in price. If there is a small increase in price, the decrease in quantity will be relatively greater, and total expenditures will fall. If there is a small decrease in price, total expenditures will rise.

These relations are shown in Figure 3–3. A straight-line demand curve for vaccinations is shown in Graph A. At a price of $10, no vaccinations are demanded, but as the price falls in $1 increments, vaccination demand increases by 100. Thus, at a price of $9, 100 vaccinations will be demanded; at a price of $8, 200 will be demanded; and so on. Graph B shows the total expenditures generated at each level of sales. Thus, if 100 vaccinations are sold, $900 in expenditures is generated, and so on (see Table 3–2 for the actual values). Over a range, total expenditures increase, but eventually the increase levels off to a maximum, and beyond that point total expenditures begin to decline.

There is a connection between the elasticity along a specific segment of the demand curve and the total expenditures specific to relevant points on the curve. At relatively high prices and low quantities on a straight-line demand curve, only a relatively small change in price (in terms of percentage) is needed to induce a relatively large change in the quantity demanded. The lower expenditures resulting from the fall in unit prices is therefore more than offset by the large increase in quantity demanded, and so total expenditures will increase. For example, in Table 3–2, for a reduction in price from $9 to $8, the arc elasticity of demand along that segment of the curve is –4.76. Demand is therefore said to be elastic, and if that reduction in price is instituted, total expenditures will increase (in this case, from $900 to $1,600). As we move down the demand curve, the relative price change

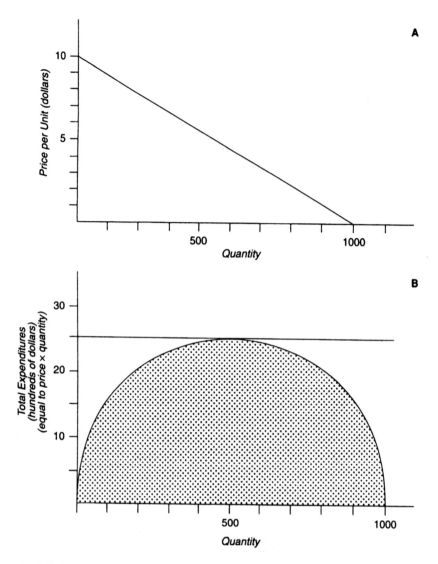

Figure 3–3 Relationship between price, quantity demanded, and total revenue. Graph A shows the basic relation between quantity demanded and price. Graph B shows the relation between total expenditures (which equal price times quantity) and quantity. Graph B is derived from Graph A.

becomes smaller in relation to the associated quantity change. Thus the absolute value of elasticity falls. But as long as this value in absolute terms is greater than 1 (i.e., we are on the elastic portion of the curve), total expenditures will increase, although not by as much as in higher priced segments. Eventually, the elasticity takes on a value of −1. At this point, price and quantity changes offset each other exactly, and total expenditures stay constant (we are at the top of the total expenditures curve). As prices fall further, we move on to the inelastic portion of the demand curve. Price reductions offset quantity increases, and total expenditures fall. Thus, along any single straight-line demand curve, the elasticity of demand will

Table 3–2 Price for Vaccinations, Quantity Demanded, and Total Expenditures

Price	Quantity Demanded	Total Expenditures
$10	0	$ 0
9	100	900
8	200	1,600
7	300	2,100
6	400	2,400
5	500	2,500
4	600	2,400
3	700	2,100
2	800	1,600
1	900	900

decrease with successive reductions in price. While elasticity is related to slope, it is not identical with the slope of the curve.

Further insight into the concept of elasticity can be gained by examining the elasticity for two different demand curves at a single price. Assume that two demand curves in two different markets for physician visits cross at a price of $3 and a quantity of 10, 000 visits, as in Figure 3–4. The consumers in Market 2 are more responsive to price reductions than arethose in Market 1. Let AD be the demand curve in Market 1 and BC be the demandcurve in Market 2. Now let the price fall by 10 cents. Consumers in Market 1 demand 10,400 visits, whereas those in Market 2 demand 10,600. The arc elasticity in Market 1 is

$$E = \frac{400/20,400}{-.10/5.90} = -1.16$$

The arc elasticity in Market 2 is

$$E = \frac{600/20,600}{-.10/5.90} = -1.72$$

As can be seen, demand curve BC is for a more responsive group of consumers, and the elasticity for a given quantity will be greater in absolute value than that of a less responsive group.

3.6 INSURANCE, OUT-OF-POCKET PRICE, AND QUANTITY DEMANDED

A major factor in considering the demand for medical care is the role that insurance plays in influencing the out-of-pocket price of medical care. There are a number of different types of insurance arrangements that consumers can obtain, and these will affect the out-of-pocket price and hence the quantity demanded in different ways. We will examine the important alternatives.

In analyzing the effect of alternative insurance arrangements, we initially specify a demand curve in which the consumers have no insurance and hence pay the full price charged by the provider (e.g., a physician). This curve, where full price equals the out-of-pocket price, is labeled D_n in Figure 3–5. Now let us introduce the first type of insurance arrangement: a copayment arrangement.

A copayment is a payment by the patient of a proportion of the charged price; the insurance company pays the remainder of the charged price. For example, with a 20-percent copayment and a charged price of $20 per visit, the patient pays the

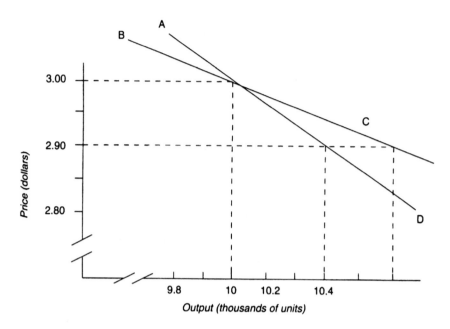

Figure 3–4 Responsiveness of quantity demanded to price for differently sloped demand curves. Curve *BC* shows a greater responsiveness of quantity demanded to price than does curve *AD*.

---

provider 20 percent of the charged price, $4, and the insurance company pays the remainder. In analyzing the impact of a coinsurance contract on demand, we assume that, even though the consumer has purchased an insurance contract, demand behavior is still governed by the demand curve D_n. What changes is that the out-of-pocket price and charged price now differ from one another. At any given charged price, the consumer faces a lower out-of-pocket price and hence will move down the demand curve D_n.

If the coinsurance rate is 50 percent, the demand curve facing the provider is D_{50} (Figure 3–5). Here, at any charged price, the out-of-pocket price is one-half the charged price, and the consumer demands a quantity determined by the out-of-pocket price and the demand curve D_n. In fact, D_n becomes the demand curve relating quantity to out-of-pocket price. Thus, if the provider's charge were $8 per visit (in Figure 3–5), the consumer with a 50-percent coinsurance contract would pay a $4 out-of-pocket price and the quantity demanded would be six visits. If the coinsurance rate was 20 percent, the market demand curve facing the providers would be D_{20}. A charged price of $10 would mean an out-of-pocket price of $2 and a quantity demanded of eight. As the coinsurance rate falls, the market demand curve facing the providers shifts out, but the curve D_n continues to represent the relation between quantity demanded and out-of-pocket price.

Next we examine the impact of an indemnity contract. An indemnity contract sets a fixed per unit amount up to which the insurer will pay in the event of a service being used. For example, if an individual has pediatric coverage, an indemnity contract might specify that the insurer will pay up to $4 per visit. If the price is greater than $4, the consumer is responsible for the balance. In Figure 3–6, D_n is again the demand curve with no insurance coverage. Now let the individual

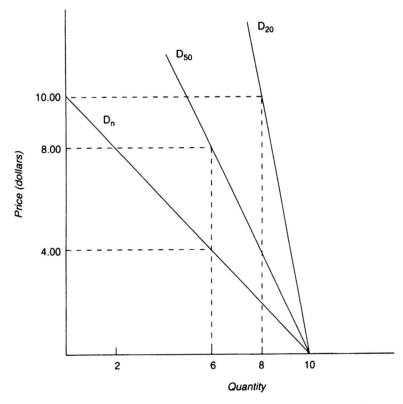

Figure 3–5 Representation of demand curves with no insurance (D_n), with a 50-percent coppayment (D_{50}), and with a 20-percent copayment (D_{20}). When there is a copayment, D_n also represents the relation between the quantity demanded and the out-of-pocket price.

purchase an indemnity contract that requires the insurer to reimburse the provider up to $4 per visit. The demand curve facing the provider becomes D_{n+i}, which is the D_n curve raised by $4 at all points. The position of D_{n+i} is such that, at each price charged, the out-of-pocket price will be $4 less than this, and the quantity demanded will reflect this lower out-of-pocket price. In Figure 3–6, a charged price of $8 means an out-of-pocket price of $4 and a quantity demanded of six. An increase in the amount by which the insurer indemnifies the consumer would shift D_{n+i} upward. The curve D_n would remain the same.

Finally, we examine the impact of a deductible. A deductible is a fixed total amount that the insurer deducts from the bill; the consumer must spend up to this amount before coverage begins. Until the consumer spends this amount, he or she pays the full price for each additional unit consumed (the price paid for the next additional unit is called the *marginal out-of-pocket price*). The marginal out-of-pocket price before the deductible is reached is the charged price. If there is no copayment in addition to the deductible, the marginal out-of-pocket price, after the deductible is met, is zero.

To analyze the impact of a deductible on demand, we will slightly reinterpret the demand curve. Assume that the curve shows the value to the consumer of each

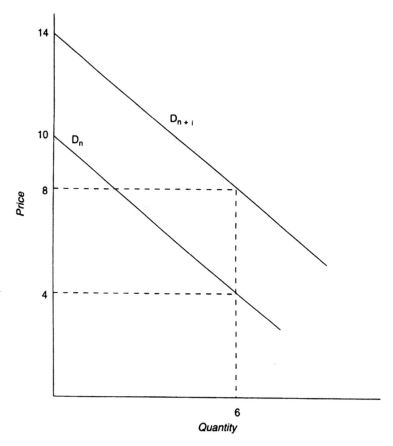

Figure 3–6 Representation of demand curves with no insurance (D_n) and with an indemnity payment of $4 ($D_{n+i}$). When there is an indemnity, D_n also represents the relation between the quantity demanded and the out-of-pocket price.

additional visit (the marginal value). If the patient consumes one visit, the value of the visit is $9. The second visit has a smaller marginal value, in this case $8. The two visits together would have a value of $17. These numbers and the value of additional visits are contained in Table 3–3. The table shows a declining marginal value for successive visits, which is consistent with what we assumed in deriving the demand hypothesis.

Let us now assume a market price of $8 and a deductible of $32. At this market price, the out-of-pocket marginal price to the consumer will be $8 per visit until (and if) the deductible is met. Thereafter, it will be zero (if there is no copayment as well). In answering the question of how many visits will be demanded, we must look at the consumer's valuation of visits in Table 3–3 and compare these with the marginal out-of-pocket price and the deductible level. At first, we might be tempted to say that only the first two visits are worth at least the marginal out-of-pocket price and so only two will be demanded. One would then conclude that, having spent $16 in total, the consumer did not meet the deductible, and so the visits will end at two.

But our consumer is truly a logical "economic person" and will look more carefully at all the options. The consumer realizes that he or she could buy the third and fourth units and, in doing so, use up the deductible of $32. Once the deductible

Table 3–3 Schedule of Value of Additional Medical Visits to Patient and Total (Summed) Value of All Units of Care

Quantity	Value of Additional Unit of Care to Consumer	Total Value of All Care Received up to Given Quantity
1	$9	$9
2	8	17
3	7	24
4	6	30
5	5	35
6	4	39
7	3	42
8	2	44
9	1	45
10	0	45

is used up, the rest of the visits demanded would be free! Indeed, if the individual consumed nine units, the value to him or her of all of them would be $45, well in excess of the outlay of $32 for the first four units. In general, we can say that, with a deductible, the amount demanded will be determined by the consumer's comparison of the additional value of all extra units with the additional out-of-pocket cost of all extra units. Even if the marginal value of the next visit (third, in this case) is less than its marginal out-of-pocket price, overall it will pay the individual to spend more in order to receive the benefits of the postdeductible units. If, however, the deductible was $100 and the charged price $8, the individual would stop consuming at two units, because there would be no other quantity of consumption at which the total value to the individual exceeded what the individual had to pay.

Frequently, a deductible and a copayment are found together in the same policy. In our example, a $32 deductible is combined with a 20-percent copayment (on units of care after the deductible has been reached). With a charged price of $8, the individual would then pay a marginal out-of-pocket price of $1.60 for each unit consumed after four. The individual would overspend the deductible in this case but would demand only eight visits, because the ninth, costing $1.60, would have a marginal value of only $1.

3.7 ELASTICITY OF DEMAND ESTIMATES

Demand responsiveness can be measured by natural experiments and controlled trials. A natural experiment (in the demand context) occurs when a change in insurance coverage is implemented by an insurer. We can use the results of such a policy action to determine demand responsiveness by conducting before-and-after comparisons of the data. Assuming all else has remained the same (e.g., that an increase in a deductible has not driven the sicker insureds to buy more complete insurance elsewhere), we can use the data to measure the degree of responsiveness. Natural experiments, unfortunately, often do not provide sufficient information. The investigators have no control over insurer policy decisions and are therefore restricted to researching the changes in price and coverage introduced by the insurers.

A more flexible but also more expensive approach is to do a controlled experiment. In this approach, study groups are selected randomly (to avoid any bias due to self-selection, such as sicker individuals choosing more complete insurance coverage) and assigned to specific categories (e.g., 20-percent copayment, 40-percent copayment, etc.). Differences in utilization (which are assumed to be caused by differences in demand) can be measured, and thus a measure of demand responsiveness can be obtained.

An example of a natural experiment in the demand field occurred in 1977, when the United Mine Workers introduced a $250 deductible for inpatient services and a 40-percent copayment for physician and outpatient visits up to a maximum family liability of $500. Prior to this, the insureds had no out-of-pocket expenses.

Scheffler (1984) conducted a study of the impact of this cost sharing on hospital admissions, average length of hospital stay, the probability that an insured would have at least one physician visit, and the number of times an insured visited a physician.

According to the analysis, in the five months prior to introduction of the hospital deductible (the comparison period), the hospital admission rate was 6.8 per 1,000 enrollees and the average length of stay per hospitalization was 5.42 days. The corresponding figures for the five months after introduction (the study period) were 4.8 per 1,000 for admissions and 6.45 days per hospitalization. The longer average length of stay in the study period may have been due to the fact that sicker cases were hospitalized. With regard to physician visits, the study's results indicated that the proportion of the population seeing a physician at least once fell from 44 percent in the comparison period to 28 percent in the study period, and the average number of visits of those who did see a physician at least once fell from 2.3 to 1.6.

The results of this experiment, like the results of other such studies, convincingly demonstrate the immediate impact of cost-sharing policies on utilization. But do the reductions in utilization last? Are there bad consequences farther down the line? One study (Scitovsky and McCall 1977) verified that reductions in physician visits did last several years, but several others have raised doubts as to whether longer term impacts occur (see Section 4.2).

By far the best known controlled experiment in this area is the six-site Health Insurance Experiment conducted by the Rand Corporation (Newhouse et al. 1981). In this study, 2,756 families agreed to participate in an experiment in which each family was assigned to one of five groups with different copayment rates. The rates included free care, 25-, 50-, and 95-percent coinsurance, and a deductible with 95-percent coinsurance (all services, such as physician visits and hospitalization, were covered under the single copayment). Those families with greater potential out-of-pocket expenses than their preexperiment coverage were compensated accordingly. Upper limits were placed on each family's out-of-pocket expenses. The families participated for three to five years.

The results dramatically indicated the differential impact of higher out-of-pocket expenses. For example, those with free care incurred average expenses for all services of $401, whereas those with 25-, 50-, and 95-percent coinsurance incurred expenses of $346, $328, and $254, respectively. Furthermore, these differentials held up over several years. Since the experiment was designed to control for all other intervening factors (e.g., health status, income, etc.), the results have had a considerable impact in health policy circles. The fact is that such controlled results are seldom obtained.

Several questions have been raised concerning the applicability of the study's results. First, the experiments affected only a small portion of the entire health care market in each of the six communities studied. If copayments were raised for the entire market or a substantial portion of the market, would providers (physicians) react and generate additional demand, thus changing the results? Furthermore, the aged (and presumably the fragile) were omitted from the study. Would their responses be any different?

Despite the unanswered questions, such studies have moved us closer toward developing a quantitative measure of the impact of out-of-pocket price on demand. As seen previously, demand elasticity depends on the starting point on an individual's demand curve, which in turn is affected by the individual's level of insurance. A rough estimate of demand elasticity when consumers have 0- to 25-percent coinsurance is −.2 (Newhouse et al. 1980).

Such an estimate can be used in the following way. If the price for a physician visit is $100, the copayment rate is 10 percent, and initially there are 120 visits, what would be the expected number of visits after the copayment rate is raised to 20 percent? The answer (assuming an elasticity of −.2) is obtained by solving for Q_2 (visits in Period 2), where

$$E = \frac{(Q_2 - Q_1)/(Q_2 + Q_1)}{(P_2 - P_1)/(P_2 + P_1)}$$

or

$$-.2 = \frac{(Q_2 - 120)/(Q_2 + 120)}{(20 - 10)/(20 + 10)}$$

The result gives a value for Q_2 of 104 visits (rounded to the nearest integer). In this case the total price did not change, although the copayment rate and therefore the out-of-pocket price did. A similar analysis could be done if the charged price and the copayment rate had both been changed.

A number of studies have been conducted analyzing demand in the nursing home market. Nursing home care is a health care service whose demand has distinct characteristics that have an impact on its elasticity of demand. First, there are a significant number of self-pay (uninsured) patients in this market; in 1994, out-of-pocket payments accounted for one-third of all nursing home expenditures. For those patients who are not covered by public insurance (primarily through Medicaid), the out-of-pocket price becomes an important variable because private insurance for long-term care is still a minor factor. Second, there are close substitutes for nursing home care. Home health care is, in many instances, a viable alternative to nursing home care. Also, some patients who are hospitalized and could be moved to a skilled nursing care facility "economize" on skilled nursing home care by remaining in the hospital longer and transferring later or not at all. The existence of close substitutes increases the elasticity of demand for nursing home care.

Lamberton and colleagues (1986) conducted a cross-county study of nursing home demand in South Dakota. In analyzing the relationship between nursing home days and variables such as price, income, and home care visits, they estimated an elasticity of demand for private patients of −.76. They also detected a significant negative relationship between home care visits and nursing home care, which substantiated the hypothesis that the two forms of care are substitutes. These results, which show that nursing home care has greater elasticity of demand than hospital care, were expected. Given the current interest in expanding long-term care insurance, an elasticity of this magnitude indicates that the demand for long-term care would increase substantially if long-term care insurance were to increase (since the out-of-pocket price of long-term care would be lowered).

EXERCISES

1. Distinguish between demand and quantity demanded.
2. State two distinct hypotheses about the relationship between price and quantity demanded.
3. Indicate how each of the following factors will change the individual demand curve for aspirin tablets:
   a. an increase in income
   b. an increase in the price of Tylenol (a substitute)
   c. an increase in the price of bottled water (a complement)
   d. an increase in the number of people with headaches
   e. the discovery that aspirin, if taken regularly, reduces the severity of heart attacks
4. Determine whether and how each of the following factors would shift the demand curve for chiropractic visits:
   a. an increase in the out-of-pocket price of chiropractic visits
   b. an increase in back problems
   c. a reduction in the out-of-pocket price for chiropractic visits
   d. an aging of the population
   e. an increase in the out-of-pocket price of back surgery (a substitute for chiropractic services)
   f. a reduction in the price of radiographs (a complement of chiropractic services)
   g. an advertising campaign that makes people more aware of the benefits of chiropractic care
5. What will be the effect on the market demand for aspirin in North Dakota if the population of North Dakota increases?
6. In a small town in Florida, a food supplement sold for $2.00 a bottle in May. In total, 2,000 bottles were sold. In June, nothing else changed but the price of the supplement, which was increased to $2.20. A total of 1,900 bottles were sold. What is the elasticity of demand?
7. Smith has insurance coverage for drugs. The insurance company will pay 50 percent of the price charged by the pharmacy. Smith went to the store in May. The price of aspirin was $0.50 per tablet. Smith bought 60 for the month. Next month, Smith found that the pharmacy had raised the price to $0.60 per tablet. Smith only bought 50 tablets. What is the elasticity of demand for aspirin?
8. Estimate the elasticity of demand for physician checkups from the following market data from a small state. The population in the state has remained the same.

Month	Average Age of Population	Persons with Flu	Out of Pocket Price	Number of Check-ups
October	40	Many	$30	5,000
November	40	Few	$35	3,000
December	45	Few	$40	2,500
January	40	Many	$35	4,800

9. Determine whether and how each of the following factors would shift the demand for home care:
   a. an increase of $10 in the price per day charged by nursing homes, with the government picking up the entire price increase
   b. an increase, from $12 to $15, in the price paid out of pocket by users of home care
   c. an increase in the number of people being discharged early from hospital
   d. an increase in productivity among home care providers
   e. an increase in the percentage of low-income people in a given population

10. A social survey taken in the town of Maple Ridge yielded the following information for five consecutive years. Determine from the results of these surveys what direct effect price has on quantity demanded (i.e., elasticity) of physician visits.

Year	Average Health	Average Income	Direct Price per Visit	Quantity Demanded visits per person)
1	Good	$10,000	$5	3
2	Good	$10,000	5	3
3	Poor	$6,000	5	5
4	Poor	$6,000	4	6
5	Poor	$4,000	4	5

11. The elasticity of demand for physician visits was determined to be –0.2. The president of the local health insurance company wants to add a copayment of $0.50 onto each physician visit. Currently there is no copayment. The number of insured people is 3,000,000, and currently the population uses 2.4 visits per capita. How many visits will they use after the introduction of the copayment?

12. Currently there is a $0.50 copayment on drugs. The HMO has decided to raise this to $1.00 per prescription. The cost of a prescription is $6.00, which means the HMO's contribution to the total cost will fall from $5.50 to $5.00. Currently the elasticity of demand is about –0.5 for prescriptions, and the HMO members use 2.2 prescriptions per capita. How much will be demanded after the new copayment is put into effect, and how much money will this save the HMO?

BIBLIOGRAPHY

Consumer Demand: Analysis and Surveys

Frech, H.E., and P.B. Ginsburg. 1975. Imposed health insurance in monopolistic markets. *Economic Inquiry* 13:55–69.

Ginsburg, P.B., and L. Manheim. L. 1973. Insurance, copayment and health services utilization. *Journal of Economics and Business* 25:142–153.

Joseph, H. 1971. Empirical research on the demand for health care. *Inquiry* 8:61–71.

Mushkin, S.J. 1974. *Consumer incentives for health care.* New York: Neale Watson Publishers.

Rice, T., and K.R. Morrison. 1994. Patient cost sharing for medical services. *Medical Care Review* 51:235–287.

Empirical Studies

Alexander, D.L., et al. 1994. Estimates of the demand for ethical pharmaceutical drugs across countries and time. *Applied Economics* 26:821–826.

Beck, R.G. 1974. The effect of co-payments on the poor. *Journal of Human Resources* 9:129–142.

Chiswick, B.R. 1976. The demand for nursing home care. *Journal of Human Resources* 11:295–316.

Coulson, N.E., et al. 1995. Estimating the moral-hazard effect of supplemental medical insurance in the demand for prescription drugs by the elderly. *American Economic Review* 85:122–126.

Davis, K., and L.B. Russell. 1972. The substitution of outpatient care for inpatient care. *Review of Economics and Statistics* 54:109–120.

Duan, N., et al. 1983. A comparison of alternative models for the demand for medical care. *Journal of Business and Economic Statistics* 1:115–126.

Eichner, M.J. 1998. The demand for medical care: what people pay does matter. *American Economic Review* 88:117–121.

Freiburg, L., and F.D. Scutchfield. 1976. Insurance and the demand for hospital care. *Inquiry* 13:54–60.

Gold, M. 1984. The demand for hospital outpatient services. *Health Services Research* 19:384–412.

Hellinger, F. 1977. Substitutability among different types of care under Medicare. *Health Services Research* 12:11–18.

Hershey, J.C., et al. 1975. Making sense out of utilization data. *Medical Care* 13:838–851.

Holtmann, A.G., and E.O. Olsen. 1978. *The economics of the private demand for outpatient health care.* Publication no. NIH-78–1262. Bethesda, MD: John E. Fogarty Center of the National Institutes of Health.

Hurd, M.D., and K. McGarry. 1997. Medical insurance and the use of health care services by the elderly. *Journal of Health Economics* 16:129–154.

Keeler, E.B., and J. Rolph. 1983. How cost spending reduced medical spending of participants in the health insurance experiment. *Journal of the American Medical Association* 249:2220–2222.

Lamberton, C.E., et al. 1986. Factors determining the demand for nursing home services. *Quarterly Review of Economics and Business* 26:74–90.

Nelson, A.A., et al. 1984. The effect of a Medicaid drug copayment program on the utilization and cost of prescription services. *Medical Care* 22:724–736.

Newhouse, J.P., et al. 1980. On having your cake and eating it too. *Journal of Econometrics* 13:365–390.

Newhouse, J.P., et al. 1981. Some interim results from a controlled trial of cost sharing in health insurance. *New England Journal of Medicine* 305:1501–1507.

Reeder, C.E., and A.A. Nelson. 1985. The differential impact of a copayment on drug use in a Medicaid population. *Inquiry* 22:396–403.

Scheffler, R.M. 1984. The United Mine Worker's health plan. *Medical Care* 22:247–254.

Scitovsky, A.A., and N. McCall. 1977. Coinsurance and the demand for physician services. *Social Security Bulletin* 40 (May): 19–27.

Warner, J., and T.-W. Hu. 1977. Hospitalization insurance and the demand for inpatient care. In *Socioeconomic issues of health*, ed. B.C. Martin. Chicago: American Medical Association.

Chapter 4

Additional Topics in the Demand for Health and Medical Care

1. Identify the wider implications of changes in the demand for health services.
2. Identify the private, external, and social demand for health services.
3. Explain how changes in the quality of care will influence the demand for health care.
4. Explain how time costs influence the demand for health services.
5. Explain the factors that influence the demand for health.
6. Explain the roles of the principal and the agent in determining the demand for medical care when the consumer has imperfect information about his or her health status and the productivity of medical care.
7. Explain the model of the demand for preventive health services when the consumer is uncertain about his or her health status.
8. Explain the concept of discounting by which the consumer places lower valuations on future health benefits than on present benefits.

4.1 INTRODUCTION

In Chapter 3, the demand for medical care was introduced as if medical care were an ordinary everyday commodity. Some types of medical care *are* ordinary everyday commodities. Pediatric visits, the consumption of aspirin, and visits to a dentist are routine occurrences for many people. However, the circumstances surrounding many types of medical care are quite unlike the circumstances surrounding the use of everyday commodities (Culyer 1971). As a result, the traditional model must be modified to incorporate special factors. This chapter brings these factors into consideration by showing how they influence the demand relation as developed in Chapter 3.

In section 4.2, we examine the economic implications of one alleged characteristic of medical care—that it is indispensable for life and health. In section 4.3, we analyze the implications for medical care demand when individuals other than direct consumers are concerned with the consumption of medical care by direct consumers. In this context we look at the relationships between private, external, and social demand. In section 4.4, we examine the influence of quality differences on medical care demand. Section 4.5 is concerned with situations when the money paid for medical care is not an adequate reflection of the total resource commitment made by the patient in acquiring medical care. In particular, patients devote a great deal of traveling and waiting time to the obtaining of medical care. This section develops a more general picture of the cost of medical care, including the role of time costs. In section 4.6, we analyze the consumer's choice behavior in terms of the demand for health rather than the demand for medical care. In this analysis, medical care and other resources are viewed as inputs in the production of a more fundamental commodity: health.

In Section 4.7, we discuss the role of the physician as an agent for the patient; under certain circumstances, the physician will participate in the process of determining demand, a situation that can lead to "supplier-induced demand." The demand for medical care is not always determined under conditions of certainty. Often the patient will not know when he or she will require medical care. Under these uncertain conditions, the individual consumer may purchase care on a prepaid basis (insurance); as well, the consumer will decide whether or not to engage in certain activities that influence health, such as exercise, smoking, and eating certain foods. In Section 4.7, we present a preliminary introduction to the topic of demand under conditions of uncertainty. Finally, many health-related activities will have effects that extend into future time periods. Individuals' valuations of benefits in future time periods will be less than those in the current time period. In Section 4.7, we introduce the concept of discounting of future benefits.

4.2 IMPLICATIONS OF HEALTH CARE FOR LIFE AND HEALTH

One of the most widely cited characteristics of the commodity medical care is its ability to improve health. In some instances, if a person does not obtain timely medical care, he or she may die or become permanently ill. Where this condition holds (e.g., after a heart attack or a serious traffic accident), the question of substitutes will have little importance. Presumably the person would be willing to disburse all of his or her wealth to receive lifesaving medical care, and the demand curve would be vertical.

However, such instances amount to a very small portion of the total number of situations that cause individuals to seek medical care. In the vast majority of cases, alternative courses of action are available and individuals have the time to consider the options. In fact, medical care should be viewed as a spectrum of services and products rather than as a commodity only sought and consumed in an emergency. The less a situation calls for immediate action and the greater the relevance of substitutes, the less steeply sloping will be the demand curve for medical care. For example, dental checkups can be given annually, monthly, or weekly. Few would consider monthly or weekly checkups to be necessary or even reasonable. Substitutes are important even in emergency situations: individuals and planners have a wide variety of alternatives they can choose in advance of dire circumstances.

Even though most medical problems are not of emergency proportions, a reduction in medical care consumption can lead to a deterioration in health. In studying such a possibility, it may be desirable to analyze medical care demand from the longer perspective of a multiperiod analysis. The imposition of a copayment on drugs or physician visits will generally lead to a reduction in the quantity demanded in Period 1. There is nothing in the theory of demand that says which units of medical care will no longer be demanded. Some units may have been unnecessary to begin with, but some may have been highly desirable (from the point of view of their effects on health status). When medical care is desirable, a reduction in its consumption in Period 1 may lead to a decline in health status in Periods 2, 3, or 4 and to possible increases in medical care demand in these subsequent periods.

This phenomenon was first examined following the imposition of a $1 copayment for each of the first two doctor's visits and $.50 for each of the first two prescriptions in the California Medicaid program. An original study (Roemer and Hopkins 1975) stated that reductions in doctor's office visits and diagnostic tests after the copayment's introduction were accompanied by increases in hospitalization rates in subsequent periods. Although the data methods of the study were questioned, with no conclusive results (Chen 1976; Dyckman 1976; Hopkins et al. 1976), the study raised the issue of the importance of examining the wider effects of demand-reducing measures. A subsequent study based on the national Rand Health Insurance Experiment (Brook et al. 1983) examined the effects of reductions in use due to copayments on subsequent consumer health status and found that they were generally not adverse except for certain groups. In particular, for poor individuals with hypertensive conditions, free care was associated with better blood pressure control and reductions in the risk of early death. There is a likelihood that, for selected groups, reductions in demand can have considerable impact on subsequent health status and medical care demand (Fein 1981; Relman 1983).

4.3 EXTERNAL AND SOCIAL DEMAND FOR MEDICAL CARE

In the analysis in Chapter 3, it was assumed that the sum of all individuals' own demands for medical care was the same as the total societal demand for medical care. Investigators have questioned the reasonableness of this assumption. For certain social goods, such as medical care and education, it has been asserted that individuals would be willing to pay something to enable others to consume them. This is not true for all commodities. Many individuals would be willing to pay something to help ensure that a heart attack victim could reach a hospital on time; they would not be so generous if a person's car had broken down and he or she "needed" $400 for repairs. Furthermore, people's generosity probably extends only to certain types of medical care. The need for medical care with substantial health implications for the recipients (e.g., inoculations or care for the aged) elicits great concern; someone's desire to undergo cosmetic surgery does not.

To formalize the analysis of this phenomenon, let us focus on the consumption of a single individual, called A. The commodity whose demand we are analyzing will now be defined as individual A's consumption of medical care. A's demand for his or her own consumption may be called *private* or *internal demand*.

Assume that the rest of society can be characterized as individual B. B may also have a demand for A's own consumption of medical care. Such a demand can be characterized in the same way as A's own demand. In particular, as the price is lowered, B's demand for A's consumption of medical care will increase. This demand is in addition to A's own demand and can be called an *external demand*, because it comes from a force external to the consumer of the commodity.

If we define society as the sum total of A and B, then society's demand for A's consumption of medical care will depend on the private demand of A and the external demand of B. This total demand can be called *community* or *social demand*.

The effect of the external demand is to increase the quantity demanded (of medical care for A) at any given price, assuming that the external demand is greater than zero at that price. (It may well be, as in the case of the external demand for auto repair, that this external demand is zero at a particular price or at all prices.) The old phrase that "society wants everyone to have a decent level of medical care" can be recast in terms of this analysis. Society is the sum of all individuals, and the social demand for an individual's consumption of a given commodity is the sum of all private and external demands. The statement that "society wants everyone to have a decent level of medical care" can be interpreted to mean that, at the given price, there is a social demand for a "decent" level of care for each person.

There are a sufficiently large number of manifestations of external demands for medical care to impress on us how real this phenomenon is. The existence of philanthropic giving to organizations such as the American Heart Association, the United Way, the American Cancer Society, and the National Research Foundation provides evidence that donors are truly committed to enabling others to consume the services of these organizations, including health education and research. The majority of hospitals in the United States began as nonprofit organizations with large charitable components. In recent years, these charitable components have decreased because of the growth of government health programs such as Medicare and Medicaid. Such programs themselves may be an expression of external demands expressed through the "political marketplace." Before the introduction of Medicare and Medicaid, physicians contended that a great deal of their medical services were provided as a form of charity.

4.4 INFLUENCE OF QUALITY ON THE DEMAND FOR MEDICAL CARE

In Chapter 3 the analysis of medical care demand was based on the assumption that each unit of the commodity medical care was like any other unit. Of course, this is not always the case. One of the more problematic tasks in analyzing resource allocation in medical care is coming to terms with quality differences.

Quality is not a single attribute but rather a series of attributes, any of which can make the product appear better or worse to the consumer (Congress of the United States 1988). We will assume, in this section, that the consumer is fully aware of how each of these attributes that determine the quality level of a product will affect him or her. Furthermore, we will regard quality as subjective, that is, in terms of how the consumer values these attributes of the commodity.

There are three attributes of the commodity medical care that are used to identify quality (Donabedian 1988): (1) the *structure* of the resources provided (e.g., the qualifications of the clinicians and the type of facilities); (2) the *process* of medical care (e.g., the thoroughness with which the diagnostic services are carried out or the comfort or luxury of the particular services provided); and (3) the *outcome* or the level of medical excellence of the services. The latter attribute is associated with the accuracy of a diagnosis, the effectiveness of a treatment in restoring health, the effectiveness of a preventive course of action, and so on. Assuming that these aspects of quality can be accurately assessed, a consumer can make a personal evaluation of the overall quality levels associated with alternative units of medical care and can rank these alternative units according to their quality levels.

How might consumers behave when faced with different overall medical care quality levels? A reasonable hypothesis is that a higher quality level will increase the importance of medical care in relation to other commodities at all levels of medical care consumption. This will result in an outward shift of the demand curve for medical care.

One qualification must be mentioned. If the quality of care is low, the demand may be less. But if low-quality care results in subsequent illness (e.g., if rheumatic fever develops from a failure to check for strep throat or if a patient with chicken pox contracts Reye's syndrome because he or she was prescribed aspirin), it may lead to a greater demand for care subsequently.

4.5 TIME AND MONEY COSTS

Until now we have measured the resource commitment necessary to obtain a unit of commodity by the per unit out-of-pocket money price of that commodity. Thus, if a unit of medical care costs $5, then $5 was treated as an accurate measure of what a person had to give up (the opportunity cost) to obtain a unit of medical care. Yet the resources devoted to consuming a commodity include more than the money price of the commodity; when obtaining medical care, people have to travel to and from the physician's office and wait to see the physician and be examined. The effort and time expended are personal resources and are part of the totality of resources committed to obtaining medical care.

The value of the time spent by a person travelling and waiting is referred to as the time cost of obtaining medical care. The associated resource commitment is equivalent to the amount that could have been earned if the person had not visited the physician (assuming the person does forgo income in undertaking this action). If the person does not forgo income, valuable time is still given up. In this case, the opportunity cost of time would be taken to be equivalent to the value to the person of the activity given up. This latter magnitude is very difficult to measure, so for our purposes we will assume that all time spent in obtaining health care can be measured in terms of the person's wage rate.

The total cost to or total resource commitment made by the person for each unit of health care can be expressed as $(w \times t) + p$, where t is the amount of time involved in obtaining a unit of health care, w is the wage that would have been earned had the person worked during this time, and p is the money price of the health care.

We can use this expression to substitute total per unit cost for money price in our demand analysis. If we regard the commodity as medical care and the total cost per unit of this commodity as $(w \times t) + p$, we can develop a more general hypothesis about the consumption of medical care. Our new hypothesis is this: as the total per unit cost (time cost plus money price) falls, more medical care is demanded. To give an example, if the time required for a visit to the doctor is 1 hour, the wage forgone is $4 per hour, and the money price of a visit is $8, the total per unit cost is $12. If the money price is set at zero by a government program, the total cost falls to $4 per visit. Medical care may still be too costly for some people, even at a zero price. If the government wishes to encourage consumption beyond this point, it might have to take steps that would lower waiting or travel time (e.g., by relocating a clinic to a more populous area).

Framing the analysis of demand in terms of total cost provides additional insight regarding issues of distribution. Even though money costs may be the same for all consumers, total costs may vary because of variations in w and t. For example, w may vary among consumers because some may have their wages docked if they take time off from work whereas others may not. And *t* may vary because of variations in distances from care providers. Our generalized demand hypothesis states that, other things being equal, the quantity demanded will vary inversely with the total per unit cost. When medical care is offered for "free," that is, at a zero money price, variations in quantity demanded will be determined by variations in time costs. In this circumstance, individuals who incur the lowest time cost will demand the greatest quantities. Perhaps those who pay the lowest time costs and hence demand the greatest quantities are not the same as those with the most acute medical conditions. In this case, medical care would be rationed to those who are willing to wait and not to the most ill. This problem arises when a program lowers the direct money price to zero while failing to increase supply sufficiently to meet the increased quantity demanded. An excess demand results and queues may form. This raises the time cost, which becomes the mechanism by which medical care is rationed.

4.6 THE DEMAND FOR HEALTH

In Chapter 1 we showed that the output of the health care sector can be regarded either as health care or as health. An alternative formulation of consumer behavior in this area has been presented in terms of the demand for health (Grossman 1972b). Health care can be regarded as an end in itself, something people want for its intrinsic characteristics, or as a means to an end. For example, better health, by enabling a person to earn more income and purchase other commodities, would function as a means for attaining a higher level of consumer consumption.

In this analysis we assume health to be an end in itself that can be created or produced by the activities individuals undertake. These activities can include receiving medical care, engaging in self-care (exercise and proper diet), and so on. Such activities are substitutes for one another, since each contributes to achieving the desired end. The cost of each alternative activity can be expressed in terms of the resources an individual would have to commit in order to produce one healthy day. Since each activity will normally require time and purchased inputs on the part of the consumer, the cost of one healthy day can be expressed as follows:

$$c = (a \times w) + (b \times p)$$

In this equation, *c* is the unit cost (cost per one healthy day produced) of the activity; *a* is the amount of time required to produce one healthy day by engaging in the activity; *b* is the amount of purchased inputs required in conjunction with *a* to produce one healthy day; *w* is the opportunity cost of the individual's time and thus a measurement of the size of the resource commitment of one unit of time; and *p* is the price of one unit of purchased input. The cost of one healthy day (*c*) depends on *a*, *b*, *w*, and *p*. For each health-producing activity, there will be a different *c*. If one activity, say self-care, is very productive (i.e., *a* and *b* are small), then the cost of producing an extra healthy day through self-care will be low. On the other hand, if self-care is not very effective in producing health, then *a* may be very high and *c* in turn will likely be high. Recall that, although the unit price of purchased inputs (*p*) may be high, the number of units required to produce a healthy day (*b*) may be low. Thus, purchased input–intensive activities such as medical care are not necessarily more costly than other health-producing activities.

One prediction of this model is that, if the value of c of one type of health-producing activity rises relative to the value of c for another type, individuals will substitute in favor of the lower cost alternative. For example, if waiting time in a doctor's office (a) becomes lengthy, the cost of medical care will rise. Self-care becomes relatively less expensive under these circumstances, and individuals will engage in more self-care activities.

It is unlikely that a and b will remain constant across all levels of an activity. Instead, it is probable that the more of an activity (e.g., physician care or self-care) is engaged in, the more a and b will increase. That is, it will take successively larger doses of personal effort and purchased inputs to yield a unit of health. For this reason, several health-producing activities will be demanded by an individual. For example, the individual will probably demand both medical care and self-care. However, if a factor changes (e.g., there is an increase in the amount of waiting time necessary to obtain medical care), this will cause a shift in demand (e.g., more self-care and less medical care will be demanded).

Viewing the demand for health-related resources in this way allows us to incorporate the full resource commitment of alternative ways of producing health. In such a framework, medical care becomes one of several alternatives, and a broader picture of health-related resources can be obtained. However, while the picture is broader, it is also more complex, and for many purposes such a broad and complex picture is not required.

4.7 AGENCY THEORY AND SUPPLIER-INDUCED DEMAND

Many consumers do not know the effect of medical care on health, and physicians have been regarded as having two main roles: (1) to act in an advisory capacity and inform patients of their level of health and the activities and treatments that might improve their health and (2) to undertake treatments their patients have decided upon. When we introduce the physicians into the demand analysis, we widen the framework, for the patient's demand is now also dependent on the interaction with the physician.

As we saw in Chapter 3, a patient's perception of the level of his or her health and the probable effect of medical care on the patient's health can influence the patient's demand for medical care. Since the physician potentially has influence over both of these factors, the physician conceivably can change the patient's demand for medical care by providing pertinent information. For example, telling a patient that he or she has a dangerous but possibly curable neoplasm will almost certainly increase that patient's demand for cancer treatment.

If we assume that the physician knows the patient's health level and the effectiveness of medical care in producing health, and if the physician has an awareness of the patient's tastes and other circumstances (prices and income), then, assuming the physician behaves as a "perfect agent," he or she will prescribe and/or provide a quantity of medical care such that the patient him- or herself, if fully informed, would have chosen. However, principal-agent relationships are such that the agent (physician) may not behave in the best interests of the principal (patient). A deviation of the agent from the principal's own interests is called *moral hazard*.

Moral hazard will arise when there is a potential divergence of interest between the principal and the agent. Despite this divergence, there must still be a basis for the two to engage in a contractual relationship. However, when the principal uses the services of the agent, he or she in effect has entered into an agreement that the agent will meet the principal's needs. Problems with the relationship will arise when there is uncertainty and information asymmetry that make it difficult for the two parties to agree on a fixed price, agree on a predetermined service that the agent will provide, and develop an adequate mechanism to monitor and enforce the agreement.

As an example of a principal-agent relationship that would not be plagued by agency problems, imagine a private home care nursing agency administering intravenous drugs on a daily basis to a bed-ridden client. The home care nurse will agree to show up at a specified time each day and administer the drugs. The client can clearly specify the contract with the agency. Also, the client can easily monitor the performance of the nursing agency, and if the nursing agency does not perform adequately, the client can terminate the contract.

When the patient interacts with a provider, there are four types of costs which he or she incurs in addition to the price and wait and travel costs:

1. search costs, or the costs of determining specifications of the services needed and the prices of these services
2. contract costs, or the costs of reaching an agreement with the provider as to what services are to be provided
3. monitoring costs, or the costs of identifying the desired outcomes, collecting data on these outcomes, and determining whether the outcomes have been achieved
4. enforcement costs, or the costs of ensuring that the provider meets the agreed criteria

These costs are especially important in the present circumstances. The patient (principal), lacking relevant information, relies on the physician (agent) to provide advice on health status and alternative treatments and in many instances to provide the therapy. In some circumstances, the physician's interests may diverge from those of the patient. The physician can then engage in moral hazard by providing advice and therapies that are in his or her own interests rather than the interests of the patient. Despite the divergences of interests, the patient may still contract with the physician because, given the costs of engaging in the medical care process, what is provided by the physician may be the best alternative (Dranove and White 1987).

Supplier-induced demand is a phenomenon that has been linked to agency theory. Supplier-induced demand may arise when the payment mechanism encourages physicians to provide more services. Fee-for-service is a payment mechanism that has been identified as encouraging supplier-induced demand. Under fee-for-service, the physician is paid for each unit of service performed, and so one of the conditions needed for principal-agent problems to arise—the divergence of interests—will be present. Monitoring and enforcement costs may be very high for the patient; therefore, the physician has both the incentive and the ability to engage in demand-inducing practices. In Chapter 7 we discuss the effect of the basis of payment on provider supply.

There are limits to such a process. For one thing, with repeated events (e.g., common colds) the patient eventually gains information that can be used to evaluate health and medical productivity. In addition, information sharing between patients, between patients and other physicians (second opinions), or on the

Internet limits the degree to which a physician can sway the patient with misinformation. That is, the patient's monitoring abilities are improved. Deliberate misrepresentation of information would be contrary to physician ethical codes. Finally, the assumption that the *physician* has perfect information about the patient's health status and the productivity of medical care is not always realistic. Diagnosis and treatment are often undertaken under conditions of uncertainty. Under such conditions, a physician experiments to obtain the best treatment. Although the physician can still generate demand, it is impossible to say with certainty how much of the "experimentation" was intentional demand generation and how much was honest experimentation.

4.7.1 Demand under Uncertainty: The Demand for Health Promotion

The simple analysis of demand for medical care in Chapter 3 was based on the assumption that the consumer knows with certainty what his or her state of health will be during the relevant time period. This underlying assumption is not plausible for many medical problems. In these cases, a consumer cannot be certain whether or not a problem will occur. The consumer does know, however, that he or she *might* be sick during a particular period and might have to visit a health care provider and even be hospitalized. Issues related to the uncertain appearance of illness have a bearing on a number of health-related activities (Kenkel 1994; Russell 1984; Scheffler and Paringer 1980). For example, people adopt healthy or unhealthy lifestyles; these lifestyles are often resource intensive and will have an impact on the likelihood that the individuals will be sick.

The basic theory of the demand for health promotion activities presents a systematic view of how certain underlying variables—tastes, wealth, the cost of health promotion, the likelihood of an illness, and the loss resulting from the illness—can influence the decision to engage in these activities. The assumptions of the model are as follows.

1. *Time frame.* All activities and consequences occur in the current time period.
2. *Level of wealth.* Our second assumption is that our individual initially has a level of wealth of $1,000.
3. *Consumer tastes.* We assume that when an illness occurs, it leads to medical care expenses that constitute a loss of wealth. To specify what this loss means to the individual, we must introduce a concept to characterize the individual's well-being at alternative levels of wealth—the concept of utility. One hypothetical individual's taste for wealth is presented in the form of an index of utility in Table 4–1. This index shows the level of utility that is associated with each specific level of wealth. Thus, a level of wealth of $1,000 is associated with a level of utility of 100, a level of wealth of $990 is associated with a level of utility of 99.8, and so on. The size of specific numbers in the utility index is arbitrary. What is important is that higher wealth gives higher utility (i.e., increased wealth makes the individual "better off"). We further assume that the function is characterized by diminishing marginal utility. That is, each additional $10 of wealth results in less additional utility than the previous $10. For example, at $850, an extra $10 will yield 3 extra units of utility; at $860, an extra $10 will yield 2.8 extra units; and so on.

Table 4–1 Relationship between Wealth and Utility

Wealth	Total Utility	Marginal Utility
$800	57.0	4.2
810	61.2	4.0
820	65.2	3.8
830	69.0	3.6
840	72.6	3.4
850	76.0	3.2
860	79.0	3.0
870	81.8	2.8
880	84.4	2.6
890	86.8	2.4
900	89.0	2.2
910	91.0	2.0
920	92.8	1.8
930	94.4	1.6
940	95.8	1.4
950	97.0	1.2
960	98.0	1.0
970	98.8	0.8
980	99.4	0.6
990	99.8	0.4
1000	100.0	0.2

If an individual has a diminishing marginal utility for wealth, he or she is said to be *risk averse*. The basic idea is that, for a given wealth level, a loss of a given amount of wealth (e.g., $10) is of greater subjective importance (utility) to the person than would be a gain of an equal amount. Utility is the subjective index of the relative importance of wealth.

In this model, a utility function is unique to an individual. Thus, it does not imply that additional wealth means less to a rich person than it does to a poor person. This kind of comparison, called *interpersonal comparison*, would involve specifying different people's utilities on the same scale.

4. *Medical expenses in the event of illness.* Our fourth assumption is that, if the individual becomes sick, he or she will face medical expenses of $150. This expenditure is assumed to fully restore the loss in health, so that $150 is the full value of the loss when the individual is sick.

5. *The cost of health promotion activities.* The consumer uses up resources when engaging in health promotion, including time, professional services, and supplies. In our example, we will assume that these costs total $20.

6. *Likelihood of illness.* A sixth assumption concerns the element of uncertainty. We will assume that we can assign probabilities to the various possible health states the individual may experience. Let us say that without any health promotion activities there is a .3 probability of illness (i.e., of 10 people in similar circumstances, 3 will become ill) and a .7 probability the individual will remain well and will not incur any medical costs. These are the only two possibilities, so the sum of the probabilities equals 1. With health promotion activities the probability of being healthy increases to 0.9 and the probability of being ill falls to 0.1.

7. *Behavioral assumption.* The final assumption is that the individual wants to maximize the expected value of his or her utility. Thus the individual will

choose that course of action from which he or she can expect to receive the highest level of utility.

The model's conclusions are obtained by determining how, under these assumed conditions, the individual will behave so as to maximize expected utility, (i.e., which of the two options, engage in health promotion or do not engage in health promotion, will be chosen). Under the first option, not engaging in health promotion, the expected utility for the individual is 92.8 [(0.7 × 100) + (0.3 × 76.0)]. This is because when the individual is healthy, he or she has a utility of 100.0 (corresponding to a wealth of $1,000), and when he or she is ill, the utility is 76.0 (corresponding to a wealth level of $850). The expected utility if the individual engages in health promotion activities will be derived from the probabilities and utility levels when he or she is healthy or ill but has spent $20 on health promotion activities (which occur whether the individual is healthy or not). Therefore, the expected utility is 95.3 [(.9 × 99.4) + (.1 × 69.0)]. The individual is better off when he or she engages in health promotion activities under these circumstances, and so we predict that he or she will choose that option.

However, this will not always be the case. If any of our basic assumptions change, so will our conclusion. The individual will be less likely to engage in health promotion when any of the following occurs: the cost of health promotion increases, health promotion has a reduced impact on illness, and the individual experiences an increase in risk aversion.

4.7.2 Limitations of the Model

The theory of the demand for health care under conditions of uncertainty has the virtue of explicitly organizing some of the variables that are central to the decision to engage in activities that promote health. As presented, however, it has an important limitation.

The reader may find it strange that the utility function, which is supposed to measure satisfaction, does not include health. This is indeed a shortcoming of the model, because well-being can depend on health status as well as wealth. The model looks only at financial aspects of the situation, in effect assuming that the care fully and instantly restores health, with no utility implications of either the illness or the process of getting care. Clearly this is an unrealistic assumption. Including health status creates a much more complicated model that is more difficult to apply, and while it is important to understand that we have abstracted from reality, this should not detract from the value of the model. The present model has the virtue of focusing on the benefits of risk shifting, which is an economic good that is distinct from medical care.

4.7.3 Discounting Future Values

Another factor that affects health-promotion behavior is the individual's valuation of benefits in different time periods. Health promotion activities, such as the use of condoms, smoking cessation, vaccinations, and clean needles (for drug users) and unhealthy activities, such as smoking, engaging in unsafe sex, and excessive drug use, generally do not have good or bad impacts on health immediately. It takes a long time, sometimes years, for individuals to experience adverse health effects. The timing of health benefits will have an influence on the demand for health-related activities that promote these benefits.

It is generally assumed that $1,000 in current benefits will be worth more to an individual than $1,000 in benefits one year from now. The value of the preference for earlier rather than later periods can be expressed in terms of a discount rate, called r. If an individual is asked how much money he or she would accept at the end of 2001 rather than have $1,000 at the beginning of 2001, the person might take $1,100 at the end of the period. In other words, $1,000 on January 1, 2001, would be worth as much as $1,100 one year later. The discount rate is .1, and the discounting equation is be expressed as $1,000 × (1 + .1) = $1,100, or symbolically as $1,000 × (1 + r) = $1,100. This may be rewritten as $1,000 = $1,100/(1 + r). This equation says that, in the individual's eyes, $1,100 one year hence will be equivalent to $1,100/(1 + r), or $1,000, now. The discount rate for an individual is derived largely from introspection—from an acceptance that a given future amount and a lesser current amount provide the same satisfaction *at the present moment.*

The same principle holds for comparisons between December 31, 2001, and December 31, 2002. That is, $1,000 at the end of 2001 is equivalent to $1,100 at the end of 2002 if the individual's discount rate is .1. By inference, then, $1,000 at the end of 2002 would be worth $1,000/[(1 + r) × (1 + r)] on January 1, 2001 (also expressible as $1,000/(1 + r)^2$). Similarly, $1,000 on December 31, 2003, would be worth $1,000/(1 + r)^3$ at the start of 2001, and so on. Generally, improved health or added life yields a stream of benefits. That is, a saved life on January 1, 2001 will yield benefits in 2001 (valued as of December 31, 2001), 2002 (valued as of December 31, 2002), 2003 (valued as of December 31, 2003), and so on. If the benefits are $2,000 each year, the *present* value of future benefits can be expressed as $2,000 + 2,000/(1 + r) + 2,000/(1 + r)^2$, and so on, for as long as benefits last. The letter usually used to symbolize the annual benefits is B, with subscripts 0, 1, 2, . . . for right now (0), one year hence (1), two years hence (2), and so on. In our current example, $B_0 = B_1 = B_2$, and the present value of benefits can be expressed symbolically as

$$B_0 + B_0/(1 + r) + B_0/(1 + r)^2$$

If the number of years that benefits will last is quite large and the value of the benefits for every year is the same, the present value of the benefits can be expressed as B_0/r. If benefits of $10,000 a year will last forever and if the discount rate is .1, the present value of these benefits will be 10,000/.1, or $100,000. Benefits lasting for long periods can be approximated using this formula.

The discount factor can be quite substantial for benefits that will not be experienced for many years. For example, hepatitis C may not be recognized for 20 years. If hepatitis C imposes health-related costs of $1,000 in 20 years, and the discount rate is 10 percent, then the present value of these imposed costs is $148.64 [$1,000/(1+.1)^{20}$].

Not everyone will have the same discount rate. An individual who has a very strong preference for current satisfaction rather than future benefits will have a high interest rate, perhaps 15 or 20 percent. On the other hand, a person who places very great importance on future satisfactions will have a very low discount rate, perhaps 2 percent or even 0 percent. In the latter case, there would be no discount rate, and present and future values would be the same.

Discounting is usually done with a hand-held calculator or with present value tables. In Table 4–2 we show a series of discounted values varying according to

Table 4–2 Calculation of Present Value of Benefits under Alternative Discount Rates

	Part A: Discounting Factors				
Discount Rate	$(1 + r)$	$(1 + r)^2$	$(1 + r)^3$	$(1 + r)^4$	$(1 + r)^5$
.04	1.04	1.08	1.12	1.17	1.22
.08	1.08	1.16	1.25	1.36	1.41
.12	1.12	1.25	1.41	1.57	1.63

	Part B: Discounted Present Value of Benefits ($10,000)					
Discount Rate	$B_1/(1 + r)$	$B_2/(1 + r)^2$	$B_3/(1 + r)^3$	$(B_4/(1 + r)^4$	$B_5/(1 + r)^5$	Present Value (row sum)
.04	8,615	9,233	8,896	8,554	8,196	44,494
.08	9,259	8,620	8,000	7,353	7,092	40,324
.12	8,928	8,000	7,029	6,275	5,602	35,834

discount rates (4, 8, and 12 percent) and time periods (one to five years). For example, in Part A, at a discount rate of 8 percent and a four-year time horizon, the value of $(1 + r)^4$ is 1.36. The present value of a benefit of $10,000 that occurred in four years, discounted at a rate of 8 percent, would therefore be $ 7,353.

Often, benefits will repeat themselves from year to year. For example, a $10,000 benefit may be experienced in each of the next five years. If the discount rate was 4 percent, then the present value of the benefits for each of the next five years would be $8,615, $9,233, and so on, for five years. The present value of $10,000 for all five years together, called the annuity value, is $44,494, as shown in Table 4–2. Annuity tables would contain present values summed over each time horizon.

EXERCISES

1. A copayment was placed on the use of physician checkups. As a result, poor people reduced their demands for checkups, and their health status was reduced. How might this affect the demand for subsequent health care?
2. Name three different ways of identifying quality. How would increased quality affect the demand for medical services?
3. Mrs. Smith earns $20 an hour. Normally she has to drive into St. Cloud from her home (150 miles away) for a medical consultation. The drive is two hours each way. Mrs. Smith usually has a one-hour wait, and the consultation takes about an hour. Mrs. Smith estimates that the cost of the transportation is 30 cents a mile. What are Mrs. Smith's travel and waiting costs for each visit?
4. Mrs. Siegal has two alternative activities to help relieve her backache. In the first, she can visit a physiotherapist. The total time for a physiotherapist visit, including travel and waiting, is two hours. Mrs. Siegal earns a wage of $20 an hour. Physiotherapists charge $50 per visit, and Mrs. Siegal does not have any health insurance. As a second alternative, Mrs. Siegal can take pain

killers. Each pill costs 50 cents, and Mrs. Siegal needs to take 30 pills per month. The two treatments are not equally effective. The physiotherapy visits yield 10 additional healthy days per month, while the pills yield 6 healthy days.

   a. If Mrs. Siegal can only choose one alternative, and if she wants to maximize the most healthy days per dollar that she gets, which option will she choose?

   b. If the price of a pill increases to $3, which option will she choose?

5. What is information asymmetry and how does it result in a principal-agent problem?

6. What are the costs that an individual or organization must incur in order to contract with another individual or organization?

7. What is supplier-induced demand? How is it related to a principal-agent problem?

8. Mrs. Backman has a utility function like that in Table 4–1. Her wealth level is $900. If she is ill, she incurs costs of $50 in medical expenses. This is a one-time expense and will leave her at a lower wealth level ($850, in this case). Without any special diet or exercise, she has a 20 percent chance of being sick. She can purchase vitamins for $20, in which case her chance of being sick will fall to 10 percent. Using expected utility as her objective, should she purchase the vitamins?

9. Mr. Manos has a discount rate of 10 percent. To him, it is worth $2,000 to be very well and $1,900 to be moderately well. It is the beginning of the year 2001. Mr. Manos can engage in exercise, which will make him very well during the year 2003 but will leave him only moderately well for the years 2001 and 2002. Alternatively, he can take medicine, which will make him very well in 2001, but its effects only last one year. Therefore, if Mr. Manos takes the medicine, he will only be moderately well in the years 2002 and 2003. What is each alternative worth to Mr. Manos as of the present?

BIBLIOGRAPHY

General

Culyer, A.J. 1971. The nature of the commodity "health care" and its efficient allocation. *Oxford Economic Papers* 23:189–211.

Donabedian, A. 1988. The quality of care. *JAMA* 260:1743–1748.

Utilization and Subsequent Health Implications

Brook, R.H., et al. 1983. Does free care improve adults' health? *New England Journal of Medicine* 309:1426–1434.

Chen, M.K. 1976. Penny-wise and pound foolish: Another look at the data. *Medical Care* 14:958–963.

———. 1976. More about penny-wise and pound foolish: A statistical point of view. *Medical Care* 14:964–968.

Congress of the United States. 1988. *The quality of medical care.* Washington, DC: Congress of the United States, Office of Technology Assessment.

Cutler, D.M., et al. 1998. What has increased medical-care spending bought? *American Economic Review* 88(2): 132–136.

Dranove, D., and White, W.D. 1987. Agency and the organization of health care delivery. *Inquiry* 24(4):405–415.

Dyckman, Z.Y. 1976. Comment on "Copayments for ambulatory care: Penny-wise and pound foolish." *Medical Care* 14:274–276.

Dyckman, Z.Y., and P. McMenamin. 1976. Copayments for ambulatory care: Son of thrupence. *Medical Care* 14:968–969.

Fein, R. 1981. Effects of cost sharing in health insurance. *New England Journal of Medicine* 305:1526–1528.

Giuffrida, A., and H. Gravelle. 1998. Paying patients to comply. *Health Economics* 7:569–580.

Hopkins, C.E., et al. 1975. Copayments for ambulatory care: Penny-wise and pound foolish. *Medical Care* 13:457–466.

Hopkins, C.E., et al. 1976. Rebuttal to "Comment on 'Copayments for ambulatory care: Penny-wise and pound foolish.'" *Medical Care* 14:277.

Keeler, E.B., et al. 1985. How free care reduced hypertension in the health insurance experiment. *JAMA* 254:1926–1931.

Knowles, J.C. 1995. Price uncertainty and the demand for health care. *Health Policy and Planning* 10:301–303.

Lichtenberg, F.R. 1996. Do (more and better) drugs keep people out of hospitals? *American Economic Review* 86(2): 384–388.

Relman, A. 1983. The Rand Health Insurance Study: Is cost sharing dangerous to your health? *New England Journal of Medicine* 309:1453.

Roemer, M.I., and C.E Hopkins. 1976. Response to M.K. Chen. *Medical Care* 144:963–964.

Stoddart, G., and R.J. Labelle. 1985. *Privatization in the Canadian health care system.* Ottawa, Canada: Health and Welfare Canada.

Demand for Health

Chaloupka, F.J. 1995. Public policies and private anti-health behavior. *American Economic Review* 85(2): 45–49.

Grossman, M. 1972a. On the concept of health capital and the demand for health. *Journal of Political Economy* 80:223–255.

———. 1972b. *The demand for health.* New York: National Bureau of Economic Research.

———. 1982. The demand for health after a decade. *Journal of Health Economics* 1:1–4.

Hay, J.W., et al. 1982. The demand for dental health. *Social Science and Medicine* 16:1285–1289.

Hellerstein, J.K. 1998. The importance of the physician in the generic versus trade name prescription decision. *RAND Journal of Economics* 29:108–136.

Lairson, D., et al. 1984. Estimates of the demand for health: Males in the pre-retirement years. *Social Science and Medicine* 19:741–747.

Mitchell, J.M., and J. Hadley. 1997. The effect of insurance coverage on breast cancer patients' treatment and hospital choices. *American Economic Review* 87(2):448–453.

Pezzin, L.E., and B.S. Schone. 1997. The allocation of resources in intergenerational households: Adult children and their elderly parents. *American Economic Review* 87, no. 2: 460–464.

Vistnes, J.P., and V. Hamilton. 1995. The time and monetary costs of outpatient care for children. *American Economic Review* 85, no. 2: 117–121.

Wagstaff, A. 1986. The demand for health: Theory and applications. *Journal of Epidemiology and Community Health* 40:1–11.

Warner, K.E., and H.A. Murt. 1984. Economic incentives for health. *Annual Review for Public Health* 5:107–133.

Wedig, G.J. 1988. Health status and the demand for health. *Journal of Health Economics* 7:151–163.

Williams, A. 1985. The nature, meaning and measurement of health and illness: An economic viewpoint. *Social Science and Medicine* 20:1023–1027.

Economics of Disease Prevention and Health Promotion

Jones, L., and Bakler, M.R. 1986. The application of health economics to health promotion. *Community Medicine* 8:224–229.

Kenkel, D.S. 1984. The demand for preventative Medical Care. *Applied Economics* 26(4):313–325.

Russell, L.B. 1984. The economic of prevention. *Health Policy* 4:85–100.

Scheffler, R.M., and Paringer, L. 1980. A review of the economic evidence on prevention. *Medical Care* 18:473–484.

Shepart, R.J. 1987. The economic of prevention: a critique. *Health Policy* 7:49–56.

Health Care
Production and Costs

1. Define fixed and variable inputs and distinguish between a short-run and a long-run time horizon in identifying whether inputs are fixed or variable.
2. Explain the concept of a production function for medical services in terms of inputs and outputs and show how it can be used to understand the substitution between inputs and the effect of changes in the volume of inputs.
3. Explain the concepts of *total cost, average cost,* and *marginal cost* and the relationships between them.
4. Explain the concept of a *short-run cost curve* and show how to derive the total, average, and marginal cost curves from basic assumptions.
5. Identify the factors that cause the cost curves to shift and show how they shift.
6. Explain the concept of *economies of scope.*
7. Explain the concept of a *long-run cost curve* and indicate a likely shape for this curve.
8. Identify the likely actual shapes of cost curves for nursing homes, hospitals, physician services, and health insurers.

5.1 INTRODUCTION

The present chapter focuses on the economic behavior of health care providers. We first examine how the resource commitment made by individual providers varies with the amount of production undertaken by these providers. We then focus on the individual providing unit. The measure that we use to weigh the magnitude of the resource commitment of each providing unit is the cost to the unit of resource services. We examine how these costs vary as the size of operations of the providing unit varies.

Before embarking on the analysis of costs, we consider, in Section 5.2, the relation between inputs (resources) and outputs (the input-output or production relation). The presentation is in purely "physical" terms and is designed to provide a brief summary of the role of production in determining cost. In Section 5.3, we explore the basic cost-output relation and examine three alternative ways of looking at this relation. Using the cost-output relation as our basic reference point, we examine, in Section 5.4, the various factors that affect this relation, such as changing technology, the quality of care given, the incentives offered to providers, and the size of the production unit.

In Section 5.5, we examine the impact of one particular organizational factor on a unit's operating costs: the relatedness of the types of services produced together in the same unit. Producing services of different types in the same unit may give rise to economies and diseconomies of scope. In Section 5.6, we examine the impact of operating scale on a unit's costs. Finally, in Section 5.7, we investigate the empirical estimation of cost curves in relation to physician practices, hospitals, nursing homes, and health insurance companies.

5.2 PRODUCTION: THE INPUT-OUTPUT RELATION

5.2.1 Basic Relationship

The economic analysis of production involves the specification of alternative combinations of inputs that yield varying levels of outputs. The production process itself, its organization, and the technology used lie in the realm of administrative practice and medicine. The production process has considerable impact on economic variables and can be influenced by economic factors as well.

The production process is partially determined by the technology used. Roughly defined, technology is a way of doing things. The production process in medical care is determined by what things are done to the patients as well as the way they are done. In this sense, there are many "technologies" even for the same illness. To bring out the essential characteristics of the production (input-output) relation, we focus initially on one technology and later introduce complicating factors and determine how they affect this relation.

The simplest production process can be illustrated by the hypothetical case of a solo private practice physician who treats patients all with the same disease—the common cold. Treatment involves an examination, diagnostic tests, and a prescription of two aspirins and a glass of water. Two simplifying assumptions should be noted. First, the patients' conditions are homogeneous (the patients have equally severe cases of a single disease). Second, the treatment provided is of the same quality (all patients receive the same examination and the same tests and listen to the same banter by the physician).

The process involves the use of various resources. These resources can be divided into two groups: fixed and variable inputs. Fixed inputs are inputs whose use is restricted to their current function for the time period under consideration. Given their specialized nature, the high costs of transferring them to other uses, or contractual arrangements in force, fixed factors cannot be used elsewhere in the economy during the current period of production. Furthermore, the producer cannot increase the quantity during this period, which we will assume to be one month. In our example, fixed factors include physician office space, test equipment, and physician time.

Office space and equipment are rented annually, let us say, and so their use for a one-year period is fixed. As for physician time, we assume that the physician has by choice decided to remain in his or her present position for at least the next month and will work 40 hours per week. Physician time is therefore a fixed factor.

Whether or not a factor is fixed depends on the time period under consideration. If the time period was five years, office space, equipment, and even physician time might vary. The variable factor of production is nursing time. This input can be purchased in varying quantities by the physician. It will be assumed that one or more nurses perform all tasks that the physician does not.

The production process consists of three types of tasks performed using the available resources. The first are the administrative tasks of setting appointments, keeping records, moving patients through the office, and billing patients. The second type are technical tasks, such as the testing of blood with the rented equipment. These tasks are performed by medical technicians. Finally, there is the examination itself, which is performed by the physician. For simplicity's sake, we will assume no patient can be processed without the involvement of a nurse. Generally, of course, the physician is able to process some patients with no help, but we will assume this is not the case. We will also assume that, within the current ranges of resource use considered, the physician can treat all patients who ask for an appointment; his or her time limitations do not create a "capacity" problem.

We now inquire into the number of patients who can be treated at different levels of variable input. The specification of this production relation will be made under the condition that, whatever the level of variable input used in conjunction with the fixed inputs, the maximum number of patients possible are being served. This condition, discussed further at the end of this section, will only hold if the human resources (nurses) have incentives to produce as much as possible. Under this condition, a production function that expresses how output will vary when inputs are changed in quantity can be specified. In specifying this function, let us use L to refer to the nurses' input, which is measured by hours worked. All other factors, which in our example are fixed, will be called F. Output, called Q, is measured by patient visits (each visit is assumed to be identical in nature). The production function can be written $Q = Q(L, F)$, which means that Q depends on L and F.

The production function is a summary of what goes into the process and what comes out. With F fixed, only L can vary. By varying L, we are in fact specifying different combinations of L and F. With few nursing hours, a single nurse will perform all the nonexamination tasks and consequently cannot afford to specialize. Few patients will thus be treated. In Table 5–1 we present this by showing only one patient treated as a result of the first eight hours of nursing input. When more patients are treated, the single nurse can begin to perform some tasks for several patients together. This concentration of tasks allows additional output to be produced with fewer additional resources. Indeed, in our example, only seven additional nursing hours are required to process a second patient.

The additional production yielded by the use of one extra unit of variable input is called the *marginal product*. It can be expressed symbolically as $\Delta Q / \Delta L$. As can be seen in Table 5–1, at the lowest level of output (one visit), an extra nursing hour adds one-eighth of a visit to the level of output. At a level of two visits, the additional output of an extra nursing hour is one-seventh of a visit. This fraction represents the marginal product. This tendency toward an increasing marginal product, created initially by the gains that the concentration of tasks allows, is reinforced by gains from the specialization of tasks as output continues to grow. As more patients are processed and more nursing hours and more nurses are used, some tasks can be divided among the nurses, resulting in gains from specialization.

Table 5–1 Relations between Cost and Output

Total Nursing Hours (L)	Total Visits (Q)	Marginal Product (ΔQ/ΔL)	Total Fixed Cost (TFC)	Total Variable Cost (TVC)	Total Cost (TC = TFC + TVC)	Average Fixed Cost (AFC = TFC/Q)	Average Variable Cost (AVC = TVC/Q)	Average Total Cost (ATC = TC/Q)	Marginal Cost (ΔTC/ΔQ)
8	1	1/8	100	16	116	100.0	16.0	116.0	16
15	2	1/7	100	30	130	50.0	15.0	65.0	14
20	3	1/5	100	40	140	33.3	13.3	46.7	10
24	4	1/4	100	48	148	25.0	12.0	37.0	8
30	5	1/6	100	60	160	20.0	12.0	32.0	12
38	6	1/8	100	76	176	16.7	12.7	29.3	16
50	7	1/12	100	100	200	14.3	14.3	28.6	24
64	8	1/14	100	128	228	12.5	16.0	28.5	28
100	9	1/30	100	200	300	11.1	22.2	33.3	72
140	10	1/40	100	280	380	10.0	28.0	38.0	80

But such gains cannot be reaped forever. Eventually, a large number of routine activities will lead to boredom. In addition, the fixed amount of equipment in the office becomes heavily taxed and nurses have to wait to perform lab tests. This changes the relation between additional output and additional input; to produce successively more units of output at these higher levels of output requires successively larger doses of nursing hours. Putting the argument in terms of marginal productivity, at higher levels of output the marginal productivity of nurses' efforts begins to decline. Thus, in our example, at a level of output of four visits, the marginal product of an additional nursing hour is one-fourth of a visit; at a level of output of five visits, the marginal product falls to one-sixth of a visit; and for six visits the marginal product is lower still, one-eighth of a visit. Production has reached the stage of diminishing marginal productivity. It should be noted that total output is constantly rising; the assumed relation in our production function stipulates that additional increases of output are harder and harder to come by as the size of output rises.

The figures used in our example were invented to illustrate the principle we are hypothesizing—that marginal productivity eventually diminishes. Other equally illuminating examples could have been chosen to elucidate this principle.

5.2.2 Shifts in the Relationship

We have now defined a production function and specified in general terms the most important property we would expect such a function to possess: the marginal product will eventually decline as more units of a variable input are added. This relation was specified on the basis of restrictive underlying conditions. We can now examine how the productive relation will be affected by changes in these conditions. These changes will be examined using the basic production (input-output) relation specified in Table 5–1 as a point of reference. A change in any of these underlying conditions either increases or decreases the amount of output obtained from given amounts of input. Either result will be regarded as a shift in the production relation. An upward shift means that at each level of input more output can be produced; a downward shift means that less output can be produced. Looking at an upward shift in marginal terms, at any level of input more additional output can be produced with an additional unit of the variable input. Expressed in output terms, at any level of output less additional input is required to produce one extra unit of output. Stating the same thing in marginal terms, we would say that the marginal product is greater at any level of output. Thus, at a level of output of eight visits, the original production relation was such that an extra nursing hour employed led to an increase in output of one-fourteenth of a visit. With an upward shift in the production function, an extra nursing hour might now produce one-tenth of a visit. Of course, the assumption that marginal productivity is diminishing still holds, but the entire relation is such that now more can be obtained at any level of output.

We will now examine how changes in some of the underlying conditions affect the production relation. The possible changes include a change in the case mix, in the severity of illness of patients, in the quality of care, in technology, in the amount of capital (F) that the employer uses, and in the underlying incentive structure.

First, a change in the case mix would occur if the physician was confronted with a number of rheumatic fever cases in addition to patients with colds. More resources would need to be expended on each of these cases, shifting the production relation downward. The same type of downward shift would occur if the physician merely had to treat some patients with especially severe colds. These cases would require more resources and would thus shift the production relation downward.

Second, the result of a change in the quality of care will depend on the precise meaning attached to *quality*. If greater thoroughness in performing an examination is an aspect of higher quality care, then the effect of providing higher quality care is to shift the production relation downward, since more resources would be required for each examination. Similarly, if more extensive patient education is an aspect of higher quality care, then the production relation will again be pushed downward.

Third, high quality is frequently associated with high technology—in other words, highly trained specialists and sophisticated equipment. Offering the benefits of advances in technology thus usually entails an increase in capital, both human and physical. More input is required to produce a single unit of output (measured as a visit), and therefore the measured relation between input and output will shift downward. However, note that more resource-intensive visits are qualitatively different than less resource-intensive ones. We cannot say that medical resources are less productive in any of these instances. Instead, a given amount of resources will produce a lower quantity of care, but this medical care is likely to be of a higher quality.

Of course, sometimes the introduction of a new piece of equipment can increase the quantity of output without changing the quality. As an example, if a computerized blood counter replaces a manually operated counter, more tests of the same quality can be processed with the same amount of variable input (technician time). The production relation shifts upward in this case.

A final factor influencing the production relation is the "management" incentive system. Our production relation was derived using the assumption that the maximum output would be obtained at any given level of resource use. Incentives enter the picture when we consider the benefits that accrue to management (the physician, in our example) as a result of the way resources are used. If management is rewarded for keeping production costs low, then management will have an incentive to use as few resources per unit of output as possible. However, incentives can be structured in such a way as to encourage use of inputs. If, for example, the management receives a fixed rate of compensation that is positively related to its costs, then it will have an incentive to use more resources to perform each task. Even though the analysis of production lies in the realm of production management and medicine, the production relation cannot be analyzed in total isolation from the economic incentives that exist within the organization.

5.2.3 Substitution among Inputs

The analysis of the previous section was based on the assumption that one variable input existed. In fact, there may be several variable inputs, and they may be substitutable for each other, at least to some degree. Let us suppose that there are two variable inputs, nursing time (P) and medical assistant time (N), in addition to the fixed inputs (F). The production function is now expressed as $Q = Q(P, N, F)$.

Substitutability among inputs is often analyzed by assuming the level of output (Q) is held constant and then examining, for example, how much medical assistant time must be added to the process to offset a unit of nursing time. We will call this the marginal rate of substitution of medical assistants for nurses.

A number of areas have been identified in health care where substitution makes sense. One study examined the use of paraprofessional surgical assistants as substitutes for physicians or surgeons in the role of assistant to the operating surgeon. The study found that trained assistants could replace physicians in this assisting role with no adverse effects on the operating surgeon's time, particularly in less complex operations (Lewit et al. 1980).

Another example of the substitutability of inputs is the use of drugs in the care of mental patients. To some extent, increased utilization of drugs reduces the amount of effort required of psychiatric hospital attendants. Also, physician assistants and nurse practitioners can perform many of the tasks that physicians traditionally perform (Reinhardt 1972), and dental technicians can perform simple tasks, such as cleaning teeth and doing easy repairs.

Frequently, substitution is feasible and even economical, but barriers exist to limit it. For example, licensing laws may limit the degree to which nurse practitioners can substitute for physicians. In such cases, one must separate what is feasible from what is legally or institutionally permitted.

5.2.4 Volume-Outcome Relationship

The production function has been specified as a relation between the volume of services provided and the quantity of inputs. As noted, there is also a relation between the quality and volume of services. This relation has usually been specified for specific surgical procedures.

In discussing the relation between volume and outcome, the focus can be on the volume of services that are provided by individual providers (surgeons or surgical teams) or the service volume of a health care organization (Garnick et al. 1989). Surgeons individually or as part of a team can maintain their skills better when they perform more of the same types of procedures during a specified time period. If they do only a few operations of a given type within a given time frame, they may get out of practice and the quality of their work may deteriorate. We would therefore expect a positive relationship between the volume of a given procedure for a given practitioner or team and outcomes of the care provided.

A positive relation between volume and outcome may also hold for an institution, but for different reasons. An institution with an especially large volume of certain procedures may hire specialized personnel and acquire specialized equipment. For example, in the area of rehabilitation, an institution with specialized personnel and equipment can return patients to normal functioning sooner. Thus, the relation between volume and outcome can work separately for the surgical (or treatment) team and for the institution where the treatment occurs.

There is a confounding factor that can make it difficult to interpret an observed relation between outcome and volume. If a surgical team is known to be more skilled, then the team will be sought out by patients. We would then observe a positive relation between outcomes and volume, but the high volume may not be the cause of the team's maintenance of its skills. Thus, a policy that encourages larger volumes for surgical teams regardless of their skill levels may not be successful in improving the overall levels of outcome. A further confounding factor may be that an especially skilled surgical team may attract the most difficult cases, which would tend to worsen outcomes irrespective of provider skills. Determining the causes of the observed relationship is important for policy reasons, though it may be difficult in practice to uncover the real causes.

5.3 SHORT-RUN COST-OUTPUT RELATIONS

5.3.1 Production and Cost

Previously we focused on the relation between output and alternative combinations of inputs. In specifying the production relation, the inputs were presented as separate entities that work together. The next step in our analysis is to present a measure of the overall commitment of resources by the provider in producing the output. One such measure, which places all inputs on a single scale measured in money terms, is cost. To a provider, cost means the value of inputs used in the production process. However, this value is not always well approximated by money outlays.

Therefore, a broader view of cost, one that measures what the provider gives up by using all the resources committed to production, not just the ones paid for, is used in this section. Of central importance is the concept of opportunity cost, which is defined as the value that the provider gave up by not committing the resources to the next highest valued use. Another way of putting it is that the cost of resources is measured by the amount for which those resources could be sold in the market. This concept is particularly important when measuring the value of resources that are not paid (e.g., resources that the producer owns) and hence that appear to be free. If the owner of these unpaid resources is giving up some return on them, then there is a cost associated with them, and this cost must be estimated by calculating the probable market value of the resources.

Since we are concerned with the functioning of an organization, the cost of resource use will be considered from the organization's point of view. Any organization can undertake a resource commitment that does not appear in its paid out costs. Nevertheless, if the organization commits its resources to a particular use, they are part of the organization's costs and should be counted as such. On the other hand, an economic unit outside the organization may make a resource commitment that allows the organization to function. For example, a person may give blood to a blood donor clinic, a benefactor may endow a hospital with an operating room, or a physician may volunteer teaching time at a medical school. In these instances, resources are used to undertake activities, but they are not part of the resource commitment of the institution. Rather, they are part of the total resource commitment required to undertake the activity. In this chapter we are concerned with the operations of health care organizations and so focus on the resource commitment made by these organizations in their activities. This leaves out the question of the total (or social) resource commitment made to perform any activity, including the commitment of donors, volunteers, benefactors, and government agencies.

In the analysis that follows, the definitions presented are placed in a time frame of one month. Given this time frame, we can divide production costs into fixed costs and variable costs. Fixed costs are defined as those that do not change with output within the relevant time frame. Variable costs, on the other hand, increase as output increases. In the physician's practice example, the fixed costs are those that do not vary during the month; they are the costs of the fixed factors, including space and equipment rental costs and the cost of physician time. We will assume the rental values to be $50 during the period. We will also assume that the physician could have earned $50 working in a clinic rather than in a private practice; this amount measures the opportunity cost the physician faced when making the decision whether to continue to practice privately. Given that the decision to practice privately has been made, the forgoing of other ways of using work time becomes a "sunk" cost, relevant more to the past than to the present. Nevertheless, it is still a cost and is classified as a fixed cost. The total fixed costs thus equal $100. (The cost curve of a company incorporates the return that the owners could normally get on their assets, including their time, the buildings they own, etc. This normal return is called *normal profit*. Any return above normal profit is called *economic profit*.)

Variable costs are costs of variable inputs. In our example, the only variable input is nursing hours. Assume that the price of nursing services is $2 per hour. Thus, 8 hours of services cost $16. We can now specify the relation between the cost to the provider and the level of output. This relation depends on the quantities of resources used (determined by the production relationship) and the money paid for, or the opportunity cost imputed to, these resource services. The relation can be viewed in three different ways. First, we can examine costs from the point of view of the total resource commitment required to maintain production at any specific level of output. In this case, we determine how total costs vary with output. Second, we can look at the average value of resource commitment, that is, the value of the resource commitment required to produce a single unit of output. The value of this average resource commitment is called *average cost*. The third way of viewing costs is to examine the value of additional resources that must be committed to the production process to produce an additional unit of output. This value is called the *marginal cost*. We will now discuss how each of these alternative measures varies as the level of output changes.

5.3.2 Total Cost

Total cost (*TC*) is the sum of all costs incurred in producing a given level of output; total variable cost (*TVC*) is the total cost of variable inputs for any level of output; total fixed cost (*TFC*) is the total cost of all fixed factors. Total cost is the sum of the total variable cost and the total fixed cost. We now look at these types of cost with regard to the data contained in Table 5–1. The total fixed cost is $100 whatever the level of output. Therefore, this cost, plotted on the graph in Figure 5–1, is represented by a straight horizontal line (*TFC*) at the $100 level.

The behavior of the total variable cost depends on two factors: (1) the relation between output and variable inputs, specified in Section 5.2, and (2) the unit cost of these variable resources. Figure 5–1 contains a total variable cost curve that reflects the data in our example.

The total cost curve (*TC*) is the vertical sum of the two curves *TVC* and *TFC* at each output level (see Table 5–1, Column 6). The level of the *TC* curve is determined in part by the fixed cost; its shape is determined by the production function and the variation of output with variable inputs. Given the fixed per unit price of the variable input ($2 an hour), the production function relation, translated into a cost-

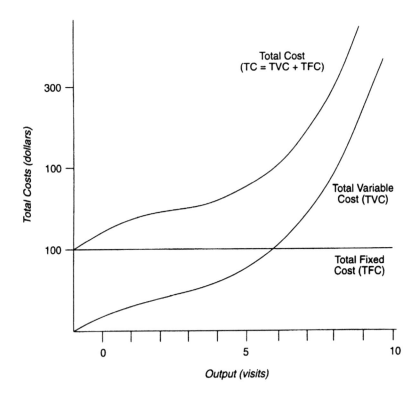

Figure 5–1 The relation between the total fixed cost, total variable cost, total cost, and level of output. At each production level, one total cost can be divided between the fixed and variable costs. The fixed cost does not vary with output. This graph is based on data from Table 5–1.

output relation, entails that the addition to total costs of the extra resource commitment levels off as output increases. Thus, the total variable cost is $16 at a scale of one visit, $30 at a scale of two visits, $40 at a scale of three visits, and $48 at a scale of four visits. This leveling off of cost is shown diagrammatically by the flattening of the section between 0 and 4 of curve *TVC* in Figure 5–1. If additional resources had been increasingly more productive beyond this scale of input, the *TVC* curve would have continued leveling off. But beyond four units of output, diminishing marginal productivity begins to set in, and in terms of costs this means that successively greater resource commitments are needed to attain successively higher levels of output. In Table 5–1, the total variable cost rises to 60, 76, 100, 128, 200, and so on, and the total cost also rises rapidly. As seen on the curve, beyond a scale of 4, *TVC* is curving upward; at the extreme, it would become almost vertical. Thus a considerable commitment in resources is required to move to a higher output level. The shape of *TC* is similar to that of *TVC*, except that *TC* is higher by $100.

5.3.3 Marginal Cost

Implicit in the total variable cost-output relation is the marginal cost-output relation. The marginal cost at any level of output is the additional cost required to move one unit higher on the output scale. It is thus defined as $\Delta TC/\Delta Q$. Since *TFC* is constant over all levels of output, the marginal fixed cost would be zero at any value, since the additional fixed resource commitment is zero at all levels of output. Thus, the marginal cost is simply the addition to total variable cost needed to produce one extra unit of output. In Table 5–1, the marginal cost (*MC*) is shown in Column 10. As can be seen, the extra cost of moving to one unit of output from zero is $16, to two units from one is $14, and so on. Until we reach four units of output, *MC* is falling. However, because of the diminishing marginal productivity of variable inputs, coupled with the fact that the additional variable inputs used are all paid the same wage, producing additional units of output eventually requires successively greater resource commitment. This is reflected in rising marginal cost after the fourth visit; the fifth visit costs $12 extra; the sixth, $16 extra; and so on. The marginal cost curve is shown in Figure 5–2. Note that beyond an output of 4, marginal costs cease falling and begin to rise.

The concept of marginal cost is central to the analysis of most economic decisions. For the most part, the types of decisions that concern economists involve determining the consequences of employing additional (or fewer) resources for a particular purpose. For example, we might be concerned with the implications of placing additional surgeon-training facilities in either Boston or Boise, we might analyze the consequences of adding one or more paramedics to an existing medical practice, or we might be interested in the consequences of decreasing the number of obstetrics beds in a particular region of the country or a particular hospital. In these instances, as in most other cases of resource allocation, the allocation decision concerns whether to expand a particular facility or service or increase the available quantity of trained personnel. The concept used to measure the added resource commitment is the marginal cost.

5.3.4 Average Cost

The third way of looking at costs is to average the costs required to obtain a given level of output. The average total cost (*ATC*) is the total cost per unit of output and is defined for any level of output. It equals *TC/Q*. It measures the value of the average resource commitment required to sustain a given scale of output. However, because it is useful in making comparisons, this variable has been frequently used in empirical studies.

The behavior of the average total cost depends on the behavior of the average fixed cost (*TFC/Q*) and the average variable cost (*TVC/Q*). The average fixed cost is lower at successively higher levels of output because the $100 in fixed cost is spread out over more output. Thus, at one visit, the average fixed cost is $100; at two visits, it is $50; and so on. The average variable cost initially falls at successively greater levels of output. At one unit of output, it is $16; at two, it is $15; at three, it is $13.30; and so on. The fall in average variable cost is made possible by the increasing productivity of additional variable inputs at low output levels.

Another way of viewing this relation is to consider that the marginal cost is initially below the average cost, which brings down the average as output increases. The marginal cost for the first visit is $16, and the average variable cost is $16. For the second visit, the marginal cost is $14. This brings down the average variable cost of the two visits to $15 (i.e., $30/2). The falling average variable and the average fixed cost together ensure that the average total cost (which is the sum of the two)

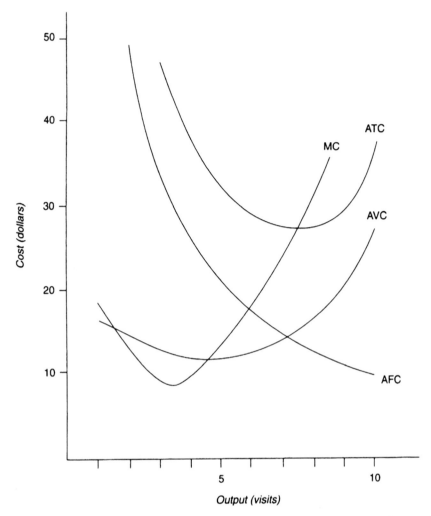

Figure 5–2 Relation between cost and output. The average cost is shown in total (*ATC*) and as separated into the two components of the total: fixed cost (*AFC*) and variable cost (*AVC*). Marginal costs (*MC*) is the addition to total cost of the next unit produced. There is a unique relation between *MC* and both *AVC* and *ATC*: when *MC* is below *ATC* (or *AVC*), the average cost is falling; when *MC* is greater than *ATC* (or *AVC*), the average cost is increasing; and when *MC* equals *ATC* (or *AVC*), the average cost is constant, that is, it has reached a minimum point.

---

will also fall as output expands. Eventually, after four visits, the marginal cost increases as output expands. Expanding output from four to five visits costs an extra $12, expanding to six visits costs another $16, and the marginal cost at seven is $24. However, as long as the marginal cost is lower than the average total cost, a further expansion of output will continue to reduce the average total cost.

For example, in Table 5–1 we can see that at five units of output the total cost is $160 and the average total cost is $32. An expansion of output by one unit to a level of output of six would cost an additional $16. The *ATC* at six units of output decreases to $29.33 because the *MC* of the sixth unit of output is lower than the

ATC, and so expanding output brings down the average. With a rising MC, this situation will not continue indefinitely. At some level of output, the MC will just equal the ATC, and at a still higher level it will exceed it. The ATC must then begin to rise. In our example, the level where the MC equals the ATC is eight visits. As seen in Table 5–1, an expansion from seven to eight visits will cost an extra $28. With an ATC of $28.57 at the level of seven visits, expansion to eight visits leaves the ATC at about the same level. An expansion to nine visits has an MC of $72. This is above the ATC at eight visits. The ATC increases to $33.33 at nine visits.

The average cost curves are shown in Figure 5–2 in juxtaposition to the MC curve. These curves are based on the data presented in Table 5–1 but have been smoothed out. The average fixed cost (AFC) curve declines over all levels of output. The average variable cost (AVC) curve declines until four visits. At five visits, the MC just equals the AVC, and so the AVC curve bottoms out. For output levels higher than five, the MC is above the AVC, and so the AVC increases with expansion of output. The AVC curve is thus U-shaped, indicating that at lower levels of output the AVC falls as output expands. The AVC curve then bottoms (where $MC = AVC$) and begins to rise. The ATC curve (remember, $ATC = AVC + AFC$) is also U-shaped. It is located above and slightly to the right of the AVC curve and also bottoms out where the rising MC cuts it.

The ATC, as already noted, has a fixed and a variable component. The relative sizes of these two components will determine at which level of output the ATC curve will begin to slope upward. The fixed cost component (AFC) always falls as output increases, because the same costs are spread over a greater output. The variable cost component (AVC) follows the rules of productivity and begins to rise, because eventually higher marginal costs will raise the average. The larger the fixed cost component, the greater the range over which the average total cost will fall. Hospitals have been identified as having large fixed cost components. If this is indeed true, then hospitals should experience a diminishing average total cost over a wide range of potential output levels.

The fixed cost component is related to the use of capital equipment. A heavy investment in capital equipment will create a large fixed cost. However, such equipment may permit additional procedures to be undertaken with a small additional commitment of resources up to high levels of output. In such a situation, although the fixed cost would be high, the marginal cost would be low, and the average total cost would fall over a wide range of output levels. In a related phenomenon, called *indivisibility*, expensive equipment, available in a large dose, cannot be divided into smaller units. It is operated at low levels of output at a high ATC and operated at high levels at a low ATC.

This section has identified three related cost-output measures: total cost, average cost, and marginal cost. Their shapes are dependent largely on the production relation. As shown in Section 5.2, the production relation is subject to shifts caused by a variety of conditions. These same conditions can cause a cost curve to change its positions, as discussed below.

5.4 COST CURVE POSITION

The position of a cost curve is determined by the same factors that influence the production relation. These factors include the case mix and the severity of cases treated, the quality of care provided, the technology used, the amount of fixed factors employed in the production process, and the incentive system under which the provider is operating. In addition, change in input prices can affect the position of the cost curve. Each factor will be considered separately.

Given fixed inputs and fixed costs, a change in the case mix toward more complicated cases and an increase in the average severity level will increase the variable resources required per unit of output and will thus increase marginal and average costs at all output levels. The positions of both the ATC and MC curves will now be higher. The shifts in position are shown in Figure 5–3. Here, ATC_1 and MC_1 are the average total cost and marginal cost relations before the change to a more complex case mix. This change results in a shift to ATC_2 and MC_2.

An increase in quality, if this entails more thorough examinations or treatments, will similarly shift the cost curves upward. The adoption of a technology that uses more resources per case will have a similar effect. Many recent technological innovations have been associated with a large capital investment for equipment as well as a larger flow of variable expenditures for the services of the highly trained personnel needed to operate this equipment. Examples of such technological innovations include open-heart surgery, a procedure that intrigued economists in the 1960s; coronary care units (CCUs) or intensive care units (ICUs), which are high-cost monitoring and life support units; computed tomography (CT) scanning; magnetic resonance imaging (MRI), a revolutionary and somewhat costly advance on radiology; and laparoscopic surgery, which allows a surgeon to perform an

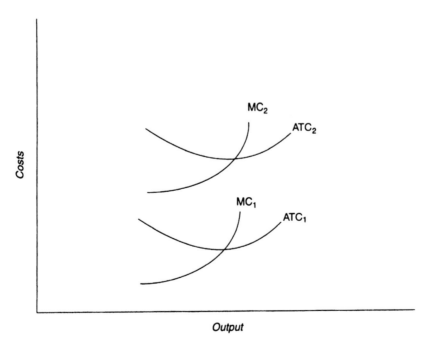

Figure 5–3 Diagrammatic representation of a shift in average and marginal cost curves. Curves ATC_1 and MC_1 indicate the initial relation between costs and output. Curves ATC_2 and MC_2 represent an upward shift in costs at every level of output.

operation through a small incision. All these examples require a heavy investment in equipment, and the effect of introducing any of them would be to shift both the fixed and variable components of the *ATC* upward, thus increasing the *ATC* for all levels of output. However, it should be remembered that an increase in the quality of services provided may accompany the introduction of new technology. One physician visit or one hospital stay is not always the same as another.

All technological innovations in medical care are not of this resource-using type, however. Innovations in pharmaceuticals have reduced the length of hospitalization required for some illnesses. Two notable examples are tuberculosis treatment and mental illness treatment. Furthermore, new laboratory equipment has allowed many tasks to be automated. This has led to falling average costs over broad ranges of output because of the low variable costs associated with the use of this equipment.

The effect of incentives that encourage resource use is to raise the level of average cost associated with any single level of output. Assuming that a single least-cost position is associated with each output level, we can identify a least-cost average cost curve. Incentives to use resources will encourage the provider to choose a position above this curve. It has been questioned whether a cost curve that measures the cost-output relation when given resources are not used to maximize output (i.e., a more-than-least-cost curve) is a meaningful concept. This is because more than one such average cost point may exist at any output level. There can only be one least-cost point, however, and in the least-cost case, a cost curve that supposedly represents a unique relation between cost and output can be uniquely determined. Once a provider chooses to use more than the least amount of resources to achieve a given output level (with no change in quality), he or she can use these excessive resources to varying degrees. There is no longer a unique cost curve (Zuckerman et al. 1994).

Another factor that might cause cost curves to shift is the price the provider pays for hired resources. In our example, if the physician had to pay $3 per nursing hour instead of $2, both the marginal and the average cost curves would shift upward. Conversely, if the price fell to $1, the curves would shift downward. A final factor that can influence the position of the average cost curves appears when two or more types of variable input exist. When these inputs can be substituted for each other, at least to some degree, then a substitution of a less costly for a more costly input can lower the cost curves, although other factors may push them the other way. For example, if a paramedic is substituted for a physician but takes much longer to do the same task, the total or average cost may not shift downward as a result of the substitution. Also, keep in mind that the quality of the product may become lower as a result of the substitution, and even though the output may cost less to produce, it might not be exactly comparable.

5.5 ECONOMIES OF SCOPE

We have proceeded with the discussion of costs as if a health care institution had a single type of output. Although this assumption helps to clarify certain relations between costs and output, it is generally false in the case of larger institutions, notably hospitals. Hospitals are multiproduct firms that offer a large number of separate product lines, such as clinical laboratory services, emergency department services, physical therapy, and intensive care (Berry 1973; Goldfarb et al. 1980).

The product line dimension of output should be distinguished from the case mix dimension. Case mix refers to the complexity of the types of diseases being treated. A hospital that treats a large number of different diseases has a different case mix than one that specializes in a few. If, as is sometimes done, severity is included as a dimension of case mix, then case mix indexes can be developed (Hornbrook and Monheit 1985). Each hospital also has a number of services or product lines. In fact, two hospitals can have very similar case mix measures but very different service scopes. As a consequence, the relation between cost and scope offers itself as a possibly fruitful topic of investigation.

Economies of scope are savings derived from producing different products jointly in the same production unit rather than producing them individually in separate production units. Let X_1 stand for one output (e.g., family planning services) and X_2 stand for a second output (e.g., pediatric services). Let $C(X_1)$ stand for the total cost of producing X_1, $C(X_2)$ stand for the total cost of producing X_2 in a separate setting, and $C(X_1, X_2)$ stand for the cost of jointly producing X_1 and X_2 in the same production unit. Economies of scope arise when the cost of jointly producing specific quantities of the two services $[C(X_1, X_2)]$ is less than the sum of the costs of producing each service separately $[C(X_1) + C(X_2)]$. In our example, economies of scope would exist if a clinic could jointly produce given quantities of family planning services and pediatric services more cheaply than the same quantities produced in sharply separated units or departments.

Economies of scope might arise when some of the tasks involved in providing two distinct services are complementary. For example, if family planning and pediatric services require a common core of testing capabilities, then providing the two types of services in separate units would cause duplication. Savings could be achieved by combining the two services into a single unit that caters to both groups of patients. Of course, it is also possible to have diseconomies of scope. This would occur when two types of output are best produced in separate units. For example, if psychiatric patients are treated with one regimen and home health service patients with a different one, combining the psychiatric and home health services in a single unit may be more costly than keeping them separate.

In one study of the economies of scope in health care, Cowing and Holtmann (1983) estimated economies of scale and scope for 138 short-term hospitals in New York State. They divided hospital output into five diagnostic categories (actually representing different case mixes rather than service scopes): medical-surgical, maternity, pediatric, other inpatient care, and emergency department care. For four of the services (pediatric care being the exception), marginal cost fell over low ranges of output and then became constant. These results indicate substantial economies of scale in these services and suggest that merging services produced on a small scale into larger units could yield considerable savings. However, with regard to the existence of economies of scope, the findings were generally negative. These findings, if they hold up in repeated trials, indicate that, on cost grounds alone, hospitals should specialize rather than become multiproduct organizations. One must be careful not to overgeneralize, because, even though economies of scope may not be widespread, specific services may have production conditions that, when combined, yield economies of scope.

5.6 LONG-RUN COST CURVES

In deriving the cost curves in Section 5.4, the assumption was made that some of the inputs were fixed. Suppose we take a longer perspective and allow enough time for the providing unit to change its "fixed" factors—to expand or contract its physical plant to buy and sell equipment and hire and fire physicians. For planning periods of sufficient length, such changes are certainly possible. An analysis of relevant issues is called a *long-run analysis*.

Indeed, the factors that are considered fixed from the perspective of the short term are no longer fixed; they, too, can vary. From the longer planning perspective, all resources are variable. Suppose a hospital board is planning to build a new facility from scratch. The board can choose either a 60-, 120-, or 250-bed facility, entailing a capital outlay of $2 million, $3 million, or $3.5 million, respectively. Associated with each size are the given annual capital cost of depreciation and the interest on the financial capital. During the planning period—up until the size decision is made—these capital costs can be varied (in three different levels) and thus are variable.

Associated with each facility under consideration is an average cost curve (either ATC_1, ATC_2, or ATC_3 in Figure 5–4) that includes capital costs (remember that, in the long run, there are no fixed costs). Now assume that each facility is least costly for a given range of output. For fewer than 1,000 annual admissions, ATC_1 is the least costly; for over 3,000 admissions, ATC_3 is the least costly. Depending on which level of output is chosen, one plant size will be the least costly. The dashed

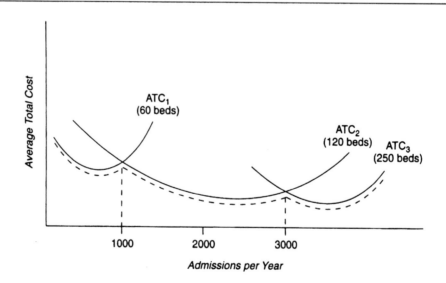

Figure 5–4 Relation between short- and long-run aveage cost curves. Short-run curves (ATC_1, ATC_2, and ATC_3) are shown for three plant sizes (expressed in terms of bed size). The long-run average cost curve (*LRAC*) is derived from these curves (shown as the dashed line). The *LRAC* is the minimum cost point at each level of output. At 1,000 and 3,000 admissions, the *LRAC* becomes associated with the different cost curves (different plant sizes), because it becomes more economical to produce successively greater outputs with larger-sized plants.

curve in Figure 5–4 represents the least cost that can be produced at any given output level (assuming we can choose the size of the facility). This is called the *long-run average cost (LRAC) curve*. It is made up of the minimum cost points at each output level. The *LRAC* is usually hypothesized, if it were represented in a smooth fashion, to be U-shaped. Such a shape would be generated by falling long-run average costs (economies of scale) at low levels of output, followed by constant and finally increasing costs (diseconomies of scale).

Before discussing such costs, it is necessary to specify whether the entity in question is a single operating unit (e.g., an individual hospital, nursing home, or ambulatory care clinic) or an entire system (e.g., a corporate chain). A single operating entity may be subject to eventual diseconomies because the gains from specialization in certain tasks eventually run out. Also, a single hospital unit may be able to expand only by the addition of diverse units (e.g., a CAT scanning unit or a physiotherapy department), and such units may be costly to manage in a single unit. For these reasons, the long-run cost curve of the single operating unit may exhibit diseconomies of scale.

A multiplant system, such as a multihospital corporation, may exhibit economies of scale as it expands by acquiring additional distinct operating units. Certain functions, such as purchasing, may be run more efficiently on a scale that exceeds that of an individual operating unit. Furthermore, a multiunit system can develop standardized procedures in patient records, accounting, and the like and can make comparisons between units. For these reasons, as a system expands, it may exhibit economies of scale, at least up to a point.

5.7 EMPIRICAL ESTIMATION OF COST CURVES

5.7.1 Background

Average or per unit cost is a convenient and accessible summary of a producer's performance. To obtain the average cost at any level of output, divide total cost by quantity. Given the convenience of this measure of performance, it is natural that analysts would use it to compare providers who produce roughly the same product but at different levels of output. Our simple, unqualified, short-run hypothesis would lead us to expect a U-shaped relation between average cost and output. However, interproducer comparisons are fraught with complications.

Quality, case mix, and technology differences among producing units may make comparisons difficult. For this reason as well as others cited in Section 5.4, producers may be operating on different cost curves, as shown in Figure 5–5, where ATC_1, ATC_2, and ATC_3 are average short-run cost curves of three producers. As compared with Producer 1, Producer 2 is producing a higher quality product or serving patients with a more severe case mix but is using the same amounts of fixed inputs. Therefore, Producer 2's cost curve (ATC_2) is above ATC_1 at all levels of output. To identify the shape of the short-run cost curve, one must control for factors that shift the curve. Assume, for example, that Producer 1's cost-output point is at *x* and Producer 2's is at *v*. Without knowing how the quality of services and other factors differed, one would not know if points *x* and *v* are on the same curve or on different curves.

In estimating long-run cost curves, one encounters even greater difficulties. Let us say that Producer 3 has a more capital-intensive operation than Producers 1 or 2

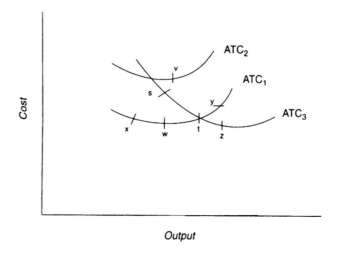

Output

Figure 5–5 Identifying points on the *ATC* curve. When data are gathered from producers on their average total costs at various output levels, care must be taken in interpreting these points. Data points collected from different producers may be on similar *ATC* curves (such as *x*, *w*, *y*, and *t*) or on different *ATC* curves (such as *v* and *y*). The key to determining which is more likely is to identify extraneous circumstances (other than output) that might have caused producers to operate on different curves. These circumstances, if identified, would lead us to conclude whether pairs such as *x* and *z* are on different or similar curves. The circumstances that shift the cost curve (or lead to different cost curves) include differences in input prices, quality of output, and capital equipment.

---

because Producer 3 has invested more heavily in capital equipment to gain economies from automation. Let us also assume that the quality and case mix of Producer 3 are similar to those of Producer 1. The true long-run cost curve for the industry (assuming that these are the only two scales of operations available) is ATC_1 up to point *t* in Figure 5–5 and ATC_3 for scales of output above and beyond point *t*. But when we start to estimate this curve, we do not know this. Among the data that are usually available for making such comparisons, we have only one observation for each producer. These observations tell us, for example, that Producer 1 is producing at 1,000 units of output with an *ATC* of $50, Producer 2 is producing at 1,200 units with an *ATC* of $80, and so on. (We may, of course, also have some information on some of the operating characteristics of each producer.) With this information, we have only one point on each producer's cost curve, which is not enough to tell us where on its cost curve each producer is operating.

   If, for example, Producer 1 is producing at point *x* and Producer 3 at point *z*, then both are on the long-run cost curve, and an estimation of a long-run cost curve with points such as these will give us a reasonably accurate picture of what the long-run cost curve looks like. But there is no reason why we should be so lucky. Producer 1 could well be producing at a high-capacity level, such as point *y*, and Producer 3 could be at a low-capacity level, such as point *s*. While both are on their short-run curves, neither is on its long-run curve. We would have no way of knowing this, and if we assumed that we were estimating a long-run curve, we would end up with biased results.

In fact, where on its cost curve each producer is producing depends on supply. It also depends on the producer's goals or objectives as well as the conditions underlying costs and revenues, which is the topic of Chapter 6. Following are brief summaries of empirical evidence on producer cost curves for several health-related activities. When reviewing this material, keep in mind the difficulties in identifying actual cost-output relations.

5.7.2 Group Practices

Group medical practices have occasionally been held up as institutions that should yield considerable economies of scale and thus help raise output while moderating increases in total costs. Since a fairly large number of group practices are in operation, it might seem that the proposition that average costs are falling would be easy to test. However, because of the considerable variation in the types of group practices, difficulties in output measurements, and problems associated with gathering appropriate data, only tentative answers have been obtained. The first statistical analysis was done using data collected on solo and group practices in the field of internal medicine (Bailey 1968). Because the study compared practices in the same field, it circumvented problems associated with the inclusion of different production techniques used by different types of practices. The data collected showed that the average volume of services provided per physician, adjusted for the type of visit (e.g., routine visit, annual examination, or complete examination), was greater for solo practices than for group practices. Although the sample size was small, it cast some doubt on the existence of economies of scale.

There are several reasons why this finding may not be so surprising. First, the technology generally used in internal medicine is such that the gains from task specialization and the use of capital-intensive techniques may be achieved at a low level of output. For the tasks involved in operating an internal medicine practice, the *ATC* curve may reach a lower point at a scale of output supportable by one practitioner. Second, an incentive factor may be at work when several practitioners combine forces. This factor, which has a tendency to shift the *ATC* curve upward when the group is formed, is operative in situations where members of the practice share revenues and costs. When this sharing occurs, the revenues that any single member of the group generates are shared and the costs that he or she incurs are borne by all the members. Because of reduced burden, the individual physician can make a heavier use of nurses' time and of equipment while feeling less impact than in a solo practice. It is hypothesized that, under cost-sharing arrangements, each physician in the group will generate more costs than in a solo practice, pushing up the cost curve for the group. Furthermore, the larger the group, the higher will be the cost curve (assuming that offsetting factors do not exist; see Scheffler 1975).

Another study analyzed interpractice variations in the relation between staff salary costs and scale of output (measured by office visits) for a sample of single-specialty practices, although they were not all of the same specialty (Newhouse 1973). The presence of cost sharing was found to shift the cost curve upward for group practices. Furthermore, after adjusting for this incentive factor, the cost curve was found to exhibit economies of scale, indicating that such economies do exist among practices with no cost sharing and also among practices with some cost sharing. Because of the small sample, the inattention paid to case mix, and technology differences among practices due to specialty differences, the results are not conclusive.

5.7.3 Hospital Marginal Costs

The importance of the topic of hospital marginal cost is related to the objective of reimbursing hospitals for the extra resource costs they incur when their volumes change. If a hospital is being reimbursed at the level of costs in 1995 and its admissions have increased by 5 percent, its additional costs may be greater than, equal to, or less than 5 percent. If the hospital is reimbursed an additional 5 percent (ignoring inflation) to cover the volume differential and actual costs had gone up by 3 percent, the hospital would incur a windfall gain. On the other hand, the hospital would lose out if its costs had increased by 10 percent.

Marginal cost variation is often measured using the ratio of marginal to average costs (M/A). Recall that if M is greater than A (or $M/A > 1$), then the average cost will increase (Section 5.3). For example, beginning from an initial output level of 1,000 admissions and an average cost of $200 per case, if output expands by 5 percent (50 admissions) and M is $220, then M/A is 1.1. Expansion has raised the average cost, and if the hospital was reimbursed for the additional cases at $200 per case, it would incur a loss. If the hospital was reimbursed on the basis of its prior year's costs plus the marginal cost of its additional cases, it would be fully reimbursed.

This problem has arisen in a number of instances. During the early 1970s, when price controls were set on hospital revenues, allowable revenues were set at the previous year's revenue levels, plus an inflation factor, plus a volume adjustment based on estimates of M/A (Lipscomb et al. 1978). In the Finger Lakes region of New York State, a regional reimbursement experiment was set up: hospitals were reimbursed based on a base year cost, plus an inflation factor, plus a volume adjustment that assumed that the value of M/A was .4 for inpatient care and .6 for outpatient care (Farnand et al. 1986). And currently under Medicare regulations, hospitals are given extra reimbursement for cases in a particular diagnostic group whose length of stay or costs are outside diagnostic limits (outliers). The additional reimbursement is based on an M/A value of .6 for the extra days.

One way of estimating hospital marginal cost is to take short-term (e.g., monthly) values of operating costs and volume for a given hospital over a period (two to three years) and find the average variation in costs with a given variation in output. Another way is to relate variation in costs and outputs across hospitals. The former method will probably give a more accurate estimate than the latter of short-run marginal cost, but there are difficulties even with it. Among these are that the cost levels of inputs must be adjusted for (assuming they have changed) and that capital equipment and operating techniques must remain the same throughout the study period (otherwise the hospital will have moved from one short-run cost curve to another).

In addition, the marginal cost will depend on the measure of output (e.g., whether it is length of stay or admissions). It will vary with the amount of the volume adjustment (e.g., 2 or 5 percent) and the relative permanence of the adjustment as estimated by the hospital administrator. For a volume increase that is small or short lived, the administrator may decide to tax existing resources for a time rather than immediately expand and thereby raise marginal cost. The estimate of *M* under these circumstances would appear to be lower than if the administrator responded more automatically.

For the preceding reasons, there is no accepted measure of the true short-run value of *M/A* (Lave and Lave 1984). Estimates range from .2 to .6, but remember that the value will vary depending on a number of factors (Friedman and Pauly 1983).

5.7.4 Hospital Economies of Scale

A large number of studies have investigated the possible existence of economies of scale in hospitals, with very mixed results (Berki 1972; Frech and Mobley 1995). Early studies identified economies of scale but subsequent studies have uncovered no evidence (Lave and Lave 1984) or conflicting evidence (Frech and Mobley 1995). There is an explanation for the differences in findings.

As discussed earlier, the typical hospital is an organization with a complex case mix and a large number of different services. Each service has its own cost-output relation, which may exhibit economies of scale. The scope of services is greater for larger hospitals (Berry 1973), but these hospitals may have more varied case types, so some services (e.g., cobalt therapy) that are devoted to specific case types may be operated at low capacity and high cost. A multiproduct hospital can be quite large yet have a number of services with considerable excess capacity (Finkler 1979b). As a result, it might exhibit a higher average cost than many smaller hospitals.

One study (Hornbrook and Monheit 1985) that incorporated both case mix and service scope variables to investigate economies of scale found no such economies at the hospital level. But a number of studies of individual services, such as open-heart surgery facilities, CT scanner units, therapeutic radiology facilities, and hospital laundries, have found evidence of economies of scale (Finkler 1979a; Gregory 1976–1977; McGregor and Pelletier 1978; Okunade 1993; Schwartz and Joskow 1980). This suggests that the economies of scale that do occur in some hospital departments are offset by diseconomies of scale in others.

5.7.5 Nursing Home Costs

A number of studies have been undertaken in the nursing home area with a view to determining the effect on costs of operating variables such as volume of operations, product quality, case mix, and organizational characteristics (e.g., for-profit or nonprofit status and membership in a chain) (Bishop 1980). The relevant variable for such studies is average cost, which is the most appropriate variable for a comparison of costs in different facilities. There is no agreement as to whether total costs (which include fixed costs such as administrative costs, interest, and depreciation) or only variable costs should be used. Using just variable costs would be appropriate when focusing on short-term operations, whereas including capital and other fixed costs would be appropriate when dealing with long-term issues. For example, one might want to find out whether a large-scale plant is more efficient than a small-scale plant. Asking which is the most efficient implies that time would be allowed to develop a plant of the appropriate size.

Studies that have examined the relationship between average cost and various causal variables have uncovered some interesting relationships. There is disagreement as to the relationship between average cost and scale of operations (Bishop 1980; McKay 1988). The fact that a nursing home is a member of a chain does not appear to influence its costs (Ullman 1986). On the other hand, for-profit nursing homes have been identified as having a lower average cost that nonprofit nursing homes (Ullman 1984).

As with all cost studies in the health care area, such studies have had to deal with difficulties in measuring and netting out the impact of patient case mix and the level of quality, two factors that influence the level of care and hence nursing home costs. For example, it has proved extremely hard to identify patient characteristics associated with specific levels of care. Patients differ considerably with regard to health status, and their different needs should translate into differences in the level of care or resource intensity. Several case mix classifications (for long-term care patients) that try to take into account resource use differences have been developed. These measures are far from perfect, but even allowing for their shortcomings, their inclusion in the cost analysis may not be sufficient to account for differences in average cost that are related to level-of-care differences. A nursing home that offers "high-quality" care as measured by resource-intensive processes (rehabilitation, nursing care) may provide more care to all patients regardless of their health status. Similarly, in a low-quality nursing home, all patients may receive fewer services than in the high-quality home, adjusting for health status. One must therefore find a quality measure that is independent of case mix or case severity in order to control for the influence of each factor on cost of care. As will be seen in the following chapter, most measures of case mix do not adequately distinguish between case mix and severity, and so it has been very difficult to identify each factor's specific impact on cost.

Average cost is not the only relevant cost measure in nursing home analysis. Marginal cost is also important when forecasting resource use or when assessing nursing home profitability. A New York study analyzed the marginal cost of nursing homes, adjusting for variables such as SNF/ICF days, average level of service in the institution, patient characteristics, input prices, and for-profit or nonprofit status. The marginal cost for the healthiest patients was $51 per patient day. For the least healthy patients, the marginal cost was $60. These rates can be compared with the reimbursement rate of $72, indicating a profit for patients at all levels.

5.7.6 Health Insurance Costs

Theoretically, health insurance administrative costs are potentially influenced by the scale of a firm's operations. Additionally, a very important factor affecting these costs is the ratio of group policies to all policies that an insurance company sells. Per policy, individual policies are more expensive to sell. Also, employers perform many of the functions for group policies that insurers perform for individual policies. This fact may influence public policy, because if individual and group policies have significantly different costs, the government may act to encourage holders of individual policies to obtain group policies.

One study examined health insurance administrative costs for a cross section of insurance companies that offer health insurance. The study found that both factors have a significant impact on these costs (Blair et al. 1975b). An unexpected finding of their study was that mutual (nonprofit) companies had lower administrative costs than stock (for-profit) companies. As will be seen in Chapter 6, one might have expected the opposite to be true.

EXERCISES

1. The Green City Hospital treated 100 patients in May with 20 nursing hour inputs, and it treated 120 patients in June with 22 nursing hour inputs. What is the total product for each month? What is the marginal product?

2. Sweetgrass Radiology Labs has a fixed amount of radiology equipment. The laboratory can hire any number of radiology technicians per hour to produce radiographs, which are displayed on a screen. The relationship between the number of technicians hired per hour and the number of radiographs produced per hour is shown in the following table. Show the total and marginal products and indicate at each level of production whether the production function exhibits increasing, constant, or diminishing marginal productivity.

Radiograph Technician per Hour	Radiograph Produced per Hour
1	10
2	26
3	50
4	74
5	94
6	100

3. Given the production function between nurse hours and patient visits per day to a community clinic, how will each of the following shift this function:
   a. a change in nurse remuneration from salary to fee for service
   b. a change in the case mix of patients, with more having leukemia and fewer having common colds
   c. a change in policy to provide more thorough examinations
   d. higher nurse wages
   e. a requirement that each patient now be told all his or her legal rights before an examination
   f. an increase in the total number of nurses who are hired
   g. an increase in the clinic's budget

4. St. Mary's Hospital owns a prime piece of real estate in the center of town. There is a small shopping center on this piece of land. Rents for each store are $4,000 per month. The benefactor of this real estate, in her endowment to St. Mary's, stated that one of the stores should be operated as a clinic for the poor and be kept open 24 hours a day. St. Mary's has agreed to these conditions. It hires three nurses monthly at $3,000 each. Furnishings are included in the estimate of the $4,000 rent. Supplies are $10 per patient; there are 800 patients a month, each of whom come in for one visit. What are the costs of operating the clinic?

5. Given the following data for a community health center, calculate the average and marginal costs for each output level and (in the case of marginal costs) between successive output levels.

Number of visits	Total cost
1	$100
2	160

3	200
4	260
5	360

6. If the total fixed cost is $1,000 at 100 visits for a clinic, what will the marginal fixed cost be for 101 visits?

7. City Home Care hires a furnished office at $2,000 per month, telephones at $200 a month, and a secretary at $2,000 per month. These resources do not change, no matter how many clients are visited. Currently CHC sees 400 patients a month, each three times (1,200 visits in total). CHC uses 30 full-time nurses with their own cars, and they are paid $4,000 per month each. There is a plentiful supply of additional nurses in town. These nurses can be hired almost on notice. Supplies are $20 per patient per month. What are the money costs of operating CHC at its current level? Approximately how much would it cost to operate CHC at a level of 1,300 visits per month?

8. The Jonesville Clinic is an inner-city clinic that provides primary care for indigent persons. Three physicians volunteer five hours a week each. Normally, physicians earn $150 per hour, but the clinic is lucky to get their services for free. The clinic hires two nurses annually at $18,000 each. Overhead, including secretarial time, is $15,000 a year. Ace Pharmaceuticals donates $2,000 worth of drugs annually, and the First Street Mall donates a small office. The mall's owners could get $400 monthly in rent for the office. What is the economic cost annually of operating the clinic.

9. For each volume of output, calculate the total fixed costs.

Clinic visits	Total costs	Total variable costs
10	$1,200	$1,000
11	1,300	1,100
12	1,500	1,300
13	2,000	1,800

10. The following is an estimate by the manager of the Centerville Nursing Home for total monthly costs at alternative operating levels, measured by patient days. Calculate the total fixed cost for the Centerville Nursing Home.

Patient days	Total cost
0	$120,000
1	150,000
2	180,000
3	210,000
4	240,000

11. The May Clinic rents a small office in Dubuque. May pays the building owner a rent of $2,000 a month, which includes all utilities. It has signed a three year lease. May hires a general practice physician at $50 an hour, a nurse at $15 an hour, and a secretary at $10 an hour. May assumes that each patient uses $10 in supplies. In September, the clinic was open for 200 hours, during which all personnel were available at all times to staff the clinic. During that time, 1,000 patients were seen. What were May's fixed and variable costs for the month?

12. Given the following monthly data for alternative operating levels at the St. Christopher's Ambulance, calculate the total fixed cost, average fixed cost, average variable cost, average total cost, and marginal cost for successive output levels. If St. Christopher's is operating at a level of three trips and it

wants to determine the resources needed to make another trip, which statistic will it use?

Ambulance Trips	Total variable cost	Total cost
0	$ 0	$1,200
1	1,300	2,500
2	1,400	2,600
3	1,500	2,700
4	1,800	3,000
5	2,400	3,600
6	3,400	4,600

13. The Grinch Clinic pays its nurses $20 an hour. It also pays $100 a week rent and has other weekly overhead costs of $50. Supply costs are $1 per patient. The short-run production function, relating patient visits and nursing hours, is shown below. Given this relationship and the other specified data, calculate the total variable, total fixed, and total costs; average costs (variable, fixed, and total); and marginal costs at each output level.

Patient visits	Nursing hours
1	2
2	4
3	8
4	14
5	22
6	32

14. The Rushmore Clinic pays nurses an hourly wage of $10. The clinic's fixed costs in 1992 were $1,000. The schedule relating visits to nursing hours is given below.

Visits	Nurse hours
1	10
2	25
3	50
4	100
5	200
6	400

   a. Determine the average, marginal and total costs at each operating level when the nursing wage is $10.
   b. Determine the average, marginal, and total costs at each operating level when the nursing wage is $20.
   c. If the clinic manager wants to compare her clinic to that of another in order to determine which was more efficient, what statistic would she use?

15. Given the following data, calculate the total fixed, total variable, and marginal costs.

Quantity	Total cost
0	$100
1	120
2	150
3	200
4	300

BIBLIOGRAPHY

Production of Medical Care

Cromwell, J. 1974. Hospital productivity trends in short-term general non-teaching hospitals. *Inquiry* 11:181–187.

Deb, P., and A.M. Holmes. 1998. Substitution of physicians and other providers in outpatient mental health care. *Health Economics* 7:347–362.

Defelice, L.C., and W.D. Bradford. 1997. Relative inefficiencies in production between solo and group practice physicians. *Health Economics* 6:455–466.

Goldfarb, M., et al. 1980. Behavior of the multi-product firm. *Medical Care* 18:185–201.

Lewit, E.M. et al. 1980. A comparison of surgical assisting in a prepaid group practice. *Medical Care* 18:916–929.

Lu, M. 1999. The productivity of mental health care: An instrumental variable approach. *Journal of Mental Health Policy and Economics* 2:59–71.

Nyman, J.A., and D.L. Bricker. 1989. Profit incentives and technical efficiency in the production of nursing home care. *Review of Economics and Statistics* 71:586–593.

Okunade, A., and C. Suraratdecha. 1998. Factor interchange and technical progress in U.S. specialized hospital pharmacies. *Health Economics* 7:363–372.

Reinhardt, U. 1972. A production function for physicians' services. *Review of Economics and Statistics* 54:55–66.

———. 1973a. Manpower substitution and productivity in medical practice. *Health Services Research* 7:200–277.

———. 1973b. Proposed changes in the organization of health care delivery. *Milbank Memorial Fund Quarterly* 51:169–222.

Rosenman, R., et al. 1997. Output efficiency of health maintenance organizations in Florida. *Health Economics* 6:295–303.

Ruchlin, H.S., and I. Leveson. 1974. Measuring hospital productivity. *Health Services Research* 9:308–323.

Scheffler, R.M. 1975. Further consideration of the economics of group practice. *Journal of Human Resources* 10:258–263.

Outcome-Volume Relation

Bunker, J.P., et al. 1982. Should surgery be regionalized? *Surgical Clinics of North America* 62:657–668.

Garnick, D., et al. 1989. Surgeon volume vs. hospital volume: Which matters more? *JAMA* 262:547–548.

Hamilton, B.H., and V.H. Hamilton. 1997. Estimating surgical volume-outcome relationships applying survival models: Accounting for frailty and hospital fixed effects. *Health Economics* 6:383–396.

Luft, H.S. 1980. The relationship between surgical volume and mortality: An exploration of causal factors and alternative models. *Medical Care* 18:940–959.

Luft, H.S., and S.S. Hunt. 1986. Evaluating individual hospital quality through outcome statistics. *JAMA* 255:2780–2784.

Luft, H.S., et al. 1987. The volume-outcome relationship: Practice makes perfect or selective referral patterns? *Health Services Research* 22:157–182.

Luft, H.S., et al. 1990. *Hospital volume, physician volume, and patient outcomes.* Ann Arbor, MI: Health Administration Press Perspectives.

Spector, W.D., et al.1998. The impact of ownership type on nursing home outcomes. *Health Economics* 7:639–654.

Tilford, J.M., et al. 1998. Differences in pediatric ICU mortality risk over time. *Critical Care Medicine* 26:1737–1743.

Tilford, J.M., et al. 2000. Volume-outcome relationships in pediatric intensive care units. *Pediatrics* 106:289–294.

Costs: Hospitals

Barer, M. 1982. Case mix adjustment in hospital cost analysis. *Journal of Health Economics* 1:53–80.

Bays, C. 1980. Specification error in the estimation of hospital cost functions. *Review of Economics and Statistics* 62:302–305.

Berki, S. 1972. *Hospital economics.* Lexington, MA: D.C. Heath.

Berry, R.E. 1973. On grouping hospitals for economic analysis. *Inquiry* 10:5–12.

Carey, K. 1997. 1997. A panel design for estimation of hospital cost functions. *Review of Economics and Statistics* 77:443–453.

Cary, K., and J.F. Burgess. On measuring the hospital cost/quality trade-off. *Health Economics* 8:509–520.

Cowing, T.G., and A.G. Holtmann. 1983. Multiproduct short-run hospital cost functions. *Southern Economic Journal* 49:637–653.

Dranove, D.1998. Economies of scale in non-revenue producing cost centers: Implications for hospital mergers. *Journal of Health Economics* 17:69–83.

Evans, R.G. 1981. Behavioural cost functions for hospitals. *Canadian Journal of Economics* 4:198–215.

Etzioni, R.D., et al. 1999. On the use of survival analysis techniques to estimate medical care costs. *Journal of Health Economics* 18:365–380.

Farnand, L.J., et al. 1986. An evaluation of the Finger Lakes Experimental Payment Program. *Inquiry* 23(2):200–208.

Feldstein, P. 1961. *An empirical investigation of the marginal cost of hospital services.* Chicago: University of Chicago Graduate Program in Hospital Administration.

Finkler, S.A. 1979a. Cost effectiveness of regionalization: The heart surgery example. *Inquiry* 16:264–270.

———. 1979b. On the shape of the hospital industry long run average cost function. *Health Services Research* 14:281–289.

Fournier, G.M., and J.M. Mitchell. 1997. New evidence on the performance advantages of multihospital systems. *Review of Industrial Organization* 12:703–718.

Fraser, R.D. 1971. *Canadian hospital costs and efficiency.* Ottawa, Ontario: Economic Council of Canada.

Frech, H.E., and L.E. Mobley. 1995. Resolving the impasse on hospital scale economies. *Applied Economics* 27:286–296.

Friedman, B., and M.V. Pauly. 1983. A new approach to hospital cost functions and some issues in revenue regulation. *Health Care Financing Review* 4:105–114.

Gregory, D.D. 1976–1977. Some evidence on the economic aspects of hospital cooperative ventures. *Journal of Economics and Business* 29:59–64.

Hadley, J., and S. Zuckerman. 1994. The role of efficiency measurement in hospital rate setting. *Journal of Health Economics* 13:335–340.

Hansen, K.K., and J. Zwanzinger.1996. Marginal costs in general cute care hospitals. *Health Economics* 5:195–216.

Horn, S.D., et al. 1985. Severity of illness within DRGs: Impact on prospective payment. *American Journal of Public Health* 75:1195–1199.

Hornbrook, M.C., and A.C. Monheit. 1985. The contribution of case mix severity to the hospital cost-output relation. *Inquiry* 22:259–271.

Kralewski, J.E., et al. 1984. Effects of contract management on hospital performance. *Health Services Research* 19:479–498.

Lave, J., and L.B. Lave. 1984. Hospital cost functions. *Annual Review of Public Health* 5:193–213.

Lee, M.L., and R.L. Wallace. 1972. Problems in estimating multi-product hospital cost functions. *Western Economic Journal* 11:350–363.

Linna, M. 1998. Measuring hospital cost efficiency with panel data models. *Health Economics* 7:415–429.

Linna, M., et al. 1998. An econometric study of costs of teaching and research in Finnish hospitals. *Health Economics* 7:291–306.

Lipscomb, J., et al. 1978. The use of marginal cost estimates in hospital cost-containment policy. In *Hospital cost containment*, ed. M. Zubkoff et al. New York: Watson Publishing International.

McGregor, M., and G. Pelletier. 1978. Planning of specialized health facilities: Size vs. cost and effectiveness in heart surgery. *New England Journal of Medicine* 299:179–181.

Newhouse, J.P. 1994. Frontier estimation: How useful a tool for health economics? *Journal of Health Economics* 13:335–340.

Schwartz, W., and P. Joskow. 1980. Duplicated hospital facilities. *New England Journal of Medicine* 303:1449–1457.

Sloan, F.A., et al. 1985. The teaching hospital's growing surgical caseload. *JAMA* 254:376–382.

Zuckerman, S., et al. 1994. Measuring hospital efficiency with frontier cost functions. *Journal of Health Economics* 13:335–340.

Costs: Medical Practice

Bailey, R.M. 1968. A comparison of internists in solo and fee-for-service group practice. *Bulletin of the New York Academy of Medicine* 44 (2nd series): 1293–1303.

———. 1970. Economies of scale in medical practice. In *Empirical studies in health economics*, ed. H. Klarman. Baltimore: Johns Hopkins University Press.

Dunn, D.L., et al. 1995. Economies of scope in physicians' work: The performance of multiple surgery. *Inquiry* 32:87–101.

Escarce, J.J., and M.V. Pauly. 1998. Physician opportunity costs in physician practice cost functions. *Journal of Health Economics* 17:129–151.

Frech, H.E., and P.B. Ginsburg. 1974. Optimal scale in medical practice. *Journal of Business* 47:23–36.

Hillson, S.D., et al. 1992. Economies of scope and payment for physician services. *Medical Care* 30:822–831.

Newhouse, J.P. 1973. The economics of group practice. *Journal of Human Resources* 8:37–56.

Rossiter, L.F. 1984. Prospects for medical group practice under competition. *Medical Care* 22:84–92.

Costs: Long-Term Care

Bekele, G., and A.G. Holtmann. 1987. A cost function for nursing homes: Toward a system of diagnostic reimbursement groupings. *Eastern Economic Journal* 13:115–122.

Bishop, C.E. 1980. Nursing home cost studies and reimbursement issues. *Health Care Financing Review* 1:47–65.

———. 1983. Nursing home cost studies. *Health Services Research* 18:382–386.

Chattopadhyay, S., and D. Hefley. 1994. Are for-profit nursing homes more efficient? *Eastern Economic Journal* 20:171–186.

Chattopadhyay, S., and S.C. Ray. 1996. Technical, scale, and size efficiency in nursing home care. *Health Economics* 5:363–374.

Dudzinski, C.S., et al. 1998. Estimating a hedonic translog cost function for the home health care industry. *Applied Economics* 30:1259–1267.

Kass, D.I. 1987. Economies of scale and scope in the provision of nursing home services. *Journal of Health Economics* 6:129–146.

McKay, N.L. 1988. An econometric analysis of costs and scale economies in the nursing home industry. *Journal of Human Resources* 23:58–75.

Nyman, J.A. 1988a. Improving the quality of nursing home outcome. *Medical Care* 26:1158–1171.

———. 1988b. The marginal cost of nursing home care. *Journal of Health Economics* 7:393–412.

Nyman, J.A., and R.A. Conner. 1994. Do case mix adjusted nursing home reimbursements actually reflect costs? *Journal of Health Economics* 13:145–162.

Okunade, A.A. 1993. Production cost structure of U.S. hospital pharmacies: Time series, cross sectional bed size evidence. *Journal of Applied Econometrics* 8:277–294.

Schlenker, R.E., and P.W. Shaughnessy. 1984. Case mix, quality, and cost relationships in Colorado nursing homes. *Health Care Financing Review* 6:61–71.

Schlenker, R.E., et al. 1985. Estimating patient level nursing home costs. *Health Services Research* 20:103–128.

Ullman, S.G. 1984. Cost analysis and facility reimbursement in the long-term health care industry. *Health Services Research* 19:83–102.

———. 1986. Chain ownership and long-term health care facility performance. *Journal of Applied Gerontology* 5:51–63.

Van Lear, W., and L. Fowler. 1997. Efficiency and service in the group home industry. Journal of Economic Issues 31:1039–1051.

Vitaliano, D.F., and M. Toren. 1994. Cost and efficiency in nursing homes. *Journal of Health Economics* 13:281–300.

Costs: Other Areas

Blair, R.D., et al. 1975a. Blue Cross-Blue Shield administrative costs. *Economic Inquiry* 13:237–251.

Blair, R.D., et al. 1975b. Economies of scale in the administration of health insurance. *Review of Economics and Statistics* 57:185–189.

Hay, J.W., and Mandes, G. 1984. Home health care cost-function analysis. *Health Care Financing Review* 5:111–116.

Chapter 6

Behavior of Supply

1. Define a supply curve in terms of the quantity of health care services supplied.
2. For a single for-profit provider, describe a model that can be used to predict the quantity of health care services supplied.
3. Define a market and describe and use a market model of health care supply.
4. For a single nonprofit provider, describe an output-maximizing model to predict supplier behavior.
5. Describe the joint "quantity-quality" output-maximizing model to predict supplier behavior.
6. Describe the "administrator-as-agent" model to predict the effect of ownership status (for-profit versus nonprofit) on operating efficiency.

6.1 INTRODUCTION

This chapter is concerned with the determinants of the quantity and quality of output of various health-related products. Our approach is to consider the behavior of the organizations supplying these products. It provides hypotheses about what causes suppliers to produce particular quantities and qualities of output. These hypotheses are formulated in terms of models of supplier behavior, and they incorporate the key causes of such behavior. The goal is to isolate the direction in which individual factors cause supply to move while keeping in mind other factors that may also be influencing supply movements.

In presenting the hypotheses about supply behavior, a distinction is made between the supply of a single producer and the supply of all producers in the market (i.e., individual versus market supply). It should be pointed out that, like in our analyses of demand, our focus is on the behavior of a group of market participants in isolation—in this case, suppliers.

In this chapter, no single model of supplier behavior is presented as uniquely appropriate. The subject is complex, and our models offer suggestions rather than definitive answers. In particular, health care providers differ with regard to type of organization. Some organizations, such as proprietary hospitals and nursing homes and physician practices, are profit-seeking institutions. Others, such as voluntary hospitals, the Red Cross, independent blood banks, and philanthropic organizations (e.g., the March of Dimes and the American Heart Association), are nonprofit. This means that their "owners" (or, more appropriately, governors or trustees) can neither appropriate for themselves any profits that the organization might make nor sell the rights to the assets of the organization for personal gain. Separate hypotheses are discussed for both types of organizations.

We start off by developing a basic model of an individual profit-seeking supplier, then develop a model of the market supply behavior of a group of such firms. Because for-profit and nonprofit organizations differ radically, the following three sections focus on the effects that the nonprofit organizational form has on the behavior of a nonprofit organization. Much disagreement exists over the analysis of nonprofit agency behavior. As a result, several alternative hypotheses about nonprofit agency behavior need to be presented.

In Section 6.4, the nonprofit agency is examined as if it were an output-maximizing agency. In the next section, we extend this analysis to incorporate the role of the agency in producing quality as well as quantity output, and we look at the organizational structure of the voluntary hospital, a peculiar type of nonprofit organization. In Section 6.6, we develop a model in which the nonprofit agency is regarded as an instrument used to the benefit of its managers.

6.2 A MODEL OF SUPPLY BEHAVIOR: AN INDIVIDUAL FOR-PROFIT COMPANY

6.2.1 The Basic Model

The assumptions of our initial supply model fall into three categories: (1) revenue assumptions, (2) cost assumptions, and (3) assumptions about the objectives of the organization. In our analysis, we will use the example of a laboratory (ABC Labs) that is owned by a pathologist and produces blood tests of a given level of quality.

We will assume that ABC Labs' revenues can come from two sources: (1) reimbursement for patient services (termed *patient* or *earned revenues*) and (2) other sources (philanthropic or government grants, endowment funds, and other non-patient-related sources). We will initially assume that all revenues are from reimbursement (i.e., non-patient-related revenues are zero). This assumption will be altered later in the analysis.

With regard to patient revenues, we make the assumption that ABC Labs is a "price taker," that is, a supplier that has no influence on the price of its output. This may be because the price is set by an independent administrative agency or because the lab is operating in a competitive situation in which the best price it can get for its product is the price prevailing in the market. The charging of high prices by one supplier in a highly competitive market will drive consumers to lower priced competitors, and lower prices will therefore not enable the higher priced supplier to achieve its goal.

We will assume that ABC Labs receives $12 for each test performed. Its marginal revenue (*MR*), defined as the addition to total revenue (*TR*) for one additional unit of output produced and sold ($\Delta TR/\Delta Q$), is $12. The total and marginal revenues for output levels 0 to 10 are shown in Table 6–1, Columns 9 and 10.

Table 6–1 Illustrative Data on Relation between Revenue, Costs, Profit, and Output

Quantity of tests	Total Fixed Costs (TFC)	Total Variable Costs (TVC)	Total Costs (TC)	Average Fixed Costs (TFC/Q)	Average Variable Costs (TVC/Q)	Average Total Costs (TC/Q)	Marginal Costs (ΔTC/QΔ)	Total Earned Revenue (P×Q)	Marginal Revenue (ΔTR/ΔQ)	Profits (TC–TC)
0	12	0.00	12.00							
1	12	6.75	18.75	12.00	6.75	18.75	6.75	12	12	–6.75
2	12	10.50	22.50	6.00	5.25	11.25	3.75	24	12	1.50
3	12	13.25	25.25	4.00	4.42	8.42	2.75	36	12	10.75
4	12	17.00	29.00	3.00	4.25	7.25	3.75	48	12	19.00
5	12	23.75	35.75	2.40	4.75	7.15	6.75	60	12	24.25
6	12	35.50	47.50	2.00	5.92	7.92	11.75	72	12	24.50
7	12	54.25	66.25	1.71	7.75	9.46	18.75	84	12	17.75
8	12	82.00	94.00	1.50	10.25	11.75	27.75	96	12	2.00
9	12	120.75	132.75	1.33	13.42	14.75	38.75	108	12	–24.75
10	12	172.50	184.50	1.20	17.25	18.45	51.75	120	12	–64.50

As for cost, we will assume that there are both fixed and variable costs. Our assumption regarding fixed costs is that the lab spends $7 monthly on equipment rental and mortgage payments. In addition, we will assume that the pathologist-owner could earn a total of $5 if she worked elsewhere. This sum is at the same time a fixed cost and an opportunity cost. That is, it incorporates a "normal" return on the investment of the owner's assets and efforts. The pathologist, once committed to work in the lab, gives up $5 per period. The total fixed costs are thus $12, and, being fixed, they do not vary as output changes. The total fixed costs are shown in Column 2 in Table 6–1; the associated average fixed costs are shown in Column 5.

Variable inputs are assumed to be employed in a least-cost manner (the total minimum variable cost for operating the lab at different levels of output is shown in Column 3). The average variable cost initially falls and subsequently rises (Column 6), and the marginal cost eventually rises (Column 8). The figures for the total cost, the sum of the fixed and variable costs, are shown in Columns 4 and 7 (total and average values, respectively). Therefore, the cost curves are shaped as hypothesized in Chapter 5 (see Figure 6–1). Whereas in Table 6–1 the values jump in discrete steps, the curves are drawn as smooth functions for geometric convenience.

These dollar figures are approximated in Graph A of Figure 6–1 for total values and Graph B for marginal revenue (MR), marginal cost (MC), average variable cost (AVC), and average total cost (ATC). Note that the TR curve rises at a rate of $12 per blood test and that MR is constant at $12. These are two different ways of saying the same thing: the revenue per unit of output sold is fixed at $12. This is a concrete expression of our assumption that ABC Labs is a price taker.

Finally, since ABC Labs is a for-profit company, it seems reasonable to assume that its main objective is to maximize profits (total revenues minus total costs).

We are now in a position to examine the conclusions of our model and answer the question that underlies our analysis: what will the quantity of output be? Our task is to present a hypothesis that will enable us to predict which quantity will be chosen and how this quantity will vary when some of the underlying variables in our model—prices and costs—themselves vary.

Referring to Table 6–1, we can now derive from our model a specific quantity of output that achieves ABC Labs' profit-maximizing objective: profits are at a maximum at six units of output (here they amount to $24.50). The reasoning used to obtain this conclusion can best be presented in marginal terms. Say that ABC Labs was initially supplying four units of output. Profits here, given the assumed revenue and cost conditions, equal $19.00. If ABC Labs produces and sells one more test, the additional revenue will be $12.00 (i.e., $MR = 12.00), and the additional costs of production (MC) will be $6.75. The additional profit obtained by expanding output from four to five tests will be $5.25, bringing total profits to a new level of $24.25. ABC Labs, being profit maximizers, would expand production to at least five units. In fact, they will move beyond this amount because profits can be further increased by doing so. The best ABC Labs can do at the given price and cost conditions is to produce six units of output. Expanding beyond six units still results in positive profits for a while, but these profits would be less than the profit at six units of output. According to our model, a profit-maximizing firm will continue to expand production as long as MR exceeds MC. If we were dealing with smooth, continuous changes, our conclusion would be that a profit-maximizing firm will expand output up to the point at which $MR = MC$, as long as MC is rising with output. At this point

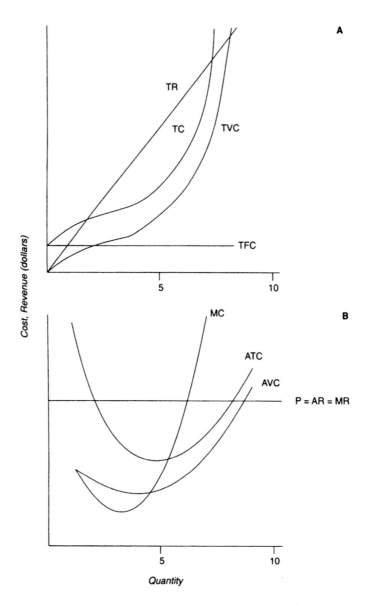

Figure 6–1 Supply relation for a profit-maximizing firm in terms of total costs and revenues (Graph A) and average and marginal costs and revenues (Graph B). In Graph A, the supplier produces where total profits, equal to the difference between total revenues (*TR*) and total costs (*TC*), are at a maximum. In Graph B, the same conclusion can be derived in terms of marginal costs and revenues. Here the profit-maximizing point is where *MR = MC*. In the diagram, since the price per unit is constant, price and *MR* are the same.

the firm is maximizing its profits, and so the quantity where $MC = MR$ is the supply position the firm should be aiming for.

This conclusion is shown diagrammatically in Figure 6–1. In Graph A, profits at each level of output are shown as the vertical distance between total revenues and total costs at that level of output. Since profits are defined as *TR − TC*, then where this vertical distance is at a maximum, profits are also at a maximum. This profit-maximizing point occurs at six units of output (allowing for small variations because we are dealing with continuous curves). In Graph B, the same conclusion is shown, but in terms of marginal costs and revenues. Here the point where *MR = MC* is the profit-maximizing quantity, that is, the quantity that will be supplied. A movement in quantity supplied in either direction would detract from total profits and so would not be consistent with the profit-maximizing objective.

The first conclusion of our model, then, is that, given revenue (i.e., price) and cost conditions and given the profit-maximizing objective, a profit-maximizing firm will produce at the quantity where *MC = MR*. Using this information, we can now derive a supply curve or schedule that shows what the quantity supplied will be at different prices. This analysis is shown diagrammatically in Figure 6–2. If the price rises from $12 to $15, the lab will add to its profits by expanding output to a sixth unit, because, even though the cost of this unit is higher, the higher extra revenue will make it profitable to expand output. The same reasoning applies to additional price increases: higher prices will bring forth greater quantities supplied until *MC = MR*. It also applies to price declines, with one major exception: eventually the price could become so low that the owner of the firm would be better off, from the point of view of profits (or losses), to shut down operations and produce nothing. For all prices below this level (represented by point *j* in Figure 6–2), the quantity supplied by the firm would be zero.

The critical price below which the firm will shut down depends on the variable costs of the firm. Recall that fixed costs are the same thing as "already committed" costs, while variable costs are those that can be avoided by not hiring the variable factors; total costs are the sum of the two at each output level. If the price falls sufficiently, it is possible that even at its best level of output (from the profitability standpoint) the firm will be incurring a loss. The criterion the firm would use in deciding whether to continue operating under such unfavorable circumstances is not whether the firm is incurring a loss but whether it is minimizing its losses. The importance of variable costs comes into play here. As long as the firm's revenues are exceeding its total variable costs, the firm will be adding to a surplus. In this case *TR − TVC* will be positive. Even though total profits (*TR − (TVC + TFC)*) may be negative, signifying a loss, the loss is less than it would be if the firm shut down entirely. For if the firm shuts down, both *TR* and *TVC* are zero and the losses would equal *TFC*. In sum, as long as the firm is meeting its variable costs and adding something to cover some or all of its fixed costs, the firm should continue to operate; in this case, its supply curve is traced out by the *MC* curve. The quantity supplied will be where price equals marginal cost. Should the price fall so low that at no level of output could the firm meet all its variable costs, then it should shut down.

We can now present a complete analysis of the firm's supply behavior using the curves in Figure 6–2. If the price is equal to or greater than the lowest point on the *AVC* curve (point *j*), then at some level of output all variable costs will be covered and the firm will produce some output. If the price is lower than this critical minimum price, the firm will shut down operations. If the price is above the critical minimum level, the firm will produce output at the quantity where *MR = MC* (i.e., where price = *MC*). The *MC* curve of the firm, then, is its supply curve, relating price to output.

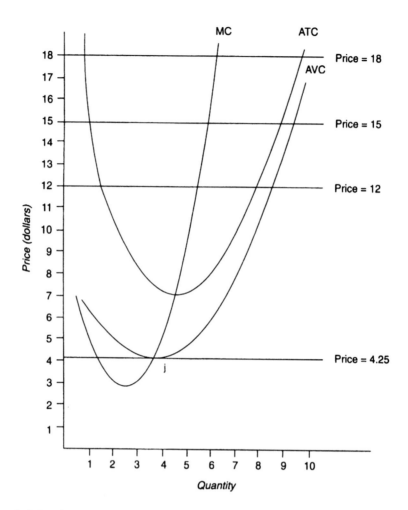

Figure 6–2 Profit-maximizing supply points at alternative prices. At each price above $4.25, the firm will maximize profits by supplying at the quantity where price = MC. If the price is at $4.25, the firm will just be meeting its variable costs. At any price below this, the firm's least unprofitable supply point will result in larger losses than if the firm shut down operations; therefore, the firm will not supply at any price below $4.25. For prices above $4.25, the firm's supply curve and its MC curve are the same.

In the context of this analysis, we can make some sense of the assumption that the costs of a for-profit firm are at a minimum. It was shown in Chapter 5 that the producer has a choice of producing a given quantity of output at the lowest possible cost or above the lowest possible cost. By choosing the lowest possible cost method of production, the firm can achieve its greatest profits, since profits are defined as the difference between total revenues and total costs. If costs were above the minimum, they would cut into profits, which is contrary to the assumed goal of the firm.

It should be noted that the supply relationship focuses on the behavior of suppliers in isolation. That is, the term *quantity supplied* refers to a distinct schedule—that of supplier responsiveness to price. As in the chapter on demand, where we studied how demanders would respond to price while ignoring suppliers, in this chapter we focus on supplier behavior in isolation from demanders. Before putting the separate forces, supply and demand, together, it is essential to understand how each operates on its own.

6.2.2 Nonpatient Revenues

Let us now introduce a new element into our analysis, nonpatient revenues. We will focus on a particular form of unearned revenue, a grant or subsidy, that is unrelated to output. Such a grant might be received from a donor or foundation. Our analytical task is to determine how it might affect the provider's supply.

The economic significance of a grant unrelated to output is that it provides a set amount of money whether output expands or contracts. Such a grant can be treated analytically in one of two ways, either as a fixed addition to revenue or as a fixed reduction from total costs (a negative fixed cost). While the rationale for the first option seems clear-cut, the rationale for the second requires some explanation. A fixed subsidy in a sense reduces by a fixed amount the total costs that the provider must meet at each output level. Operationally, it will have the same impact on profits. We can therefore treat it as a reduction in total costs.

Let us say that ABC Labs received a fixed subsidy of $5. This would increase revenues in Table 6–1 by $5 at each and every level of output. Profits would also increase by $5 at each level of output. In Figure 6–1, the increase would appear as an upward parallel shift in the *TR* curve.

What is important from a supply standpoint is that neither patient revenues (including *MR*) nor variable costs are affected. Thus, while profits are higher by $5 at every output level, the maximum profitability level of output remains at six units. The fixed subsidy does not affect the most profitable level of output; it only affects the level of profits at that and every other level of output.

This conclusion would not hold if the subsidy was related to output. For then, as output expanded, the marginal revenue would be the additional revenue from patient sources plus the additional (output-related) grant revenues. When estimating the most profitable output level, the firm would have to consider both sources of additional revenue and relate them to marginal cost.

The conclusion, then, is that a grant that is not output related will not influence the supply decisions of a profit-maximizing firm; the firm's supply position will still be where marginal patient revenue equals marginal cost.

6.2.3 Shifts in the Supply Curve

In this section, we consider what happens to the supply curve of the firm when factors that influence the position of the *MC* curve change. In general, as shown in Figure 6–3, any factor that causes the *MC* curve to shift upward from MC_1 to MC_2 will amount to a leftward shift in the supply schedule of the firm (a decrease in supply). The quantity supplied at any price will be reduced from Q_1 to Q_2. Such shifts might occur because of higher input prices or a higher quality of product being produced, to cite two of the factors discussed in Section 5.4 that might cause the firm's cost curve to shift. In the case of the production of a higher quality product, for example, the net result is that a lower quantity will be produced by the firm at any given price.

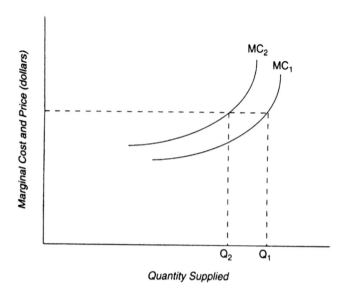

Figure 6–3 Shifts in the marginal cost curve for a profit-maximizing supplier. An upward shift in the *MC* curve of a profit-maximizing firm will mean a lower quantity supplied at any price. In this figure, a shift from MC_1 to MC_2 means a decrease in supply level indicated by the dotted line (the quantity supplied decreases from Q_1 to Q_2).

The same reasoning in reverse holds for downward shifts in the *MC* curve. For example, an increase in the capacity of the firm to produce output, caused by additional capital expansion, will cause the *MC* and thus the supply curve to shift to the right, indicating a willingness on the part of the firm to supply more output at any given price. Such expansion is likely when the firm is operating on the downward-sloping part of its long-run average cost curve. An expansion in output would allow it to move to a lower point on the *LRAC* curve (i.e., to a lower cost short-run curve).

6.3 MARKET SUPPLY

We now demonstrate how the analysis of individual supply movements can be extended to form a hypothesis about movements in product supply in a specific market. To do this, we will add two new assumptions concerning individual supply behavior:

1. There is a set number of suppliers in the market.
2. There are no agreements on the part of suppliers to restrict supply.

In the present model, two groups of factors influence market supply: the number of suppliers and the factors that influence individual supplier behavior. In other words, the market supply schedule can be obtained once we know the number of suppliers and their individual supply schedules. Let us assume the market consists of three suppliers: ABC Labs, XYZ Labs, and GHI Labs (see Figure 6–4). Each has a given

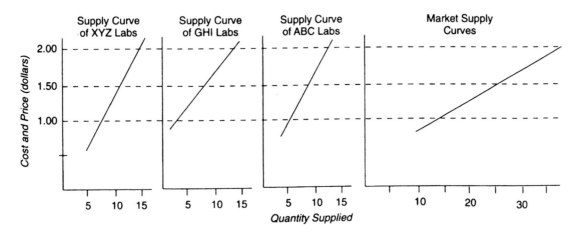

Figure 6–4 Derivation of the market supply curve from individual supply curves. The market supply curve shows the quantity supplied by all firms supplying the product to the market at each price. It is obtained by summing individual suppliers' quantities at each price.

supply schedule. XYZ Labs supplies 5 tests at $1.00, 10 tests at $1.50, 15 at $2.00, and so on. GHI Labs supplies 3, 6, and 9 tests at these prices, respectively, and ABC Labs supplies 6, 9, and 12 tests. Given these schedules and the fact that these three labs are the only ones in the market, the market supply curve is the sum of these individual supply curves at each price. At $1.00, the market supply of tests is 14 (5 + 3 + 6); at $1.50, 25 tests are supplied, and at $2.00, 36 tests are supplied. The market supply curve is shown as the horizontal sum of all individual supply curves. Given a particular price, our model predicts the quantity that will be supplied in the market.

The market supply curve will shift outward (to the right) (1) if, given the number of producers, any factors cause the individual supply curves to shift outward, or (2) if the number of suppliers increases. In either case, more will be supplied at any given price. Our model has enabled us to classify these influences and separate their effects on supply. The same type of analysis applies to reductions in supply.

With regard to the number of suppliers, just as profits are the motivating force behind the expansion (or contraction) of output by an individual firm, so are they a driving force behind the expansion of the market—the entry of new firms into the market. At any particular time, there are a number of prospective suppliers capable of acquiring the techniques and equipment needed to supply a product (e.g., blood tests). If profits are high in the market, prospective suppliers will be motivated to enter the market and thus will shift the supply curve to the right. Of course, in real life, existing firms, protective of their high profits, may act to keep potential suppliers out, but this type of behavior is ruled out of the model.

6.4 SUPPLY BEHAVIOR OF NONPROFIT AGENCIES: THE OUTPUT MAXIMIZATION HYPOTHESIS

Nonprofit suppliers abound in the health care field. One reason appears to be the existence of external demands for health care products and services. These external demands arise when people are concerned about, and willing to pay for the health care of others. To satisfy these external demands, individuals may form nonprofit agencies whose purpose is to provide products and services to those perceived to be needy, usually on a less-than-cost basis. Health-related philanthropies, such as the American Heart Association, give away educational services that are financed by donors who want others to consume the services. The Red Cross blood program exists because there is sufficient concern on the part of blood donors about the health of those requiring transfusions. Voluntary hospitals were, until recently, providing free and subsidized hospital care to the needy in substantial amounts; this care was financed largely through philanthropic donations, which can be regarded as payments to satisfy the donors' external demands for care of the needy. Public health departments attempt to satisfy external demands for health care through government-provided services.

There are, no doubt, other reasons for the formation of nonprofit agencies. For example, these agencies may be formed as "captives" of other nonprofit groups. During the 1930s and 1940s, Blue Cross plans began under the auspices of nonprofit hospitals to ensure that hospitals were paid. The scope of our inquiry does not encompass the conditions under which health service agencies become organized on a voluntary basis (see Culyer 1971). Rather, we will treat the existence of this type of organization as a given and restrict our attention to the supply behavior of these agencies once they are formed.

To ensure that the services offered by a nonprofit agency are provided in a reasonable manner, a board of trustees is formed. The members of a board of trustees cannot gain direct financial benefit from the organization either in the form of profits or of proceeds from the sale of the enterprise. Furthermore, they are frequently banned from garnering indirect gains, such as might occur if a board member's law firm provided legal services to the organization. The board of trustees is primarily responsible for setting organizational policies, but many of their responsibilities are delegated to a full-time, salaried administrative staff. The actual responsibilities of each (the trustees and the staff), including the making of supply decisions, vary from organization to organization.

Several approaches can be taken in forming hypotheses about the supply behavior of nonprofit agencies. One approach is to regard the trustees as being in charge. Following this approach, we would hypothesize goals the trustees are likely to pursue and then develop a model of the organization that incorporates these goals. Another approach is to regard the salaried executives as the people who maintain control, make hypotheses about their goals, and develop a model of organizational supply based on *these* goals. No doubt the supply behavior of a real nonprofit firm is influenced by trustees and staff, but to keep our analysis simple we will pursue each approach separately. We begin with the trustee dominance model. We will assume that the trustees' objective is to maximize the output of the agency, that is, to carry out their mandate to the fullest extent possible.

Now, let us imagine a nonprofit lab initially financed by a public-spirited benefactor. Cost and revenue conditions are the same as in the ABC Labs example, with the exception that the pathologist is under contract and receives an explicit payment of $5 per month for her services. From the point of view of the lab, once the contractual commitment is made, this is a fixed cost, and so the total fixed costs of the laboratory are $12. The quality of the product is the same as in the previous example and is constant. Revenues are $12 per test, but now the reimbursement may be made by a third party. (Reimbursement may be collected through individual donations or from a united agency.) The major difference between the two examples is that the nonprofit lab seeks to maximize output rather than profits.

According to our model, since revenues come only from reimbursement for services, output will be expanded to the point where the firm breaks even, that is, where $TR = TC$. In Table 6–1, given a price of $12, output will be expanded to eight units. In Graph A of Figure 6–1, the break-even point at eight units of output is shown in total terms. In Graph B, the lab's operating point is where price per unit equals average total cost. The lab just covers costs for all units when it operates at this level.

Given our assumptions, output for a for-profit firm will be lower than that for a nonprofit firm that behaves as we have hypothesized (i.e., maximizes output). The supply curve for an output-maximizing firm is its ATC curve for prices above the minimum point on the curve. If the revenues do not total at least this minimum amount, the firm runs a deficit and must raise the funds from nonpatient sources. For the moment we will assume that nonpatient revenues are zero and that the firm has no reserves to meet a deficit. If it does not meet all its obligations, it will go out of business.

As long as the price is above the minimum point on the ATC curve, the supply curve of the nonprofit agency that maximizes output is the ATC curve. As the price rises, so will the supply. Any factor that shifts the ATC curve downward (lower unit costs at any level of output) will cause output to increase at any price.

The response of an output-maximizing nonprofit firm to a fixed subsidy is very different from that of a profit-maximizing firm. Recall that a fixed subsidy will not influence a profit-maximizer's supply (Section 6.2). Let us assume that a donor gives our nonprofit lab a $25.00 subsidy unrelated to output. Analytically, we can treat this as an overall increase in total revenues or as an overall reduction in total costs (and a reduction in average fixed costs of $25.00/Q). In the former case, the analysis in Table 6–1 would be altered to show TR and profits higher at every level of output by $25. Whereas, formerly, the output-maximizing output level was 8, with the subsidy an output level of 9 will show an overall (operating and nonoperating) profit of $0.25 ($25.00 – $24.75). The lab would be in the red at an output level of 10, but it could now meet all its costs at a level of 9, and this is where it would maximize output (subject to the fact that it must break even).

Graphically, if the fixed subsidy is treated as a reduction in fixed costs, it would appear as a downward shift in AFC and also ATC (because AFC is part of ATC). It will appear as an outward shift in the firm's supply curve, which is identical to the ATC curve. The conclusion in either case is the same: a non-output-related grant will shift the supply curve of the output-maximizing firm and thus will lead to increased output. In this respect, the output-maximizing firm is very unlike the profit-maximizing firm.

The market supply analysis in the case of nonprofit organizations is somewhat more complicated than in the case of for-profit organizations. If we make the assumption that each separate nonprofit supplier has a vested interest in providing output to the needy, the market supply curve will be made up of the sum of what all the individual suppliers would be willing to supply at each price or reimbursement rate. That is, the market supply curve is the sum of the individual producers' supply curves for prices above the minimum ATC.

Individual nonprofit suppliers might act competitively if the trustees developed some sense of identification with the organizations of which they were board members. However, if this sense of identification did not develop, trustees would not care which organization supplied the output to the needy as long as it was supplied by someone. In this situation, market supply would consist of a far more complicated set of arrangements, since trustees would pull their organizations out of the market when other organizations supplying the same product appeared. We will assume that in our example organizational pride develops to the point that the standard market supply model is appropriate.

6.5 SUPPLY DECISIONS INVOLVING QUALITY

Until now we have assumed that quality of output was held constant and thus did not enter the supply decision. In fact, quality is an extremely important supply variable for suppliers. In particular, it has frequently been asserted that hospitals seek to supply output of the highest quality. In this section, a model is developed to incorporate quality of care into the supply picture.

To understand the bias of nonprofit hospitals toward high-quality supply, it is necessary to examine their unusual management structure. Like other nonprofit firms, a nonprofit hospital includes a board of trustees and a group of salaried administrators. However, physicians have a special relationship to the hospital: They are in charge of the medical activities of the hospital, and yet for the most part they are unsalaried staff members. Because their services are so crucial (indeed the hospital's activities revolve around them), physicians have enormous influence over hospital supply decisions, and hospital supply policies are set by an informal arrangement between physicians, trustees, and administrators. This type of arrangement has been termed a "management triangle," and hospital activities are the result of directives (sometimes conflicting) issued by two lines of authority, medical and administrative. In particular, the medical influence in the decision-making process has been held to be responsible for the bias toward quality in hospital objectives, since physicians benefit considerably from high-quality inputs.

A supply model that is based on the preceding analysis but incorporates the bias toward quality can be developed. Assume a given level of reimbursement, say $200 per patient day (see Figure 6–5). ATC curves are drawn for three different levels of quality of service; each higher level is produced with more resources. ATC_1 represents an ATC curve for a specific level of output and level of quality. ATC_2 and ATC_3 are similar curves for successively higher levels of quality.

An output-maximizing hospital will choose Q_1 (12,000) units of output at Quality Level 1, Q_2 (10,000) units at Quality Level 2, and Q_3 (9,000) units at Quality Level 3. Indeed, a trade-off between quality and quantity of care typically occurs. Such a trade-off is shown in Figure 6–6, with quality of care represented on the vertical axis and the quantity on the horizontal. Curve XY shows the maximum output that can be achieved for each level of quality given the reimbursement rate of $200 and thus reflects the constraints or the choices facing the hospital. The actual combination of quality and quantity supplied will depend on the hospital's policies. A highly quality oriented hospital will choose a quality level close to Qu_3, whereas an output-oriented hospital will choose a level closer to Qu_1. If the assertion that hospitals are quality oriented is correct, it might be expected that Qu_3 would be more frequently observed. That is, of the various output combinations that a

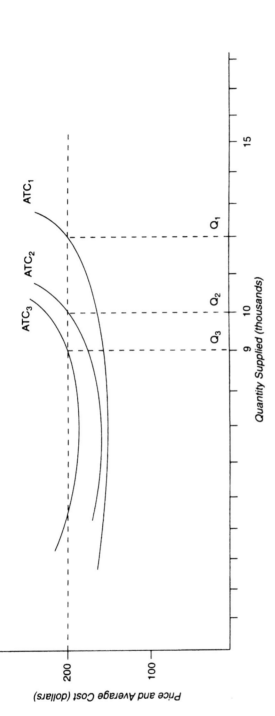

Figure 6–5 Representation of alternative quantities and qualities supplied by a nonprofit supplier. The *ATC* curves represent relations between *ATC* and output at various quality levels. ATC_3 represents the highest quality level, ATC_2 the intermediate level, and ATC_1 the lowest level. A nonprofit producer who maximizes the quantity of output (given the quality level) will produce where the unit reimbursement rate or price equals *ATC*. For the lowest quality level, the output will be 12. Higher quality levels entail a reduction in the maximum output levels achievable given the reimbursement rate.

nonprofit hospital can choose, it will tend to provide care of a higher quality level. By itself, however, this does not mean that we will observe such high-quality care in the market. For it must be remembered that we are currently examining only the supply side of the market. The quality of care actually produced will be determined by what the suppliers are willing to supply and what the consumers are willing to take. Determining what output actually is produced and utilized requires that we examine the market in its entirety.

6.6 SUPPLY BEHAVIOR OF NONPROFIT AGENCIES: THE ADMINISTRATOR AS AGENT MODEL

An alternative theory of resource allocation and product supply in nonprofit agencies focuses on the behavior of the executive or administrator of the organization. The underlying assumption is that the administrator, even though just an agent of the trustees, has considerable control over the organization's resources. This seems a plausible assumption given that trustees of a nonprofit agency

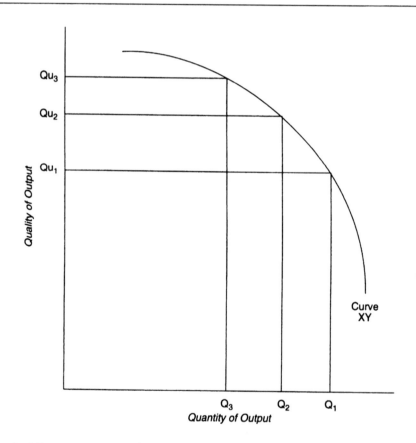

Figure 6–6 Representation of the trade-off between quality and quantity. Based on Figure 6–5, for any given reimbursement rate, a higher quality level can be achieved only with a lower quantity of output. The curve shows alternative levels of quantity and quality that can be achieved at a given reimbursement rate.

typically can devote only a small portion of their time to trustee-related activities, whereas the administrator is usually a full-time employee. As part of this approach, a comparative analysis can be done that examines how the same administrator would behave if operating the same agency as a profit-seeking enterprise and as a nonprofit enterprise. The differences in behavior, which are due solely to the different incentive structures of the two types of organization, create differences in the use of the agency's resources and in the agency's output.

The theory can be viewed as simply an extension of the basic demand hypothesis presented in Chapter 3. According to this hypothesis, the lower the direct cost of a commodity or other benefit to an individual, the more the commodity will be demanded. The extension of the hypothesis involves identifying the commodities that are desired by the administrator of an agency as well as their relative prices or costs under varying institutional circumstances. Since we are focusing on the administrator's behavior, we will identify two types of benefits that can be obtained in the context of the job. First, there are the pecuniary benefits, especially the administrator's salary. In addition, if the administrator is a part or full owner of the agency, the pecuniary benefits will encompass the profits that accrue. Benefits of the second type, sometimes called *on-the-job benefits*, are nonpecuniary. These include high-grade office furniture, a relaxed work atmosphere, "business" trips to exotic places, and so on. Both types of benefits are wanted by the administrator, but because their supply is limited, the administrator cannot have everything he or she would like.

Before developing the hypothesis about how much of each type of benefit will be demanded, we will look at the implications for resource use of obtaining the two types. First, when a smaller amount of resources is used to obtain a given output, an opportunity to increase profits is created. Nonpecuniary benefits also require the commitment of resources. Better office equipment, more liberal working conditions, and other on-the-job benefits are obtained from the expansion of the total resource commitment and result in an increase in costs and a contraction of profits. In a nonprofit enterprise, this reduction in profits does not detract from the manager's pecuniary benefits since he or she will not be rewarded on the basis of the profits the enterprise earns.

The hypothesis as to how the administrator will behave under these alternative incentive structures is based on the constraints facing the administrator in the two different environments. In a nonprofit environment, since the administrator cannot convert profits into take-home pecuniary benefits, they must be converted into organizational resources if any benefit is to be obtained. On the other hand, the use of these extra resources in a for-profit organization will detract from profits and hence from take-home pecuniary benefits, assuming these are related. The personal costs of on-the-job benefits are lower for the administrator of the nonprofit agency, and we thus hypothesize that more will be demanded.

The implications of this hypothesis for nonprofit resource allocation are considerable. The hypothesis implies that the nonprofit agency will use more resources to get a given job done, and so its costs will be higher. The absence of incentives for efficiency has been the target of investigation, including its effect on nonprofit agency operating costs, particularly in the case of nonprofit health insurers (Frech 1976), nursing homes (Borjas et al. 1983; Frech 1985), and dialysis units (Lowrie and Hampers 1981). Similar analyses comparing nonprofit and for-profit hospital behavior have not been as conclusive for several reasons. First, to compare operating costs between nonprofit and for-profit hospitals, variables such as case mix, case severity, and quality must be adjusted for. Assertions have been made that nonprofit hospitals have a more complex case mix because for-profit hospitals engage in "cream skimming" by encouraging the admission of low-cost cases. Evidence on this score seems mixed (Bays 1977a, 1979b; Renn et al. 1985; Schweitzer and Rafferty 1976). Even more difficult to determine is whether quality differentials exist by ownership category. Nonprofit managers do have an incentive to produce quality care (which will show up in higher costs). The role of quality in pushing costs higher has yet to be fully explored.

Another difference that has been uncovered when comparing nonprofit and for-profit hospital behavior lies in the pricing area. Charges are the prices set by the hospital for its services. Two California studies found that for-profit hospitals had higher charges (relative to costs) for ancillary (lab, radiology, pharmacy) services (Eskoz and Peddecord 1985; Pattison and Katz 1983). Generally, markups (charge-to-cost ratios) for ancillary services were found to be higher than basic room charges. For-profit hospitals also provided more (high-profit) ancillary services per patient than nonprofits in the studies and were more profitable, although cost levels were similar. One possible explanation of this finding is that nonprofit managers (or trustees) can gain nonpecuniary benefits from encouraging the use of hospital services by keeping patient charges low (which may result in lower profits) as well as by providing more free care to indigents.

However, relying solely on the incentives identified in the administrator as agent model to explain cost and price differences between for-profit and nonprofit hospitals would be a mistake. The incentive differences are but one factor operating to influence costs (and possible cost differences) in the two types of organization. The reimbursement system is another major influence on cost and supply behavior. Indeed, the absence of cost differences between nonprofit and for-profit hospitals that was uncovered by the investigators in California may have been partly due to the reimbursement system, which, at the time of the studies, encouraged cost inflation in all types of hospitals. It is to this factor that we turn to next, in Chapter 7.

EXERCISES

1. Over 4,000 individuals called up Dr. Kalikorn and asked him to perform a new surgical procedure. Dr. Kalikorn booked 2,000 of these and told the rest to seek care from another physician. What is his quantity supplied?
2. One thousand patients called up Dr. Kalikorn and asked him to perform a new surgical procedure. Dr. Kalikorn booked all 1,000 and told them that he could perform twice as many procedures if only he had more patients. What is his quantity supplied?
3. The state Medicaid agency sets the price for nursing home care. The unit price is $80 per day. This price is beyond the control of any nursing home. What is the marginal revenue for another patient day at Holly Head Nursing Home?
4. The following is a cost function for clinic visits in a small inner city clinic:

Quantity of Visits	Total Cost per Week
0	$10
1	15
2	25
3	45
4	75
5	115
6	165

a. Determine the marginal cost for each level of output.
b. If the price per visit is given to be $25, at what level of visits will the maximum profit position be? What are the profits at this level? What is the quantity supplied?
c. If the price per visit increases to $45, what will be the quantity supplied (assuming maximizing profits)?

5. Given the following data, answer questions (a) and (b). The total fixed cost for the Grand Forks Clinic is $30 per month. The total variable cost is given as follows:

Quantity of Visits	Total Cost per Week
1	$10
2	25
3	45
4	70
5	105
6	145

a. If the price per visit is $30, what is the quantity supplied?
b. If the total fixed cost increases to $40 and the price per visit is $30, what is the quantity supplied?

6. Given the following cost schedule for a regional hospital that seeks to maximize its profits, answer the following three questions:

Days of Care Supplied	Total Cost
0	$10
1	20
2	40
3	70
4	110
5	160
6	220

a. If the price per day is $22, what is the quantity supplied?
b. If the price per day increases to $32, what is the quantity supplied?
c. If the price per day is $45, what is the quantity supplied?

7. Given the following cost schedule for a clinic, determine the quantity supplied at alternative prices of $10, $20, and $30 per visit.

Quantity of Visits	Total Cost	Marginal Cost
0	$10	
1	25	$15
2	43	18
3	75	32
4	125	50

8. The following is a marginal cost curve and an average variable cost curve for the White River Hospital. The government is considering setting prices for White River's output (days of care), but it is unsure what per diem to set. It has asked you to evaluate the following per diem rates, assuming that the hospital has the objective of maximizing its profits.
   a. What is the quantity supplied if the price per diem is $10?
   b. If the price is $20?
   c. If the price is $40?

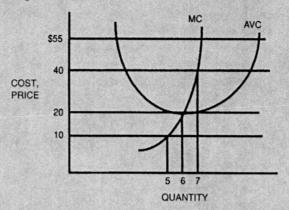

9. A clinic receives a per visit payment of $20. It has an upward sloping supply curve. Indicate the net effect on the quantity of visits supplied if the following occur:
   a. The wage rates for the clinic nursing staff increase.
   b. The fixed overhead costs (rent, electricity) increase.
   c. The clinic patients become sicker.
   d. The clinic increases productivity.
   e. The clinic decides to increase "quality" (defined as a more thorough examination for each patient).
10. Given the supply curve for radiographs by a radiology practice, predict how this curve will shift (supply will increase or decrease) if the following occur:
    a. an increase in the wages of radiological technicians
    b. a reduction in productivity
    c. a decrease in the wages of technicians
    d. an increase in the price of radiographs
    e. an increase in the quality of services (radiologists spend more care in reading and interpreting radiographs)
    f. an increase in the price of film
    g. an increase in the number of patients with multiple and rare problems

BIBLIOGRAPHY

Supply Functions

Glied, S. 1998. Payment heterogeneity, physician practice, and access to care. *American Economic Review* 88, no. 2:127–131.

Goldfarb, M., et al. 1980. Behavior of the multi-product firm. *Medical Care* 19:185–201.

Hornbrook, M., and M. Goldfarb. 1983. A partial test of a hospital behavior model. *Social Science and Medicine* 17:667–680.

Thornton, J., and B.K. Eakin. 1996. The utility-maximizing self-employed physician. *Journal of Human Resources* 32:98–127.

Nonprofit Organization Behavior

Banks, D.A., et al. 1997. Uncompensated hospital care: Charitable mission or profitable business decision? *Health Economics* 6:133–144.

Culyer, A.J. 1971. Medical care and the economics of giving. *Economica* 38:295–303.

Gaskin, D.J. 1997. Altruism and moral hazard: The impact of hospital uncompensated care pools. *Journal of Health Economics* 16:397–416.

Harris, J.F. 1977. The internal organization of hospitals. *Bell Journal of Economics* 8:647–682.

Lee, M.L. 1971. A conspicuous production theory of hospital behavior. *Southern Economic Journal* 38:48–58.

Luksetich, W., et al. 2000. Organizational form and nursing home behavior. *Nonprofit and Voluntary Sector Quarterly.* 29:255–279.

McGuire, A. 1985. The theory of the hospital: A review of the models. *Social Science and Medicine* 20:1177–1184.

Pauly, M., and M. Redisch. 1973. The not-for-profit hospital as a physicians' cooperative. *American Economic Review* 63:87–100.

For-Profit and Nonprofit Comparisons

Bays, C. 1979a. Case-mix differences between nonprofit and for-profit hospitals. *Inquiry* 14:17–21.

———. 1979b. Cost comparisons of for-profit and nonprofit hospitals. *Social Science and Medicine* 13C:219–225.

Borjas, G.J., et al. 1983. Property rights and wages: The case of nursing homes. *Journal of Human Resources* 17:231–246.

Clarkson, K.W. 1972. Some implications of property rights in hospital management. *Journal of Law and Economics* 15:363–384.

Eskoz, R., and K.M. Peddecord. 1985. The relationship of hospital ownership and service composition to hospital charges. *Health Care Financing Review* 6:51–58.

Frech, H.E. 1976. The property rights theory of the firm: Empirical results from a natural experiment. *Journal of Political Economy* 84:143–152.

———. 1985. The property rights theory of the firm: Some evidence from the U.S. nursing home industry. *Zeitschrift fur die Gestamte Staatswissenschaft* 141:146–166.

Lewin, L.S., et al. 1981. Investor-owneds and nonprofits differ in economic performance. *Hospitals,* 1 July, 52–58.

Lowrie, E.G., and C.L. Hampers. 1981. The success of Medicare's end-stage renal disease program. *New England Journal of Medicine* 305:434–438.

Pattison, R.V., and H.M. Katz. 1983. Investor-owned and not-for-profit hospitals. *New England Journal of Medicine* 309:347–353.

Relman, A.S. 1980. The new medical-industrial complex. *New England Journal of Medicine* 303:963–970.

Renn, S.C., et al. 1985. The effects of ownership and system affiliation on the economic performance of hospitals. *Inquiry* 22:219–236.

Rice, T., and J. Gabel. 1996. The internal economics of HMOs: A research agenda. *Medical Care Research and Review* 53 (suppl.): S44-S64.

Ruchlin, H.S., et al. 1976. A comparison of for-profit investor-owned chains and nonprofit hospitals. *Inquiry* 10:13–23.

Schweitzer, S.O., and J. Rafferty. 1976. Variations in hospital product: A comparative analysis of proprietary and voluntary hospitals. *Inquiry* 13:158–166.

Provider Supply under Managed Care Contracting

Debrock, A., and R.J. Arnould. 1992. Utilization control in HMOs. *Quarterly Review of Economics and Business* 32, no. 3:31–53.

Feldstein, P.J., et al. 1988. The effects of utilization review programs on health care use and expenditures. *New England Journal of Medicine* 318:1310–1314.

Hillman, A.L. 1987. Financial incentives for physicians in HMOs. *New England Journal of Medicine* 317:1743–1748.

Hillman, A.L., et al. 1989. How do financial incentives affect physicians' clinical decisions and the financial performance of health maintenance organizations? *New England Journal of Medicine* 321:86–92.

Pauly, M.V., et al. 1990. Managing physician incentives in managed care. *Medical Care* 28:1013–1024.

Robinson, J.C. 1993. Payment mechanisms, nonprice incentives, and organizational innovations in health care. *Inquiry* 30:328–332.

Scheffler, R.M., et al. 1991. The impact of Blue Cross and Blue Shield plan utilization management programs, 1980–1988. *Inquiry* 28:276–287.

Wickizer, T.M., et al. 1989. Does utilization review reduce unnecessary hospital care and contain costs? *Medical Care* 27:632–647.

Provider Payment

1. Explain the principal-agent framework as it relates to provider reimbursement in health care.
2. Identify the major types of physician reimbursement and compare their incentives using the principal-agent framework.
3. Explain the Resource-Based Relative Value Scale as a fee-for-service funding instrument.
4. Identify the alternative bases for the reimbursement of hospitals.
5. Using the principal-agent framework, explain the incentives associated with each of the major types of hospital reimbursement.
6. Explain the diagnosis-related group reimbursement system for Medicare.
7. Identify the major methods for reimbursing long-term care facilities.
8. Explain the method by which capitation rates are set for health maintenance organizations in Medicare.
9. Explain the impact of alternative provider reimbursement methods on HMO performance.
10. Identify the different methods that can be used by payers to monitor and regulate provider behavior.

7.1 INTRODUCTION

In the health care field there are a wide variety of services, the major ones being hospital, physician, outpatient drug, long-term care facility, and home care services; in addition, there are combined service units, such as health maintenance organizations. For each of these types of services, there are alternative ways of paying the provider. For example, physicians can be paid on a fee-for-service basis or by salary, and hospitals can be reimbursed on the basis of a global budget, on a per case basis, or for costs already incurred (retrospectively). In recent years, there has been a swing toward prospective reimbursement (that is, predetermined rates) and away from retrospective payment.

It was shown in Chapter 6 that the rate of payment will influence supplier behavior. In addition, payment bases are not neutral with respect to their impacts; that is, the basis of payment will have an impact on the quantity and quality of services provided. The theory of agency can shed light on the effect of the different types of payment. In this chapter we provide a description of the key forms of provider reimbursement in the health care field.

7.2 PRINCIPAL-AGENT RELATIONSHIPS AMONG PAYERS AND PROVIDERS

In the area of provider reimbursement, the provider, acting as an agent, faces two principals: the patients and, when there is health insurance, the insurers (Blomquist 1991). Our primary focus is on the relationship between payers (insurers) and providers (physicians, hospitals, long-term care facilities, and home care agencies).

Insurers must reimburse providers a given amount when the providers provide services. The reimbursements include the costs incurred by the providers and any profits they may make. In addition, as will be seen presently, some payment bases impose higher risks on the providers than others. Providers may demand a risk premium to compensate them for incurring these risks, and if they are risk averse, these risk premiums can be considerable, thus adding to the insurer's costs. In addition to the reimbursement to providers, insurers and other payers will incur costs of transacting with the providers. These costs, already discussed in Chapter 4, include the costs of searching for product availability, characteristics of the products, and prices; costs of negotiating and preparing contracts; costs of monitoring the providers' performance; and costs of enforcing the terms of the contracts. These transactions costs will vary according to the basis of payment. For example, if a particular payment basis encourages the provision of low-quality care or of excessive services, then additional monitoring and enforcement costs will be imposed on the insurer. In this chapter, we will examine the economic implications of different reimbursement systems in light of these concepts.

7.3 PHYSICIAN REIMBURSEMENT

There are four major types of physician reimbursement: fee-for-service, per case, per capita, and salary reimbursement.

7.3.1 Fee-for-Service Reimbursement

The fee-for-service method of reimbursement is similar to a piece-rate method. The physician is paid a specific sum for each individual service he or she provides to the patient. The services are broken down into units, such as a complete physical exam, a follow-up visit, a tonsillectomy, and so on.

There are several ways in which the fees can be set by the third party. One, which most closely corresponds to the assumption of an absence of control by the provider over the fee, is the relative value scale (Havighurst and Kissam 1979; Hsiao and Stason 1979). In this method, each category of service is assigned a relative value in accordance with some criterion (e.g., the number of minutes required to perform the procedure). For example, in the frequently used California Relative Value Scale (surgical component), a single coronary bypass operation would have an index number of 25. This relative value can be converted to fees by applying a conversion factor. If the conversion factor for surgery was $50 per point on the relative value scale, the surgeon would be reimbursed $1,250 for the bypass operation. A recent version of this mode of payment is discussed below.

A second type of fee setting does not really correspond to the assumption that fees are beyond the control of the individual provider. This method is referred to as the UCR (usual, customary, and reasonable) form of reimbursement. *Usual* refers to the usual or typical fee charged by the billing physician, *customary* refers to fees charged by all physicians in the community, and *reasonable* refers to allowances for particular circumstances (Epstein and Blumenthal 1993). Suppose Dr. Welby performed 100 varicose vein injections and charged an average of $100. Her usual fee for the procedure would then be $100. The customary fee would be derived from the frequency distribution of the fees charged by all physicians in the community for the procedure (e.g., the physicians in the 10th percentile might charge an average of $55, those in the 20th percentile might charge $63, and so on). The insurer then decides which percentile to use to set an allowable maximum fee. If the reimburser used the 70th percentile, then the associated charge might be $87. Dr. Welby would then be reimbursed her usual fee or the customary fee, whichever was lower (in her case, the customary fee, since her usual fee is $100).

The reason why the provider is not a mere price taker in this approach is that the provider's fee partly determines the customary fee prevailing in the market. If all physicians (or even some) raise their fees, the customary fee will increase as well. Each physician thus exerts some degree of influence over the market's fees. When there are many physicians in the market, the degree of influence may be small, and for analytical purposes the physicians might take the customary fee as a given fee. (Note that the fee in this case is also beyond the control of the insurer.)

The profit-maximizing model is useful for analyzing the effects of the level of rates in a fee-for-service payment system. Since the physician is paid a fixed rate per unit of service provided, the number of units produced will depend on what the reimbursement rate is and on the physician's marginal costs for the specific service. If the marginal cost schedule slopes upward steeply, only a slight addition to supply will result from an increase in the fee (Phelps 1976). Another important factor is the composition of fees. If surgical fees are high relative to general checkup fees—that is, surgical operations yield considerable profits relative to checkups—then surgeons will have an incentive to operate more. Physicians, on the other hand, will not have an incentive to perform checkups (which might be marginally profitable, if at all). Indeed, fee-for-service reimbursement is believed to encourage physicians to provide more medical care. As we have just seen, however, the degree of encouragement, if any, will depend on the relation between the fee and the service's marginal cost. Some analysts have taken the argument one step further and claimed that fee-for-service reimbursement encourages many unnecessary practices (Klarman 1963). In the context of the present analysis, we can only say whether additional services are likely to be offered; we cannot determine whether they would be necessary.

The fee schedule is a potentially powerful tool that third parties can use to influence both the type of practices performed and where they are performed. For example, tonsillectomies are thought to be unnecessary in many instances. If a third party wanted to discourage this procedure, it could lower the amount of reimbursement. Also, if a third party wanted to encourage certain procedures to be performed on an outpatient rather than an inpatient basis, it could reimburse physicians differentially for the same procedure. For example, the South Carolina Preferred Personal Care Plan reimbursed physicians $675 for a colonoscopy performed in an outpatient setting and $515 for the same procedure performed in a hospital.

The profit-maximizing hypothesis can be altered to take into account alternative possible behavior patterns of the physician-owners of medical practices.

7.3.2 Per Case Reimbursement

The second type of physician reimbursement is payment per case. In this type of reimbursement, the physician is paid a fixed amount for each type of case treated, much like the DRG system. In fact, the DRG system is among the systems considered as a basis for per case reimbursement (Mitchell 1985). In per case reimbursement, the physician bears the cost of any services he or she provides and is paid a sum for the entire case. If the physician reduces the number of services, more money will be left over as profit.

Per case reimbursement for physicians is not widely being considered at this time, in part because studies have indicated that there are wide variations in services for a single case type (DRG), which would result in difficulties in establishing rates or fees and would give providers greater leeway to select cases with potentially low costs and to refer potentially high cost cases.

7.3.3 Per Capita and Salary Reimbursement

The incentives for physicians who are paid on a per capita or a salary basis are decidedly different than the incentives in fee-for-service reimbursement. In both cases, there is some incentive for physicians to provide no more than the basic minimum level of services. However, a physician who intends to remain in practice a long time could not afford to allow the quality of services to fall to a low level. Considerable evidence exists regarding the impact that the payment system has on physician practices. Reference has been made to the large difference in surgical operations in the United States and England, and the difference in general payment patterns is considered one underlying factor. In England, surgeons were traditionally paid on a salary basis, while in the United States the usual payment basis is fee-for-service (Aaron and Schwartz 1984), although the fee schedule has been changed considerably since the introduction of the Resource-Based Relative Value Scale (RBRVS). In the United States, several reimbursement experiments have been undertaken (Eisenberg and Williams 1981; Myers and Schroeder 1981). In one, primary care physicians were given financial responsibility for the entire health care expenditures of their patients; they shared in any surpluses of premiums over total medical care costs (including hospitalization costs, laboratory fees, radiology fees, etc.) as well as in any deficits. The incentive was for them to reduce the expenditures paid out so that the surpluses would be greater. This experiment was based on a view of the physician as "gatekeeper" to the health care system, someone who has the ability to control a good deal of the patient's cost. The results showed a considerable reduction in overall expenses relative to a fee-for-service comparison group (Moore 1979). Another study examined how physician prescribing behavior was affected by an ambulatory care center's introduction of monetary incentives to generate additional business. The findings showed there was a substantial increase in radiographs (Hemenway et al. 1990).

7.3.4 Agency Theory and Physician Reimbursement

Many investigators have linked the fee-for-service payment system with the generation of a high volume of services and consequently with high expenditure levels. Usually, fee-for-service is compared with capitation funding.

Under any payment system, the physician has the ability to generate additional services because of the information asymmetry between physician and patient. Under fee-for-service, the physician has the incentive to generate more services, especially if the fee exceeds the marginal cost of the service. By comparison, the physician will not have such an incentive under capitation. If the physician is not concerned about repeat visits, then he or she will have an incentive to reduce the volume of visits. However, if the physician has a desire to encourage repeat visits by patients, then he or she will not want to reduce services to the point where quality of care is compromised.

The capitation imposes risks on the provider; the provider must incur the costs of all services for all patients, including the very high cost ones. In determining his or her capitation rates, the provider will add a risk premium that will vary with his or her degree of risk aversion. This will be very high if the provider is risk averse.

A third-party payer will incur contract costs under both fee-for-service and capitation funding. Under fee-for-service funding, the insurer must monitor for excessive services, while under capitation funding, the insurer must monitor for low quality of care due to inadequate provision. There is no predetermined answer as to which funding system is more costly once societal costs are included, although most commentators would say that fee-for-service costs more.

7.3.5 A Resource-Based Relative Value Scale

Medicare adopted a variant of the UCR system called *customary, prevailing,* and *reasonable* (CPR), but it had regulated these fees since 1984. Recently, a new fee schedule has been adopted to replace the old fee system. The new schedule has fixed fees that are based on resource use measures. This system, called RBRVS, attempts to classify the costs that would be incurred by physicians operating in a competitive environment. Based on the classification, a questionnaire was developed to capture the costs incurred in the classification scheme. The questionnaire was applied to national samples of physicians in 18 specialties to develop a relative cost schedule for physician procedures or services. The cost categories include costs related to actual work done by a physician, costs of operating practices, and the "amortized" cost of physician training (an annual amount derived from averaging training expenses over the period of a standard career). A fee schedule was developed that reflected these costs.

The national survey interviewed a sample of physicians about the time, mental effort and judgment, physical effort, technical skill, and stress associated with each procedure. These elements were combined into work indexes. For example, an office visit for internal medicine had a work index of 100, whereas a resection for rectal carcinoma had an index value of 445. To these work indexes were added practice cost factors and the opportunity cost of training. Practice costs were determined by specialty based on a survey of costs and revenues by physicians in each specialty.

The results of the calculations indicate the value of the services relative to each other, not their value in dollars. The relative valuations must then be assigned a dollar value in order to be translated into a fee schedule. For example, if the dollar value assigned to the schedule was $1 per index point, then the physician would receive $445 for a resection for rectal carcinoma (which was given an index value of 445 points).

Table 7–1 presents simulated fees for selected office visits under the old Medicare system and under the RBRVS. These numbers, which reflect the direction the RBRVS is taking, show that surgical fees would be cut substantially under the RBRVS whereas evaluation and management fees would increase substantially (Hsiao et al. 1988a, 885).

The effects of such changes can be analyzed in terms of the supply analysis presented in this chapter. An increase in the fee for a procedure should increase the quantity supplied of that procedure, and a reduction should reduce the quantity supplied. Thus, for those procedures whose fees are increased, the quantity supplied will increase. This is shown in Figure 7–1, where S_1 is a supply curve for a single profit-maximizing physician (ignore S_2 for the moment). Initially the fee for an office visit is $40, and at this level the physician will be willing to supply 210 office visits. An increase in the fee to $100 will result in a supply of 500 visits. According to this analysis, a fee increase will increase the quantity of procedures and a fee reduction will reduce the quantity. The RBRVS, according to this analysis, will have substantial supply effects in favor of primary care and away from more intensive and invasive procedures.

We should note that this discussion is restricted to the issue of supply. The number of services actually provided will depend on the quantity of services *demanded*.

There are some other qualifications that should be kept in mind. The first is the appropriateness of this analysis for dealing with labor supply issues. After all, the physician's labor is a key factor in the supply of physician visits. Individual physicians have limitations on their work time, and the supply model needs to be modified to take this into account.

At lower income and wage levels, the propensity to substitute leisure for work may be strong enough to more than offset the income effect. An upward-sloping supply curve would result. However, at higher wage levels, the income effect may more than offset the substitution effect, and a backward-bending supply curve would result. In Figure 7–1, the supply curve of S_2 begins to bend back just beyond 200 office visits. Up to the fee of $40, the physician behaves as in curve S_1. If the fee rises above $40 per visit, the physician's supply will increase in smaller amounts and

Table 7–1 Simulated Charges for Selected Procedures According to Medicare and Simulated RBRVS, 1986

Procedure	Mean Medicare Charge (dollars)	RBRV Fee (dollars)	Ratio of Medicare Fee to RBRV Fee
Extended office visit, medical	37	130	0.27
Coronary bypass surgery	4,663	2,871	1.62
Interpretation of chest film	20	22	0.91

Source: Data from W.C. Hsiao, et al., Results and Policy Implications of the Resource Based Relative Value Study, *New England Journal of Medicine*, Vol. 319, pp. 881–888, © 1988.

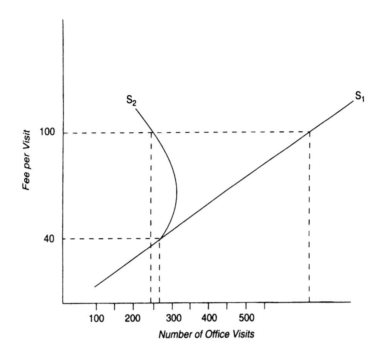

Figure 7–1 Supply curves for physician services are shown under two sets of assumptions. Curve S_1 shows a situation where higher fees result in more labor (and less leisure). Curve S_2 shows a case where higher fees result in physician's taking more leisure time and cutting back on work.

eventually begin to decrease. If this is the way physicians behave, then raising fees above the maximum point will cause physicians to cut back on the number of services they are willing to provide. An increase in primary care fees, then, may not necessarily cause an increase in the quantity of primary care supplied. However, there is little evidence to support the notion of a backward sloping supply curve of labor.

7.4 HOSPITAL REIMBURSEMENT

7.4.1 Alternative Bases of Reimbursement

Until the early 1980s, hospitals were reimbursed on a retrospective basis. That is, a third-party insurer would reimburse a hospital for the expenses it had already incurred (if reimbursement was on a cost basis) or the charges it had already billed (if reimbursement was on a charge basis). There are numerous variations of retrospective reimbursement. The third party can pay on a cost-plus basis, which means it can reimburse the hospital for its allowable operating costs plus a specified amount (say, 2 percent of costs) for capital equipment. In another method of reimbursement, the third party pays the hospital whichever is lower, costs or charges. There is also considerable variation in how costs are defined. Allowable costs could exclude costs not directly related to patient care (e.g., teaching costs). Whatever the arrangement, retrospective reimbursement has one overriding effect on supply and on costs: it encourages an organization to expand. Increases in both the scope and quality of services tend to occur, and if the provider is a maximizer of anything (e.g., profits or perquisites), retrospective reimbursement can lead to higher costs, more services, and higher quality services.

In response to this recognized bias in retrospective reimbursement, a number of prospective reimbursement plans have been introduced. Prospective reimbursement involves setting the basis of reimbursement before the reimbursement period. As a result, this sort of payment scheme puts the provider "at risk" for any excess of cost over revenue. There are many different bases for setting the rate of prospective payments and an infinite number of rate levels. We will examine several of the alternatives and their hypothesized effects on cost and quantity.

To help classify the effects of different types of reimbursement, we will use the following formula to break out the components of total cost:

$$\frac{\text{Total}}{\text{Cost}} = \frac{\text{Cost per}}{\text{Service}} \times \frac{\text{Services per}}{\text{Patient Day}} \times \frac{\text{Days of Stay}}{\text{per Admission}} \times \frac{\text{Number of}}{\text{Admisisons}}$$

Let us now explore the likely effect of three types of prospective reimbursement—per service, per diem (per day), and per admission—on an output-maximizing hospital.

In per service reimbursement, the hospital will receive a fixed amount for each service performed (e.g., an operation, a radiograph, or kidney dialysis). The amount for each service is set in advance (e.g., $45 for a specific lab test, $300 for a complete CT scan, etc.). The second method of payment is per diem reimbursement. Under this method, an amount is arrived at by multiplying the per diem cost for the particular service by the number of days of care provided. The third prospective payment method, per admission reimbursement, rewards the hospital only for adding more patients. Under the per admission method, payers usually adjust the payment by a case mix or severity index because cases differ considerably by diagnosis and severity. For a discussion of a diagnosis-adjusted per admission payment system, see the section below entitled "Diagnosis-Related Groups." Even cases within a diagnosis group may differ from one another; in such circumstances, the per admission and per diem bases of payment may be combined. This will be discussed below.

7.4.2 Agency Theory and Hospital Reimbursement

We can use the agency framework to analyze the effects of the different hospital payment systems. As usual, the key issues include uncertainty, information asymmetry, and monitoring and other transactions costs.

7.4.2.1 Retrospective Payments

Retrospective payment is the funding of costs that were actually incurred. Under retrospective funding, the payer incurs all of the financial risks. The provider has an incentive to increase the quality and volume of services, as it will be reimbursed for these; it bears no financial risks. In order to protect itself financially, the payer must incur expenses to set standards and monitor and enforce them. These contracting costs can be quite high because of the technical nature of medical care, including the wide variety of diagnoses and treatments; the complexity of the product leads to information asymmetries, such that the provider may have considerably more technical and detailed knowledge of the patient than does the payer.

7.4.2.2 Prospective Fee-for-Service System

Prospective payment means the setting of the rate in advance of the service. Fee-for-service means that a fee for each service is set before the services are provided. Under this type of reimbursement, almost all of the financial risk is imposed on the payer. This is because all services provided by the hospital will be paid for. As long as the per service rate exceeds the hospital's marginal cost, the provider will have an incentive to add additional services. The payer would have to set standards and monitor and enforce them, thus incurring costs. The detailed knowledge possessed by the providers would create considerable information asymmetries. Information asymmetries would add considerably to the costs incurred by the payers.

7.4.2.3 Per Diem Fees

Under a flat per diem fee, there will be a sharing of financial risks between the payer and the hospital. The longer the hospital keeps the patient, the more it will be reimbursed. Since the latter part of most hospital stays are less costly than the earlier portion, the per diem rates are likely to exceed the marginal costs of the latter part of a stay.

The actual rates paid in relation to cost will be very important incentives. The per diem cost of a case depends on the diagnosis. For example, a liver transplant case will have daily costs that are well above the average. A hospital that performs transplants could lose money on such operations. The provider would require a risk premium if a flat per diem payment system were implemented, since the hospital might demand compensation if it treats high-cost cases. In addition, the payer would incur the cost of monitoring the stays. The hospital will have considerable leeway in extending stays; because the hospital has considerably more information on the patients and their conditions than the payers, information asymmetries will arise. The payer would have to develop standards, write contracts, monitor these, and enforce them. These costs could be substantial.

7.4.2.4 Per Case Payment

Because of the wide range of diagnoses and treatments, all per case payment systems make use of case mix groups. Each group contains cases that use roughly the same amount of resources, and payers reimburse the hospitals the same sum of money for all cases within each group. Under such a system, the risk to the payer is reduced considerably. However, there is still a wide range of costs within each diagnosis group; sometimes the within-group variation in resource use is said to be due to "severity." Hospitals that attract higher severity cases, either because they are referral centers or inner-city hospitals, may lose money due to the higher costs. They may therefore refuse to accept such cases without some kind of severity adjustment.

In addition to these additional costs, a case mix system contains considerable informational asymmetries. The providing hospitals have considerable discretion in assigning patients to diagnosis groups. In order to counteract this tendency, the payer will have to develop an adequate reporting system and ensure that it is being followed. The development and maintenance of such a system will impose considerable costs on the payer.

7.4.2.5 Per Case Reimbursement with Adjustment for Outliers

In order to reduce the costs imposed on providers who accept more severe cases under a flat per case reimbursement system, payers have developed a two-part system. Cases within each diagnosis group are divided into two groups, typical cases and outliers. Using the distribution of stays within each diagnosis group, a trim point is established that separates long-stay outliers from typical cases. The actual setting of the trim point is arbitrary and depends on how much pressure the payer wants to impose on the provider to reduce its stays. Outliers are reimbursed in two parts: a per case portion to cover those days inside of the trim and an additional per diem payment to cover the additional days. Thus the risk of very high cost cases due to very long stays will be borne in a large part by the payer. Such a system has been adopted by the Medicare payment system.

7.4.3 Other Hospital Reimbursement Issues

When evaluating types of hospital reimbursement, several things have to be kept in mind. First, one must distinguish between an all-payer system and a multipayer system. In an all-payer system, each payer pays the same rate. For example, assume that Medicare, Blue Cross, and commercial insurers each have one-third of the overall caseload of 300 cases in a hospital and that the case mixes and severities of the patient groups are identical (so there is no objective basis for differential payments). Assume, further, that the regulatory authority in the state has determined that the hospital's allowable revenues should be $900,000. This means that each insurer "should" pay $300,000, and this is what it would pay in an all-payer system.

A multipayer system is more like a free-for-all, with each payer setting up its payment rules unilaterally or based on market principles. Let us say that, in the preceding example, the regulatory agency only regulates Medicare and Blue Cross rates and that it allows each to pay $270,000. The commercial group rates are unregulated. In this instance, the hospital must charge the commercials more to cover its deficit. Whether or not it collects all its bills is another issue. What is significant here is that the hospital is no longer a price taker, and so a more complex model that can incorporate the reaction by the hospital to the regulated rate is needed.

A second important fact to keep in mind is that other parts of the health care system may be affected by the reimbursement type and level. For example, if a system penalizes a hospital for keeping patients hospitalized for more than a specified time, this will most certainly reduce length of stay. It may have other effects as well. For instance, if home health care or long-term care facility care are reimbursed separately, the hospital may open up a long-term care facility or begin a home health care program to which it could discharge its patients.

A considerable number of experiments with prospective reimbursement have been conducted at the state level (Bauer 1977; Carter et al. 1994). Most of these have occurred in multipayer systems, and so their effects are harder to identify than they would be in an all-payer system. One such experiment, conducted by the New York State legislature, set rates on a per diem basis for Medicare- and Blue Cross–reimbursed patients according to a preestablished formula beginning in 1970. This had the effect of rewarding hospitals for longer stays. In testing for the effect of this type of reimbursement, a comparison was made between length of stay and occupancy rates after 1970 in New York State and those in several comparison states, where prospective per diem rates were not in force (Ohio and the New England states). Between 1970 and 1974, New York showed a slight increase in the average length of stay and no net change in the occupancy rate (i.e., the average percentage of beds filled). Both of these indicators of hospital supply decreased considerably in the control states during the same period of time. This suggests that the reimbursement mechanism had its expected effect (Berry 1976).

7.5 DIAGNOSIS-RELATED GROUPS

In 1983 the federal government introduced a new prospective payment system (PPS) for Medicare hospital patients. In this system, reimbursement for all Medicare discharges is on a per diagnosis basis. Here, we review how diagnoses are grouped into separate DRGs and how rates are set for each DRG.

The DRG system is one of many possible ways of classifying patients according to common elements (Hornbrook 1982). There is the presumption that, if the classification system is to be used for reimbursement purposes, all cases in each group must be similar with regard to resource use. Based on several patient characteristics (the major diagnostic group, the presence of comorbid diagnoses, the presence of a surgical procedure, and discharge status), an algorithm was developed to assign individual cases to groupings that exhibit common resource-use tendencies (as measured by length of stay) (Fetter et al. 1980). The component characteristics of one set of DRGs is shown in Figure 7–2. As can be seen, DRGs for breast disorders were developed based on the major diagnostic groups the disorders fell into and on factors such as the need for surgery, the patient's age, and the presence of complicating diagnoses. The criteria were selected so that cases in each category would use similar amounts of resources and thus could be reimbursed with a single rate. There are 511 categories in the 2001 DRG classification system. A sample list of DRGs, along with their relative weights, is presented in Table 7–2.

Based on cross-hospital studies, an average cost for each DRG was estimated. Factors in the calculation included the lengths of stay (within the DRG) in routine and special care, per diem costs in routine and special care, and the estimated per case cost of ancillary services (laboratory, radiology, drugs, medical supplies, anesthesia, and other services) (Pettengill and Vertrees 1982). Each DRG was then assigned a relative weight intended to approximate the relative amount of resources used by an average case in the group. For example, a cardiac arrest (DRG 129) has an assigned weight of 1.0969 and a coronary bypass (DRG 106) has an assigned weight of 7.5203. This means that, in comparison to an "average" diagnostic group (with a weight set equal to 1), a typical case of DRG 129 uses 1.0969 times the amount of resources and a case of DRG 106 uses 7.5203 times the amount.

Using these weights and the frequency of types of cases, a hospital can develop a case mix–adjusted admissions measure. This measure would presumably be a better approximation of the resources required to serve the hospital's patient population than mere admissions or patient days (which have traditionally been

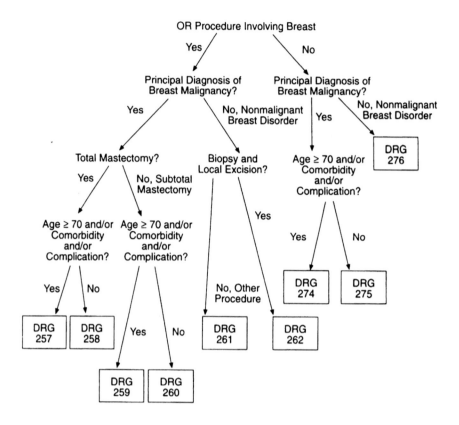

Figure 7–2 Derivation of diagnosis-related groups (DRGs) for breast disorders. Among the criteria used to separate the various DRGs are the use of operating room (OR) procedures, the principal diagnosis, the type of OR procedure (if used), the age of the patient, and complications and/or comorbidity.

used). For example, let us say that both Aiken and Bethesda General Hospital treated 200 patients in 1990, with an average length of stay of 6 days. Both would have a measured output of 1,200 patient days. Let us say, however, that of Aiken's 200 cases, half were inguinal hernia cases (DRG 162, with a weight equal to 0.6229) and half were complicated peptic ulcer cases (DRG 176, with a weight equal to 1.1052). Then Aiken's case mix–adjusted measure of admissions would be equal to 172.71 [(0.6229 × 100) + (1.1052 × 100)]. Bethesda's case mix included 100 cases of DRG 106, bypass surgery, with a weight equal to 7.5203, and 100 kidney transplants (DRG 302, with a weight equal to 3.4241). Bethesda's adjusted output would be equal to 1,076 [(7.5203 × 100) + (3.4241 × 100)].

With the hospital's output being measured in terms of case-weighted admissions, a reimbursement rate (called a *standardized amount*) must be set for each single point (relative weight = 1.00). Originally, this rate had national, regional, and hospital-specific components. In 1989 Medicare went to a national rate, although the rate for each hospital is affected by its location (urban or rural), the number of residents per bed (for teaching hospitals), and the number of low-income patients treated (Russell 1989). For example, in 2000 the national standardized amount for

Table 7–2 Relative Weights for Selected Diagnosis-Related Groups (2001)

DRG	Description	2001 Relative Weight (average = 1.0000)
039	Lens procedure	0.5778
060	Tonsillectomy	0.2087
070	Otitis media	0.4628
106	Coronary bypass with PTCA	7.5203
211	Hip and femur procedures	1.2647
302	Kidney transplant	3.4241
373	Normal vaginal delivery	0.4169

Source: Data from Health Care Financing Administration.

hospitals in large urban areas was $3,951. An urban hospital with no teaching facilities would be reimbursed $1,647 for a vaginal delivery (0.4169 points times $3,951 per point). These amounts are also adjusted for geographic location and share of low-income cases.

If the hospital was a teaching hospital, it would be entitled to an "indirect" teaching adjustment to pay for additional services (lab tests, radiographs, etc.) consumed in the process of teaching interns and residents. This additional amount is based on the hospital's intern-resident per bed ratio (Lave 1984). The indirect teaching adjustment equals about a 7 percent increase in the basic rate for each .1 interns and residents per bed. A large teaching hospital with a ratio of .4 residents per bed would have a 28-percent increase added to its basic rate. This hospital, if it was in a large urban area, would receive $5,057 (1.28 × $3,951) per point.

As an example, let us say that a typical teaching hospital, Denver City Hospital, with 200 beds and .4 residents per bed, had 24,000 admissions last year, one-quarter of which were Medicare patients. Assume, further, that one-half (3,000) of the Medicare cases fell into DRG 39 (lens surgery, with a weight equal to 0.5778) and one-half into DRG 211 (hip procedures, with a weight equal to 1.2647). Since this hospital is in a large urban area, it was reimbursed at a rate of $5,057 per point (after the adjustment for its intern-resident population). Denver's receipts for its 6,000 Medicare patients would be about $26.8 million (3,000 cases with a weight equal to .5055 and 3,000 cases with a weight equal to 1.2647).

Medicare also reimburses the hospitals for certain additional costs that fall outside of the basic case-mix formula: outlier-related costs and direct medical education costs. An *outlier* is a case whose cost or length of stay is sufficiently high that it falls outside certain predetermined limits. There are two kinds of outliers— day and cost outliers. A day outlier for a specific DRG is a case whose length of stay exceeds a preset number of days (e.g., 24 days); all days in excess of this trim point are called *outlying days*. For example, if the trim point for DRG 103 is 24 and a case has a stay of 32 days, then 8 of these days will be deemed outlying days. In 1997 Medicare stopped paying for long-stay outliers and provided extra funding only on the basis of high-cost cases. A high-cost outlier is one whose adjusted charges exceed the Medicare payment rate for the DRG by over $14,050.

Outlier rules were developed to reimburse hospitals for cases that used an unusually high amount of resources. Rates for reimbursing hospitals for outlying portions of cases are set by Congress. Outlier payments cover about 5 percent of total per case reimbursement, and their importance will vary depending on the degree of complexity of the hospital's cases.

7.6 LONG-TERM CARE FACILITY REIMBURSEMENT

Because there is such wide variability in long-term care facility lengths of stay, it is not feasible to reimburse long-term care facilities on a per case basis. They are therefore funded on a per diem basis. Medicaid state agencies, being the largest third-party payers of long-term care facilities, have traditionally paid long-term care facilities in two different ways: with a flat per diem (per day) rate or with a facility-specific per diem rate. Facility-specific rates are largely retrospective and consequently result in high costs. In flat rate reimbursement, a single rate is paid to all long-term care facilities regardless of patient characteristics, quality levels, and so on. Often a separate rate will be paid by level of facility—SNF or ICF. One virtue of the flat rate is that, at least in the case of for-profit long-term care facilities, the facilities have an incentive to minimize costs. This may lead to some problems, however. Long-term care facilities might seek to attract patients who are healthier or who need less care (and hence cost less to treat), or they might compromise on quality (which would also lower costs and increase profits). As long as long-term care facilities seek profits to some degree (they might also have other objectives), they will tend to lower costs when such a payment mechanism is in place. It is primarily to balance the incentive to select patients with fewer needs that case mix measures have been introduced (Schlenker 1986). The primary purpose of case mix reimbursement in long-term care is to relate reimbursement rates to required levels of care and help ensure that patients receive appropriate care.

One case mix measure that has been developed is called *Resource Utilization Groups* (RUGs) (Fries and Cooney 1985). This measure has now been superseded by RUGs II (Micheletti and Shlala 1986) and RUGs III (Fries et al. 1994). The RUGs case mix measure is based on a set of hierarchical groups related to levels and types of services (rehabilitation, extensive services, special care, clinically complex cases, impaired cognition, behavioral problems, and reduced physical functioning) and, within these hierarchical groups, scores on the activities of daily living (ADL) scale. The ADL scale assigns numerical scores according to the degree of physical functioning an individual can attain in each of six categories: bathing, dressing, toileting, feeding, transferring between locations, and continence (Katz et al. 1963). RUGs III uses four of these categories: eating, transferring, bed mobility, and toileting. Based on the points assigned to each of these, in combination with the hierarchical groups, the patient is assigned to 1 of 44 RUGs III categories. The categories are assigned weights according to their relative costs (see, e.g., Schlenker et al. 1985), and reimbursement is made in accordance with these relative weights.

Such a system overcomes the first disadvantage mentioned above—that case mix selection creates a bias in favor of light-care patients. Indeed, if the weights of each category are in line with the relative costs of treating patients, then the selection bias should be removed. This does not mean that other selection biases do not exist. Indeed, three other types of biases that result from a RUGs type of payment system have been identified (Butler and Schlenker 1989). The first of these is a bias against patient rehabilitation. If a patient improves, he or she moves into another payment category and the long-term care facility loses revenue. Particularly if the case mix reimbursement system is oriented toward patient condition rather than services, the long-term care facility will incur higher costs by rehabilitating patients. An incentive not to rehabilitate would therefore be present (Smits 1984). To counteract this, a reimbursement program might pay long-term care facilities on the basis of outcomes or pay at the higher reimbursement level for a limited period even when the patient improves. A second bias in such a system involves the provision of unnecessary care. If the reimbursement system pays more for certain services (e.g., rehabilitation), then this might give the long-term care facility an incentive to provide such services, sometimes unnecessarily. As for the third bias, the long-term care facility has a motive to misreport patient status, thus acquiring a higher reimbursement rate.

The best way to eliminate these biases may be to adopt regulations and institute a monitoring system. New York State, which adopted the RUGs II system, had a regulatory system to monitor the quality of care in long-term care facilities (Micheletti and Shlala 1986). Such a monitoring system was developed because the reimbursement system was not sufficient to achieve all of the public policy goals of the long-term care facility system.

7.7 HEALTH MAINTENANCE ORGANIZATIONS

The major characteristics of an HMO from a supply standpoint are that it is responsible, simultaneously, for two types of services—health insurance and health care. Health insurance coverage is sold to customers on a per capita basis. The medical care itself is provided, or contracted for, by the HMO directly. The HMO assumes all the financial risk for providing this care. At the same time, its physicians act as "gatekeepers" and therefore have some degree of control over the patients' utilization of care.

In discussing the supply incentives inherent in such an organization, we must recognize that an HMO can make a number of different types of arrangements with the physicians that it contracts with and the hospitals to which it sends its patients.

The per capita funding formula provides an incentive for any for-profit HMO to minimize costs (all other factors being held constant). An HMO can reduce its costs by lowering the use of services by existing patients, encouraging the enrollment of members who are at low risk, and disenrolling high-risk patients. Lower cost enrollees would include younger members, nonsmokers, individuals who exercise, and so on. In order to encourage healthy enrollees to select it, the HMO can design a product with this end in mind. It might, for example, have more pediatricians and fewer gerontologists on staff, specialize in sports medicine, and open more branches in the suburbs and few or no branches in the inner city (Enthoven 1988; Hellinger 1995; Luft 1986). Indeed, the likelihood of an HMO's encouraging self-selection and thus having an enrollee mix that does not reflect the demographics of the general population has resulted in the development of adjustment formulas to compensate for potential differences in enrollee risk and the cost of utilization (Anderson et al. 1986). These formulas are used to calculate higher payment rates for higher risk individuals, thus inducing HMOs to enroll these individuals.

One such adjustment formula, Medicare's former average adjusted per capita cost (AAPCC) formula, was used to determine the rates at which Medicare pays HMOs. The rates are based on Medicare's own current payment rates for hospital and physician services in the fee-for-service system. AAPCCs were calculated for separate groups of patients (factors used in constructing the groups included sex, age bracket, county, welfare status, and institutionalization). For example, the monthly AAPCC for noninstitutionalized females aged 70–74 who were not on welfare in Washington County, Oregon, was $62 for hospital services and $30 for medical services. The Medicare rate to be paid to the HMOs for these individuals was 95 percent of the AAPCC of $92. The rationale behind this payment rate was that, for those individuals who did shift from fee-for-service coverage to HMO coverage, Medicare would save 5 percent of its average cost. The HMO would benefit if it could provide coverage at a cost lower than this.

One criticism of this payment system was that it did not pinpoint risk categories accurately enough and that HMO cream skimming was a distinct possibility even with the AAPCC adjustments. For example, the AAPCC did not take into account the amount of prior health services used, which is a good indicator of future utilization of services. If an HMO could use this information to supply a product with characteristics that appeal to low-risk individuals, then it could obtain a large share of low-cost users even allowing for AAPCC adjustments. The result could be costly to Medicare, whose 95 percent rule was designed to achieve savings for the program.

Assume that there are 100 individuals in Washington County who are enrolled in Medicare and who have the characteristics specified above (70–74 years old, female, noninstitutionalized, nonwelfare). If they were in the fee-for-service program, Medicare would pay on average $92.00 a month for each. For each such individual attracted by an HMO, the HMO will receive 95 percent of the AAPCC, or $87.40 monthly. If the HMO is successful, through careful design of product characteristics, in drawing 10 very healthy, low-risk females from this group of 100, its average costs for these members will likely be below the $87.40 rate. The total cost to Medicare will be $87.40 times 10. The fee-for-service sector will now be left with a higher cost pool, having lost 10 lower-than-average-cost members, and its costs will rise. It is thus possible that this payment scheme could end up costing Medicare more money.

A second problem with this system was that it created a wide regional variation in rates. Medicare paid low rates for residents who lived in counties where costs were low, and HMOs would not offer services in counties with low AAPCC rates.

In order to address these problems, Medicare instituted a new risk-premium–setting mechanism in 2000. This system was called "Medicare + Choice" and was instituted under a new Part C of Medicare. The risk-adjustment factors included prior hospitalization and demographic factors. The demographic factors included age, sex, disability status, Medicaid eligibility, and institutional status. As an example, an HMO that newly enrolled a male aged 66 would receive a payment of $2,921 annually. If the person was also Medicaid eligible, the HMO would receive an additional $3,297.

If the individual had been hospitalized in the previous year, and if his or her diagnosis fell into a serious category, the HMO would receive an additional payment to cover a higher risk status. There are 15 illness categories that are based on reason for hospitalization. The new categorization system is called Principal Inpatient–Diagnostic Cost Group (PIP-DCG). As an example, PIP-DCG 8 is asthma, and if a person has been hospitalized for asthma, Medicare will add an additional $4,192 annually onto its rate (Health Care Financing Administration, 1999).

In developing a single rate, Congress hopes that HMOs will increase supply in areas currently underserved because of low rates. The new system seems to better address risk factors, but it may overserve low-cost areas and underserve areas where costs are high.

7.8 PROVIDER SUPPLY UNDER MANAGED CARE

7.8.1 Agency Theory and Incentive Contracts

The quantity and quality of services that an HMO supplies to its members are determined to a large extent by the health care providers that the HMO contracts with. The HMO is reliant on these providers to assess the HMO members' conditions and to provide appropriate levels of care. The manner in which the HMO compensates these providers will affect their supply behavior.

The HMO management does not usually know its members' health status, nor what treatments are appropriate. The providers have the best information about these matters, and so there is an "information asymmetry" between the two groups. Consequently, it is possible for the providers to act strictly in their own interest. In order to encourage the providers to act in the interest of the HMO, the HMO management can design a compensation scheme for the providers. Agency models can be used to analyse such compensation schemes. The two contracting bodies in such models are the *principals* (HMOs) and their *agents* (providers). We will set out a model in this section to examine how alternative compensation schemes influence the supply behavior of providers.

The principal, or HMO, contracts with its members (on a per capita payment basis) to provide them with care.

- *HMO objectives.* We assume that the HMO's objectives are to maximize profits. However, we also assume that there is a minimum profit level that is acceptable to the HMO; in our example, this will be $500,000. Profits are equal to total revenue minus total cost.
- *HMO revenues.* The HMO's revenues depend on the capitation rate applied to its members and the number of members who join the HMO. In our model, we will hold the capitation rate constant.
- *HMO costs.* The HMO's costs include those that are incurred in treating the HMO members who become patients.
- *HMO-provider interaction.* In many respects, the HMO is dependent on its agents, the providers of care (physicians, physical therapists, hospitals, etc.), for the achievement of its profit targets. Providers can influence HMO profits by varying their levels of effort. If providers function at very low effort levels, patients will be dissatisfied with the heath care they receive and will switch to other health plans. As a result, HMO profits will be low. As physician efforts increase, quality of care will improve and more members will join. However, additional physician effort means more lab tests, more procedures, and so on. While this will bring in more members to the HMO, it will also increase costs. Eventually, the additional effort will work against profitability, and profits will fall. Graph A of Figure 7–3 shows the relationship between the HMO's profits and the effort of the agents. At some effort level (E_3), profits will be at a maximum level. At other effort levels (E_1 and E_4), profits will be at minimally acceptable levels. HMO profits, then, are directly tied to the efforts of its contracting physicians. The physicians know how much effort they are providing and how much is required to treat their patients. The HMO cannot directly observe this effort. This is another way of saying that there is an information asymmetry between the principal and its agents. While the HMO cannot directly observe physician efforts, it can observe its profits. This perfor-

mance indicator will come in useful when the HMO sets compensation policies for the physicians.

- *Physician objectives.* We turn now to the assumptions about the behavior of the physicians. The objective of each physician is to maximize net income (profits), which is equal to revenues from the HMO minus the personal costs of supplying care (or exerting effort). With a rising marginal cost curve for effort, the maximization point (which indicates what level of effort will be chosen by the physician) occurs where the marginal revenue (MR) equals the marginal cost for the physician.
- *Physician costs.* We will assume that all provider revenues come from the HMO (i.e., that each provider has no additional source of revenue). The relationship between alternative payment schemes that the HMO can institute and physician revenues will be discussed below. The physician costs in this model are the opportunity costs to the physician of engaging in productive practices. The physician places a value on his or her time, and this value is based on alternative uses of the time spent on care. We assume that the marginal cost to the physician of time spent on patient care increases as more time is spent. Put another way, as more time is taken away from leisure activities, the value of the last unit of time increases. This rising marginal cost curve of effort is shown in Graph B of Figure 7–3.
- *Physician revenues.* The proposition being established in this section is that the level of effort selected by the physician will be influenced by the basis and level of reimbursement.

We will now examine three alternative forms of compensation: salary, fee-for-service reimbursement, and incentive compensation based on the HMO's profits.

If the physician is paid a straight salary, any additional effort by the physician results in costs but yields no extra revenue. There is a minimum acceptable level of effort that the physician must put in—the level that corresponds to the minimum profit target of the HMO (level E_1). The physician will provide this level but no more.

We will now assume the physician is paid a fee of \$35 per service. Extra effort on the part of the physician will result in extra services provided. These extra services result in marginal revenues of \$35 per service (see the straight line at \$35 in Figure 7–3). The physician would maximize net income at a level of effort of E_5. However, because the HMO's profits are below those that are acceptable to the HMO, the physician will reduce his or her effort level to E_4. If the fee falls below \$35, then the physician will choose an effort level below E_5. If the fee level increases, then the effort level will also increase. It is quite possible, therefore, to have a low effort level under fee-for-service reimbursement if the fee levels are low enough.

The HMO can set a contract that provides specific incentives. Recall that the HMO does not know how much effort is provided by the physician. The HMO only has a proxy for this—mainly HMO performance (in this case, HMO profits). The HMO can pay the physician a fixed percentage of HMO profits. The MR curve for the physician will appear like that in any demand situation—it will decline to a level of zero as profits increase to their maximum. Beyond this point the MR to the physician will be negative because HMO profits are falling. However, in these circumstances the physician will not choose the level of effort that corresponds to maximum HMO profits but will choose instead level E_2, where the MR and marginal

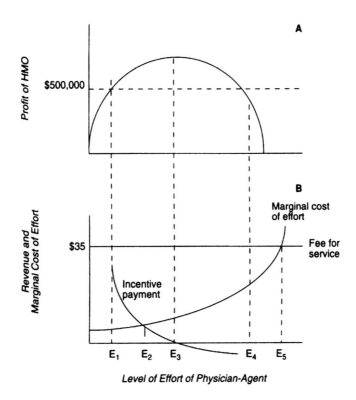

Figure 7–3 Optimal compensation of health care providers by an HMO. Graph A, the top diagram, shows the relationship between the providers' average effort and the HMO's profits. The minimum acceptable profit level for the HMO is $500,000. Graph B indicates each provider's level of effort under alternative payment schemes. The marginal cost of additional effort is the same under all payment schemes. Under a straight salary payment scheme, the provider will supply the minimum level of effort acceptable to the HMO, E_1. Under a fee-for-service scheme, at the assumed wage of $35 the provider will supply up to E_5, but only E_4 is acceptable. Under a profit incentive arrangement, E_2 will be provided. This is slightly less than the HMO's maximum profit because the incentive scheme is not "perfect."

---

cost curves intersect. This will provide the HMO with lower than maximum profits but more profits than under a salary compensation scheme.

There are numerous other compensation schemes that can be selected, some of which are more complicated but may motivate the physician to supply an effort close to the optimal level from the point of view of the HMO.

7.8.2 Management of Provider Behavior

In addition to setting contracts, insurers can engage in the direct management of provider supply behavior with the objective of influencing utilization patterns. The direct management of providers is an activity that is most closely associated with HMOs because of their close association with physicians. However, in recent years the management of care has become widespread under all types of payment

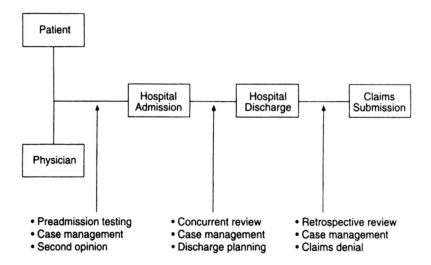

Figure 7–4 Techniques for managing provider behavior. Provider behavior can be regulated before, during, or after hospital admission. Prior to hospitalization, insurers can require providers to seek permission; during hospitalization, insurers can monitor length of stay; and following hospitalization, insurers can conduct reviews and deny claims.

arrangements. Most of these practices have been focused on the use of inpatient care, primarily because of the expense of this mode of care.

There are a number of different measures that insurers can use to influence providers' supply of hospital care (Scheffler et al. 1991). They include overall case management, preadmission management (e.g., second opinions and preadmission testing), concurrent management (e.g., concurrent review and discharge planning), and posthospital review (e.g., retrospective review and claims denials). Figure 7–4 indicates where the measures are applied. Each measure involves the setting of standards and the review of patients in accordance with these standards.

Many of the regulations set by HMOs carry financial penalties, such as nonpayment for a claim. For example, if a second opinion is required for surgery, payment might be denied if the surgeon operated without a confirming opinion. Probably for this reason, the private regulation of providers has been quite successful in containing utilization and costs. One study indicated savings of about 7 percent overall (Feldstein et al. 1988; Wickzier et al. 1989), although the savings will depend on the type of program and types of penalties imposed (Scheffler et al. 1991).

EXERCISES

1. Which costs are incurred by insurers when there is information asymmetry between payer/insurer and provider?
2. What are four different methods for reimbursing physicians?
3. How will each of these methods of paying physicians influence the volume of services supplied?

4. What "perverse" incentives must an insurer guard against in fee-for-service and per capita funding?

5. What is the Resource-Based Relative Value System and how were fees set in order to influence the volume of surgical and medical services?

6. What is retrospective hospital reimbursement and what incentives are created by this type of reimbursement?

7. What is prospective reimbursement? List three alternative bases of prospective hospital reimbursement.

8. How will each of the following bases for hospital reimbursement affect the number of admissions, the average length of stay, the volume of services per day, and the unit cost of services (cost per service):
   a. fee-for-service reimbursement
   b. per diem reimbursement
   c. fixed fee per admission

9. Indicate the effect of each of the following hospital reimbursement systems on the relative risks of the insurer and the hospital:
   a. retrospective reimbursement
   b. prospective fee-for-service reimbursement
   c. per diem fees
   d. per case reimbursement
   e. per case reimbursement plus outlier adjustments

10. What is the benefit of a diagnosis-related grouping system over a flat per diem reimbursement system?

11. If DRG001 (craniotomy) had a weight of 3.0970, how much would the hospital receive for a craniotomy case if the hospital was a teaching hospital in a large urban area?

12. How can a hospital influence its case mix?

13. What methods can be used to fund a long-term care facility on a prospective basis?

14. What indicators are used to place long-term care facility patients in a RUGs group?

15. If a single rate is set for all HMO members, what basis can the HMO use to recruit less costly members?

16. What criteria can be used to develop groups for HMOs who are paid for by Medicare?

17. What incentives do HMOs have with regard to
    a. recruiting members
    b. providing services to its members

BIBLIOGRAPHY

Per Capita Reimbursement

Anderson, G.F., and J. Knickman. 1984. Adverse selection under a voucher system: Grouping Medicare recipients by level of expenditure. *Inquiry* 21:135–143.

Anderson, G., et al. 1986. Paying for HMO care: Issues and options in setting capitation rates. *Milbank Quarterly* 64:548–565.

Anderson, G.F., et al. 1990. Setting payment rates for capitated systems: A comparison of various alternatives. *Inquiry* 27:225–233.

Beebe, J.A. 1992. Outlier pools for Medicare HMO payments. *Health Care Financing Review* 14 (fall): 59–63.

Ellwood, P. 1972. Models for organizing health services and implications for legislative proposals. *Milbank Quarterly* 50:73–100.

Enthoven, A. 1988. *Theory and practice of managed competition in health care finance.* Amsterdam, The Netherlands: North-Holland.

Giacomini, M., et al. 1995. Risk adjusting community rated health plan premiums. *Annual Review of Public Health* 16:401–430.

Hellinger, F.J. 1995. Selection bias in HMOs and PPOs: A review of the evidence. *Inquiry* 32:135–142.

Hornbrook, M.C. 1984. Examination of the AAPCC methodology in an HMO prospective payment demonstration experiment. *Group Health Journal* 5 (spring): 13–21.

Hornbrook, M.C., and S.E. Berki. 1985. Practice mode and payment method. *Medical Care* 23:484–511.

Hornbrook, M.C., and M.J. Goodman. 1991. Health plan case mix: Definition, measurement, use. *Advances in Health Economics and Health Services Research* 12:111–148.

———. 1995. Assessing relative health plan risk with the RAND-36 Health Survey. *Inquiry* 32:56–74.

Klarman, H.E. 1963. The effect of prepaid group practice on hospital use. *Public Health Reports* 78:955–965.

Luft, H.S. 1978a. How do health maintenance organizations achieve their "savings?" *New England Journal of Medicine* 298:1336–1343.

———. 1978b. Why do HMOs seem to provide more health maintenance services? *Milbank Quarterly* 56:140–168.

———. 1981. *Health maintenance organizations.* New York: John Wiley.

———. 1986. Compensating for biased selection in health insurance. *Milbank Quarterly* 64:566–591.

———. 1995. Potential methods to reduce risk selection and its effects. *Inquiry* 32:23–32.

Manton, K.G., and E. Stallard. 1992. Analysis of underwriting factors for AAPCC. *Health Care Financing Review* 14 (fall): 117–132.

Newhouse, J.P., et al. 1989. Adjusting capitation rates using objective health measures and prior utilization. *Health Care Financing Review* 10 (spring): 41–54.

van de Ven, W.P.M.M., et al. 1994. Risk adjusted capitation. *Health Affairs* 13:120–126.

Reimbursement and Supply: Physicians

Aaron, H., and W.B. Schwartz. 1984. *The painful prescription.* Washington, DC: Brookings Institution.

Blomquist, A. 1991. The doctor as double agent: Information asymmetry, health insurance, and medical care. *Journal of Health Economics* 10:411–432.

Burney, I.L., et al. 1978. Geographic variation in physicians' fees. *JAMA* 240:1368–1371.

Clark, D., and J.A. Olsen. 1994. Agency in health care with an endogenous budget constraint. *Journal of Health Economics* 13:231–251.

Cromwell, J., et al. 1997. Cost savings and physician responses to global bundled payments for Medicare heart bypass surgery. *Health Care Financing Review* 19 (fall): 41–57.

Eisenberg, J.M., and S.V. Williams. 1981. Cost containment and changing physicians' practice behavior. *JAMA* 246:2195–2201.

Epstein, A.M., and D. Blumenthal. 1993. Physician payment reform: Past and future. *Milbank Quarterly* 71:193–215.

Feldstein, M. 1970. The rising price of physicians' services. *Review of Economics and Statistics* 52:121–133.

Gabel, J.R., and M.A. Redisch. 1979. Alternative physician payment mechanisms. *Milbank Quarterly* 57:38–59.

Gruber, J., et al. 1999. Physician fees and procedure intensity: The case of cesarean delivery. *Journal of Health Economics* 18: 473–490.

Havighurst, C.C., and P. Kissam. 1979. The antitrust implications of relative value studies in medicine. *Journal of Health Politics, Policy and Law* 4:48.

Hemenway, D., et al. 1990. Physicians' responses to financial incentives. *New England Journal of Medicine* 322:1059–1063.

Holahan, J. 1989. The potential effects of an RBRVS-based payment system on health care costs and hospitals. *Frontiers of Health Services Management* 6:3–37.

Hornbrook, M.C. 1983. Allocative medicine: Efficiency, disease severity and the payment mechanism. *Annals of the AAPSS* 468:12–29.

Hsiao, W.C., and W.B. Stason. 1979. Toward developing a relative value scale for medical and surgical services. *Health Care Financing Review* 1:23–39.

Hsiao, W.C., et al. 1987. The resource based relative value scale. *JAMA* 258:799–802.

Hsiao, W.C., et al. 1988a. Results and policy implications of the resource based relative value study. *New England Journal of Medicine* 319:881–888.

Hsiao, W.C., et al. 1988b. Resource based relative values: An overview. *JAMA* 260:2347–2353.

Hsiao, W.C., et al. 1988c. Estimating physicians' work for a resource based relative value scale. *New England Journal of Medicine* 319:835–841.

Levy, J.M., et al. 1990. Impact of the Medicare fee schedule on payments to physicians. *JAMA* 264:717–722.

Lowenstein, S.R., et al. 1985. Prospective payment for physician services. *JAMA* 254:2632–2637.

Lu, M., and C. Donaldson. 2000. Performance-based contracts and provider efficiency. *Disease Management and Health Outcomes* 7:127–137.

Ma, A., and T.G. McGuire. 1997. Optimal health insurance and provider payment. *American Economic Review* 87:685–704.

Mitchell, J.B. 1985. Physician DRG's. *New England Journal of Medicine* 313:670–675.

Monsma, G. 1970. Marginal revenue and the demand for physicians' services. In *Empirical studies in health economics*, ed. H.F. Klarman. Baltimore: Johns Hopkins University Press.

Moore, S. 1979. Cost containment through risk sharing of primary-care physicians. *New England Journal of Medicine* 300:1359–1362.

Myers, L.P., and S.A. Schroeder. 1981. Physician use of services for the hospitalized patient. *Milbank Quarterly* 59:481–507.

Phelps, C.E. 1976. Public sector medicine. In *New directions in public health care*, ed. C.M. Lindsay. San Francisco: Institute for Contemporary Studies.

Schreiber, G.I., et al. 1976. Physician fee patterns under Medicare: A descriptive analysis. *New England Journal of Medicine* 294:1089–1093.

Showstack, J.A., et al. 1979. Fee-for-service payment: Analysis of current methods and their development. *Inquiry* 16:230–246.

Sisk, J., et al. 1987. Analysis of methods to reform Medicare payment for physician services. *Inquiry* 24:36–47.

Sloan, F.A. 1975. Physician supply behavior in the short run. *Industrial and Labor Relations Review* 28:549–569.

Sloan, F.A., and J.W. Hay. 1986. Medicare pricing mechanisms for physician services. *Medical Care Review* 43:59–100.

Stano, M., et al. 1983. Fee or use? What's responsible for rising health care costs? *Michigan Medicine* 82:228–234.

Wilensky, G.R., and L.F. Rossiter. 1986. Alternative units of payment for physician services. *Medical Care Review* 43:133–156.

Yip, W.C. 1998. Physician response to Medicare fee reductions. *Journal of Health Economics* 17:679–699.

Reimbursement and Supply: Long-term care facilities

Adams, E.K., and R.E. Schlenker. 1986. Case-mix reimbursement for nursing home services. *Health Care Financing Review* 8 (fall): 35–45.

Butler, P.A., and R.E. Schlenker. 1989. Case-mix reimbursement for nursing homes. *Milbank Quarterly* 67:103–136.

Fries, B.E., and L.M. Cooney. 1985. Resource utilization groups. *Medical Care* 23:110–122.

Fries, B.E., et al. 1994. Refining a case mix measure for nursing homes: Resource utilization groups (RUG-III). *Medical Care* 32:668–685.

Holahan, J., and J. Cohen. 1987. Nursing home reimbursement. *Milbank Quarterly* 65:112–147.

Katz, S., et al. 1963. Studies of illness in the aged. *JAMA* 185:914–919.

Micheletti, J., and T.J. Shlala. 1986. RUGs II: Implications for management and quality in long-term care. *Quality Review Bulletin* 12:236–242.

Rosko, M.D., et al. 1987. Prospective payment based on case-mix: Will it work in nursing homes? *Journal of Health Politics, Policy and Law* 12:683–701.

Schlenker, R.E. 1986. Case mix reimbursement for nursing homes. *Journal of Health Politics, Policy and Law* 11:445–461.

Schlenker, R.E., et al. 1985. Estimating patient level nursing home costs. *Health Services Research* 20:103–128.

Smits, H.L. 1984. Incentives in case-mix measures for long-term care. *Health Care Financing Review* 6 (winter): 53–59.

Reimbursement and Supply: Hospitals

Bauer, K. 1977. Hospital rate setting—this way to salvation? *Milbank Quarterly* 55:117–118.

Berry, R.E. 1976. Prospective reimbursement and cost containment. *Inquiry* 13:288–301.

Bradford, W.D., and C. Craycraft. 1996. Prospective payments and hospital efficiency. *Review of Industrial Organization* 11:791–809.

Dowling, W.L. 1974. Prospective reimbursement of hospitals. *Inquiry* 11:163–180.

Dranove, D., and W.D. White. 1987. Agency and the organization of health care delivery. *Inquiry* 24:405–415.

Eby, C.L., and D.R. Cohodes. 1985. What do we know about rate setting. *Journal of Health Politics, Policy and Law* 10:299–323.

Feldman, R., and F. Lobo. 1997. Global budgets and excess demand for hospital care. *Health Economics* 6:187–196.

Foster, R.W. 1982. Cost-based reimbursement and prospective payment: Reassessing the incentives. *Journal of Health Politics, Policy and Law* 7:407–420.

Horn, S.D., and P.D. Sharkey. 1983. Measuring severity of illness to predict patient resource use within DRGs. *Inquiry* 20:314–321.

Hornbrook, M. 1982. Hospital case mix: Its definition, measurement, and use. Parts 1, 2. *Medical Care Review* 39:1–43, 73–123.

Ligon, J.A. 1997. The capital structure of hospitals and reimbursement policy. *Quarterly Review of Economics and Business* 37:59–77.

Zuckerman, S., et al. 1984. Physician practice patterns under hospital rate-setting programs. *JAMA* 252:2589–2592.

Reimbursement and Supply: Pharmacies

Brooks, J.M., et al. 1999. Varying health care provider objectives and cost-shifting: The case of retail pharmacies in the U.S. *Health Economics* 8:127–150.

Diagnosis-Related Groups and Case Mix

Anderson, G., and P.B. Ginsburg. 1983. Prospective capital payment to hospitals. *Health Affairs* 2: 52–63.

Aronow, D. 1988. Severity of illness measurement. *Medical Care Review* 45:339–366.

Broyles, W.W., and M.D. Rosko. 1985. A qualitative assessment of the Medicare prospective payment system. *Social Science and Medicine* 20:1185–1190.

Carter, G.M., et al. 1994. Use of diagnosis-related groups by non-Medicare payers. *Health Care Financing Review* 16 (winter): 127–158.

Conrad, D.A. 1984. Returns on equity to not-for-profit hospitals. *Health Services Research* 19:41–63.

Cotterill, P.G.1991. Prospective payment for Medicare hospital capital. *Health Care Financing Review* (annual suppl.): 79–86.

Donaldson, C. 1991. Minding our Ps and Qs: Financial incentives for efficient hospital behavior. *Health Policy* 17:51–76.

Donaldson, C., and J. Magnusson. 1992. DRGs: The road to hospital efficiency. *Health Policy* 21:47–64.

Ellis, R.P., and T.G. McGuire. 1986. Provider behavior under prospective reimbursement. *Journal of Health Economics* 5:129–151.

———. 1988. Insurance principles and the design of prospective payment systems. *Journal of Health Economics* 7:215–237.

Ellis, R.P., and C.J. Ruhm. 1988. Incentives to transfer patients under alternative reimbursement mechanisms. *Journal of Public Economics* 37:381–394.

Fetter, R.B., et al. 1980. Case mix definition by diagnosis-related groups. *Medical Care* 18 (suppl 2): 1–53.

Fitzgerald, J.F., et al. 1987. Changing patterns of hip fracture before and after implementation of the prospective payment system. *JAMA* 258:218–221.

Fitzgerald, J.F., et al. 1988. The care of elderly patients with hip fracture. *New England Journal of Medicine* 319:1392–1397.

Gilman, B.H. 2000. Hospital response to DRG refinements: The impact of multiple reimbursement incentives on inpatient length of stay. *Health Economics* 9:277–294.

Hart AC, and B. Richards, eds. 2000. *DRG guidebook: A comprehensive resource to the DRG classification system, 2001.* 17th ed. Reston, VA: Ingenix Publishing Group.

Hsiao, W.C., and D.L. Dunn. 1987. The impact of DRG payments on New Jersey hospitals. *Inquiry* 24:212–220.

Lave, J.R. 1984. Hospital reimbursement under Medicare. *Milbank Quarterly* 62:251–268.

———. 1985. *The Medicare adjustment for the indirect costs of medical education.* Washington, DC: Association of American Medical Colleges.

———. 1989. The effect of the Medicare prospective payment system. *Annual Review of Public Health* 10:141–161.

Long, M.J., et al. 1987. The effects of PPS on hospital product and productivity. *Medical Care* 25:528–538.

McCarthy, C. 1988. DRGs—five years later. *New England Journal of Medicine* 318:1683–1686.

Morrisey, M., et al. 1988. Medicare prospective payment and post-hospital transfers to subacute care. *Medical Care* 26:685–698.

Muller, A. 1993. Medicare prospective payment reforms and hospital utilization. *Medical Care* 31:296–308.

Mullin, R.L. 1985. Diagnosis-related groups and severity. *JAMA* 253:1208–1210.

Neumann, B.R., and J.V. Kelly. 1984. *Prospective reimbursement for hospital capital costs.* Chicago: Healthcare Financial Management Association.

Omenn, G.S., and D.A. Conrad. 1984. Implications of DRG's for clinicians. *New England Journal of Medicine* 311:1314–1317.

Pettengill, J., and J. Vertrees. 1982. Reliability and validity in hospital case-mix measurement. *Health Care Financing Review* 4 (December): 101–128.

Russell, L. 1989. *Medicare's new hospital payment system.* Washington, DC: Brookings Institution.

Sloan, F.A., et al. 1988. Cost of capital to the hospital sector. *Journal of Health Economics* 7:25–45.

Vladeck, B.C. 1984. Medicare hospital payment by diagnosis-related group. *Annals of Internal Medicine* 100:576–591.

———. 1988. Hospital prospective payment and the quality of care. *New England Journal of Medicine* 319:1411–1413.

Wennberg, J.E., et al. 1984. Will payment based on diagnosis-related groups control hospital costs? *New England Journal of Medicine* 311:295–300.

Young, D.W., and R.B. Saltman. 1982. Medical practice, case mix, and cost containment. *JAMA* 247:801–805.

Other Case Mix Classification Systems

Kelly, W.P., et al. 1990. The classification of resource use in ambulatory surgery. *Journal of Ambulatory Care Management* 13, no. 1:55–63.

Optenberg, S.A., et al. 1990. A specialty-based ambulatory workload classification system. *Journal of Ambulatory Care Management* 13, no. 3:29–38.

Starfield, B., et al. 1991. Ambulatory care groups: A categorization of diagnoses for research and management. *Health Services Research* 26:53–74.

Steinman, M.G., et al. 1994. A case-mix classification system for medical rehabilitation. *Medical Care* 32:366–379.

Tenan, P.M., et al. 1988. PACs: Classifying ambulatory care patients and services for clinical and financial management. *Journal of Ambulatory Care Management* 11, no. 3:36–53.

Weiner, J.P., et al. 1991. Development and application of a population-oriented measure of ambulatory care-mix. *Medical Care* 29:452–472.

Provider Supply under Managed Care Contracting

Blough, D.K., et al. 1999. Modeling risk using generalized linear models. *Journal of Health Economics* 18:153–171.

Burgess, J.F., et al. 2000. Medical profiling: Improving standards and risk adjustments using hierarchical models. *Journal of Health Economics* 19:291–309.

Debrock, A., and R.J. Arnould. 1992. Utilization control in HMOs. *Quarterly Review of Economics and Business* 32 (3):31–53.

Feldstein, P.J., et al. 1988. The effects of utilization review programs on health care use and expenditures. *New England Journal of Medicine* 318:1310–1314.

Health Care Financing Administration. 1999. *Medicare + Choice rates—45 day notice*. Baltimore, MD: Health Care Financing Administration. <http://www.hcfa.gov/stats/hmorates/45d-02.htm>.

Hillman, A.L. 1987. Financial incentives for physicians in HMOs. *New England Journal of Medicine* 317:1743–1748.

Hillman, A.L., et al. 1989. How do financial incentives affect physicians' clinical decisions and the financial performance of health maintenance organizations? *New England Journal of Medicine* 321:86–92.

Hirth, R.A., and M.E. Chernew. 1999. The physician labor market in a managed care–dominated environment. *Economic Inquiry* 37:282–294.

Keeler, E.B., et al. 1998. A model of the impact of reimbursement schemes on health plan choice. *Journal of Health Economics* 17:297–320.

Pauly, M.V., et al. 1990. Managing physician incentives in managed care. *Medical Care* 28:1013–1024.

Robinson, J.C. 1993. Payment mechanisms, nonprice incentives, and organizational innovations in health care. *Inquiry* 30:328–332.

Rubin, P.H., and J.L. Schrag. 1999. Mitigating agency problems by advertising, with special reference to managed health care. *Southern Economic Journal* 66:39–60.

Scheffler, R.M., et al. 1991. The impact of Blue Cross and Blue Shield plan utilization management programs, 1980–1988. *Inquiry* 28:276–287.

Wickizer, T.M., et al. 1989. Does utilization review reduce unnecessary hospital care and contain costs? *Medical Care* 27:632–647.

Competitive Markets

1. Specify the assumptions of a competitive market model.
2. Use the competitive model to predict movements in price and utilization due to changes in factors that influence supply and demand for health services.
3. Use the supply-demand framework to predict the factors that influence shortages and surpluses.
4. Identify the evidence for and against the competitive model.
5. Describe the factors that influence how the competitive bidder sets the price for a contract.
6. Define the concept of supplier-induced demand and describe the influence of supply on price in a market in which supplier-induced demand exists.

8.1 INTRODUCTION

In previous chapters a number of hypotheses about the behavior of demanding and supplying units were developed. These hypotheses that dealt with demand behavior and supply behavior were examined in isolation. As a result, although we developed a way of predicting what quantity would be demanded (supplied) at any price, our model did not incorporate simultaneous consideration of the behavior of the supplying and demanding units and thus could not tell us whether the same quantity would be both demanded and supplied.

Beginning with this chapter, our focus shifts to models in which demanders and suppliers interact. The setting in which this interaction occurs is called a *market*. A market in economics should not be thought of as a physical location; rather, the term *market* denotes the web of interactions between those who have commercial relationships or the potential to have such relationships with other buyers and sellers of similar commodities. For example, we can think of a market for psychiatric services as consisting of a group of consumers and a group of providers who have the potential to enter into commercial relations with all members of the other group. Central to the analysis of the functioning of a market is the price that the buyer pays and the seller receives. In previous expositions, the price was taken as given for both groups; variations in price were beyond the control of any one buyer or seller. Yet, as a consequence of the related interactions of these groups, prices are set; as a result of some change in demand or supply behavior, prices change.

The market analyses that we will examine involve two categories of concepts:

1. *Phenomena to be explained.* These are objective events, such as changes in the price or the quantity of medical care utilized. The phenomenon of interest might be a rise in prices, and our models would be used to explain why the phenomenon occurred.
2. *Behavioral relationships.* The economic "forces" influencing these phenomena have been referred to as *demand* and *supply*. The strength of these forces can be increased or decreased by individual factors, such as incomes and tastes on the demand side and input prices on the supply side. Demand can be increased, for example, by higher consumer incomes, and supply can be decreased by higher input costs. As a consequence of changes in causal factors, demand or supply will change, as will price and quantity. Our models should be able to predict such causal chains of events.

In this chapter, one particular market model is developed and used to explain the outcome of price and quantity in the medical care market. This is the competitive market model, which treats the market as an interactive mechanism with many suppliers competing for consumer business. Such a model is helpful in explaining a broad range of phenomena. It offers hypotheses to explain rising prices; increasing or decreasing utilization; shortages in commodities such as physicians' services, nursing services, and blood; and surpluses in commodities such as hospital beds. Thus it is a valuable starting point for any analysis of markets. The competitive market model is presented in Section 8.2, and the predictions of the model are discussed in Section 8.3. Although the competitive model is able to generate a large number of predictions, not all the predictions are borne out by actual events. Indeed, several events are either at odds with or fail to corroborate the predictions of the competitive model. Since accurate prediction is the bottom line of explanatory economics, Section 8.4 is devoted to a discussion of corroborating evidence relating to the competitive hypothesis. Section 8.5 discusses a recent application of the competitive hypothesis in the health care field, in particular, the use of the model to explain selective contracting. Section 8.6 concerns a deviation from the competitive market that involves the notion of supplier-induced demand.

8.2 THE COMPETITIVE MODEL: ASSUMPTIONS

In our exposition of the competitive model, we will use a market for physician services as our example. The product is physician visits, which we will assume to be of constant quality, each characterized by the same accuracy of diagnosis, effectiveness of treatment, and personal attentiveness.

- *Individual demand.* Our initial demand assumption is that each consumer has a normal demand curve. This includes the stipulation that consumers are fully informed about the nature of the services they require and the benefits that they can obtain. This stipulation implies that physicians cannot *directly* influence consumer demand for medical care.

- *Market demand.* We further assume that there are many consumers in the market and that they are competing for physician services. This assumption rules out the possibility that buyers are large enough or can join together to have any influence over price. The market demand curve (*D*) in our model is shown in Figure 8–1. Here conditions are assumed to be such that, at a price of $2.50 per visit, the quantity demanded is 500 visits: at $2.40, the quantity demanded is 600 units; at $2.00, the quantity demanded is 1,000 units; and so on. Curve *D* traces out this relationship. Any change in the underlying causal factors (tastes, for example) will shift demand. These causal factors are listed in the diagram for the purpose of reminding the reader of the underlying assumptions of the model.
- *Individual supply.* Our supply assumptions can similarly be separated into assumptions about individual suppliers and about the supplier group. Individually, each supplier has an upward-sloping marginal cost curve. Assuming supplier profit maximization and no supplier influence over price (a market assumption), the marginal cost curve is the supply curve.
- *Market supply.* With regard to the supplier group, we assume there are many suppliers, they do not collude with each other to influence price, and none is large enough by itself to influence price.

Consumers are assumed to be aware of the price offers of alternative suppliers and so can compare prices when making purchase decisions. Because of consumer knowledge, any supplier charging a higher price than what would prevail in a competitive situation will sell no units. Charging a lower price will mean forgoing some intramarginal profits. And so, in such a market, each supplier will take the price as given and supply the quantity at which price equals *MC*. The market supply will be the summed individual suppliers' marginal cost curves. Market supply is shown in Figure 8–1 as curve *S*, with 700 units supplied at $1.70, 800 at $1. 80, 1,000 at $2.00, and so on. The factors influencing the position of the supply curve are also shown.

Under these conditions of supply and demand, bargaining occurs between consumers and producers. An equilibrium is reached when the quantity demanded equals the quantity supplied. The next section is devoted to the predictions of the model. That is, it presents what we would expect the market outcome to be (in terms of prices and quantities) if such conditions were approximated in reality.

8.3 THE COMPETITIVE MODEL: PREDICTIONS

8.3.1 Overview

Several important groups of conclusions can be drawn from the competitive model regarding how resources are allocated in the health care sector. These conclusions are presented next. Keep in mind that these conclusions are presented as possible explanations whose usefulness is determined by how well they conform to actual experience.

8.3.2 Market Price

In a competitive market a single price will emerge that clears the market. Competitive bidding will lower the price if a surplus of output exists (i.e., if there is

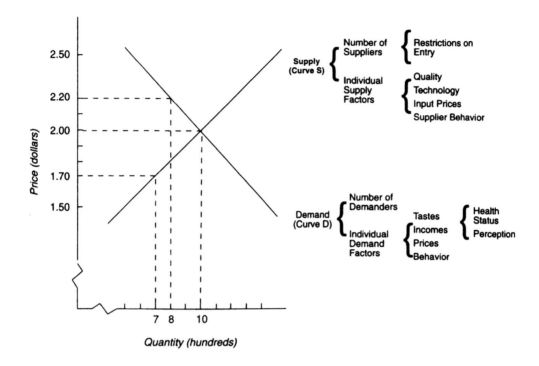

Figure 8–1 Representation of the interaction of behavioral relationships. The phenomena, price and quantity, are influenced by supply and demand. These, in turn, are affected by a number of individual causal factors (listed in the diagram). The positions of the supply and demand curves have been set based on the assumption that supply and demand are at given levels. Changes in the magnitude of any of the underlying factors will cause a shift in supply or demand (or both).

---

unsold output or excess capacity) and will raise the price in the case of a shortage. Only when buyers are satisfied with the quantities they purchase at the established price and sellers are making maximum profits will market equilibrium be established (i.e., quantity supplied equals quantity demanded). In our example, equilibrium will be reached at a price of $2.00 and a supply of 1,200 visits.

If the price is higher, say, $2.10, then 900 units of service will be demanded, whereas the suppliers will be prepared to supply 1,100. To eliminate this excess capacity, physicians will lower prices and the amounts supplied. The quantity demanded will increase at the same time. The process goes on until both groups are simultaneously satisfied. The quantity supplied will just equal the quantity that consumers demand. The same process will occur in reverse if the price is below $2.00, in which case prices will be driven up to the equilibrium point.

It can be shown that the end result of this process is a single price charged by all producers. If any single physician charged more than the equilibrium price per visit, then his or her patients, who we assume to possess full knowledge of prices charged by other physicians, would obtain medical care elsewhere. The physician would be forced to bring his or her price down to the price other physicians are charging. On the other hand, if a physician sets fees below the equilibrium level, patients will flock to this physician, creating an overload of work. Given a rising *MC* schedule for this physician, if he provides service for the additional patients, the profits gained from the sale of each additional unit will in fact be negative. The physician with such an *MC* schedule would have been better off profitwise to accept the highest price, which is the market price. That a single market-clearing price will emerge is thus one conclusion of the competitive model.

8.3.3 Price and Quantity Movements Caused by Demand Shifts

Additional conclusions based on the competitive model can be drawn regarding price and quantity movements when there is a change in any of the factors that influence demand. This set of conclusions is illustrated in Figure 8–2. Assume D_1 to be the demand curve consistent with given initial values of underlying causal factors of demand. Let *S* be the supply curve, which remains stable because all supply shift factors are assumed constant. The equilibrium price for these conditions is P_1 ($2.00), and the equilibrium quantity for the market is Q_1 (1,000 visits). If any of the initial conditions that influence demand change, causing an increase in demand to D_2, for example, there will be a new equilibrium price ($2.10) and a new quantity (1,200 units). The willingness of consumers to buy more at each price allows the producers to increase profits by producing more output (up to 1,200 units). Such a shift in demand can be caused by higher consumer incomes or a greater degree of illness in the population. Or it can be caused by an increase in the amount of health insurance purchased, which also causes demand to shift out (see Section 3.6). In either case, the result is the same—higher prices and quantities. The

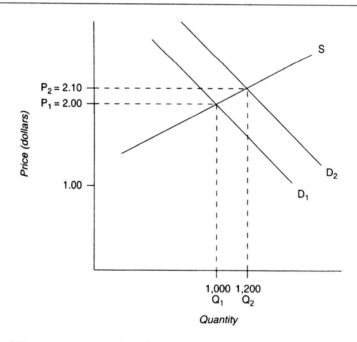

Figure 8–2 Representation of shift in demand with stable supply. An initial set of supply and demand forces, characterized by D_1 and *S*, will produce given price and output levels. An increase in demand to D_2, with a stable *S*, will cause price and output to increase.

opposite situation, lower prices and quantities, would be the consequence of factors shifting demand downward.

If the quantity utilized is to increase, additional quantity must be available. *Utilization* refers to the actual quantity traded in the market. This should not be confused with the amount demanded, because when there is disequilibrium, more (or less) might be demanded than is supplied. Nor should it be confused with the quantity offered by the supplier, because at any one price more (or less) might be supplied than consumers are willing to take at that price. Disequilibrium situations occur when the price does not adjust to allow the quantity demanded and the quantity supplied to equalize.

8.3.4 Price and Quantity Movements Caused by Supply Shifts

Another set of conclusions based on the model concern changes in factors that cause the supply to shift. What occurs if there is an increase in supply is shown in Figure 8–3. In this example, the commodity becomes less scarce and the supply shifts from S_1 to S_2. If the demand remains the same, the supply increases relative to the demand and the price falls. As a result, a new lower price ($1.00) and a higher

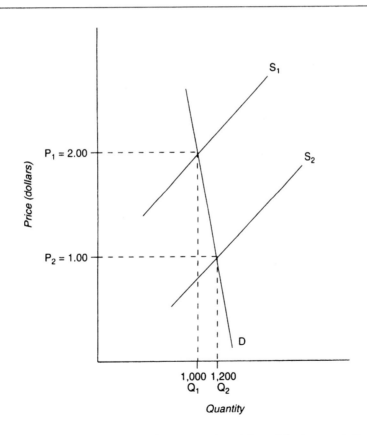

Figure 8–3 Representation of shifting supply with stable demand. Beginning with an initial demand and supply levels D and S_1 and resulting price and output levels, an increase in supply to S_2 will cause output to increase and price to fall.

level of utilization (1,200 units) are predicted. Of course, a factor that causes a reduction in supply will have the opposite effect on the price and the quantity utilized.

Changes in supply can occur because of changes in circumstances that are beyond the control of supplying firms (and to which they react) or because of changes that the present or potential suppliers themselves initiate. For example, if hospitals or public health departments decide to hire medical technicians, they will enter the market and bid for the existing supply of technicians. This will raise the price of technicians that all market participants have to pay, because the supply will initially remain relatively stable while the demand will increase. An increase in the price of technician services (or for that matter of any input) will shift the supply curve of all producers who use this input to the left. Thus, the market supply curve will shift leftward as well, and the price of physician services will increase.

Provider-initiated changes in supply will be undertaken by for-profit suppliers when these changes have the potential to add to profits. Three types of situations are discussed below:

1. a change in input combinations brought about by existing suppliers
2. an increase in the capital stock of existing suppliers
3. entry into the market by new suppliers

An example of the first situation, a change in input combinations, might occur if physicians were to hire nurse practitioners to perform, at a lower cost, services previously performed by the physicians themselves. Such a change might be the result of the passage of a law allowing such substitution to occur. The effect would be to shift the average total cost curve downward and the marginal cost curve to the right. In a competitive market, one supplier making such a change would not cause a large shift in the market supply curve. Prices would remain about the same, and that one supplier would reap an increase in profits. However, if all suppliers made a change, the market supply curve would shift to the right considerably, and the price of medical care would then fall. Consumers would reap the benefits from such actions. The net profit position of each provider after all suppliers have acted may not be any greater than before, because the price of output has fallen, but it is important to note that the providers make their decisions to undertake cost-reducing activities based on preexisting prices. Providers do not collude with their fellow suppliers, and they do not always anticipate that prices will fall as a consequence of their concerted actions. The end result of their actions, however, is lower prices and greater utilization.

The same process occurs when existing suppliers invest in plant and equipment. Additions to capital are often made in anticipation of additions to profits because of lower unit costs. If these investments cut costs, and if they are sufficiently widespread in the industry, the net effect will be to lower prices and raise utilization. As a result, after these effects have worked themselves out, profits may be no greater than before (they may even be less). These effects are presented in a before-after manner here. In actuality, they take a considerable time to occur. The potential for profits must first be realized, planning for the additions and financing them must occur, and the additional capital equipment and plant must then be constructed and put into use. As a result, the increase in supply and the fall in price may take months and even years. For this reason, the analysis of provider behavior involving capital additions, with resulting shifts in average and marginal cost curves, has been referred to as *long-run analysis.* (It is generally difficult to decide when a change in supply conditions is long run and when it is short run. Short-run changes are usually taken to be changes in quantity supplied that occur without changes in capital equipment.)

The third type of variation in supply occurs when new (profit-seeking) suppliers enter an industry or a market in response to high profits. Such a movement results in an increase in supply and a consequent fall in price and an increase in utilization. In this instance, since the cost conditions of existing suppliers remain the same, the profit levels must fall for all existing suppliers.

The conditions that determine how easily potential providers can actually enter the industry and place their products on the market are referred to as *conditions of entry.* These conditions depend on existing productive techniques as well as on legal impediments. In some industries, extensive capital requirements preclude many firms from entering because of the large financial commitment necessary to undertake the capital investment and commence production. Such requirements may exist for some types of medical care, such as intensive surgery, although the financial impediments are not nearly as great as they are, for example, in the automobile industry. For many types of medical care, financial impediments are not relevant to entry. More relevant are the legal impediments, such as the licensing requirements for medical personnel and facilities. Licensing regulations frequently amount to restrictions placed on potential entrants into an industry.

8.3.5 Simultaneous Demand and Supply Shifts

In addition to creating movements in either demand or supply alone, where the effects are readily predictable, underlying factors may cause shifts in both demand and supply at the same time. We must be careful at this stage of the analysis to specify that we are referring to separate factors causing changes in demand and supply. That is, an increase in the number of ill people occurring at the same time as an influx of physicians into the market will cause both demand and supply curves to shift; the increase in the illness level will cause demand to increase, and the increase in the number of physicians will cause supply to increase. In Figure 8–4, this is shown as a shift in demand from D_1 to D_2 and, at the same time, a shift in supply from S_1 to S_2. Although quantity increases, the net effect on price is ambiguous and will depend on how much each curve shifts, that is, on the changes in the values of the causal variables and the degree to which they cause demand and supply to shift. In the specific case illustrated in Figure 8–4, price will fall. But if we do not know the extent to which both curves are shifted, our model fails us as a predictive device.

A second type of simultaneous shift may occur when the same factor that causes demand to shift independently causes supply to shift. An increase in quality, for example, will cause supply to decrease and demand to increase. When demand increases and supply decreases, price will increase, but quantity will increase, fall, or remain the same depending on the extent of the shifts. (Another type of simultaneous shift that does *not* belong in this category is when the factors affecting supply and demand are not independent, such as when physicians can induce consumer demand. This phenomenon is discussed in Section 8.6.)

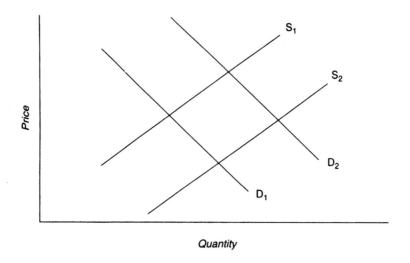

Figure 8–4 Representation of the simultaneous shifting of demand and supply curves. Beginning with initial demand and supply levels D_1 and S_1 and resulting price and output levels, a simultaneous shift in demand and supply curves (to D_2 and S_2) will have an ambiguous effect on price and will increase output. The extent of both shifts determines the effects on price and quantity. Some directional shifts, such as a decrease in demand and a simultaneous increase in supply, will lower the price but have an ambiguous effect on quantity traded.

8.3.6 Shortages

Our predictions so far have been concerned with what happens to the equilibrium price when one or several factors change. Not all situations are such that the quantity demanded is the quantity supplied. The medical care market often experiences shortages. A shortage occurs when the quantity demanded exceeds the quantity supplied at the current price. Our model shows that in a competitive market with free bidding, a shortage will cause the price to rise. Then the suppliers will offer more services and the consumers will reduce their demand, making the shortage disappear. That is the theory, although persistent shortages have been observed in the blood market, the market for nurses, the physician services market, and, in some countries, the hospital market. A slight modification of the competitive model allows us to predict why these shortages occur and how they can be eliminated.

Refer to the example in Figure 8–1. Assume that, because of a government regulation, the price cannot rise above $1.70 per visit. Perhaps the regulation is passed and enforced to help low-income consumers, who may go without medical services if the price is $2.00. The consequences of the passage of the regulation can be determined using the competitive model. At $1.70, consumers will be more willing to visit their physicians, and according to our figures 1,300 will call for appointments. But at this price it would be unprofitable for physicians to see 1,300 patients. Indeed, they will reduce quantity supplied and will see only 700 patients. A queue will form of untreated patients; in this case, 600 patients who want treatment will be untreated. Some shortages are the result of such price ceilings. In a competitive market, a shortage can only persist if the price is somehow administered to remain below the market-clearing price. This will usually be done by an official or semiofficial agency that can overrule the price that market forces set.

A shortage can also occur when insurance is purchased or when a government program "guaranteeing" medical care is instituted. In such situations, the consumers may face a zero money price, which will mean a high quantity demanded (e.g., 10,000 units, as shown in Figure 8–5). The reimbursed price to the provider may be only $20 per unit, and at this price 7,000 units are provided. In our example, it would take a price of $100 to bring forth a supply of 10,000 units. At the administered reimbursement rate of $20, there is a shortage of 3,000 units.

The situation requires a mechanism to ration the 7,000 available units, assuming that the quality produced remains the same. One tactic is to make the prospective patients wait in line; those who are willing to pay the "time costs" will receive the service (Buchanan 1965; Culyer and Cullis 1976; Sloan and Lorant 1976). Another possibility is for the providers to lower the quality of their product, for example, by reducing the time devoted to providing the service. This action would reduce demand, since the commodity would not have the same worth as before, and it would increase supply. As a result, the shortage would be reduced and perhaps even eliminated.

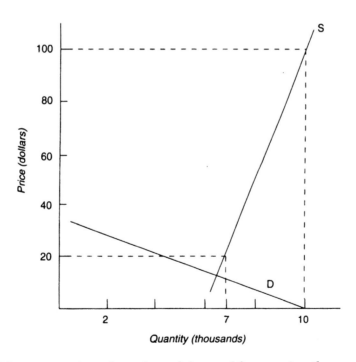

Figure 8–5 Representation of supply and demand forces using the example of full-service coverage by a third-party. Full-service (zero out-of-pocket price) coverage with a reimbursement rate of $20 will lead to a quantity demanded of 10,000 and a quantity supplied of 7,000. To reach a quantity supplied of 10,000, the reimbursement rate would have to be $100 (curve *S*).

8.3.7 Surpluses

The usual definition of a surplus is an excess of quantity supplied over quantity demanded at a given price. For a surplus to persist, some factor must keep quantity supplied above quantity demanded. If the price in the market was kept permanently above the equilibrium price, a surplus would persist: Suppliers would be willing to provide more units than consumers would be willing to purchase. In Figure 8–1, if the suppliers' reimbursed price and the consumers' out-of-pocket price were both $2.10 and could not be lowered, a surplus would appear. In this case, suppliers would be willing to supply more units at that price than demanders would want, and the suppliers would find themselves with excess capacity.

For a surplus to persist, something must prevent the market price from falling, because in a normal competitive situation an excess supply would induce suppliers to lower their prices to induce demanders to buy more. If the government pegged or supported an above-equilibrium price in the market, a surplus would occur. In the case of health care, where insurance exists, a surplus can occur if the reimbursement rate suppliers receive induces a greater quantity supplied than the quantity demanded by consumers at the price they have to pay out of pocket. In Figure 8–1, if the reimbursement rate was $2.50 and the out-of-pocket price was $1.50, a surplus would exist.

In the early 1990s there was much talk of a "physician surplus" (Schwartz and Mendelson 1990). In discussions of this topic one heard talk of falling physicians' fees and incomes (although this not always borne out by the data). To the extent that the fees and incomes of physicians were falling during that period, this situation was not a surplus in the technical sense. Falling fees are characteristic of prices responding to a shift in supply en route to a new equilibrium point. For a surplus to develop, the market cannot be allowed to move to a new equilibrium; it must remain in *dis*equilibrium.

The surplus in hospital beds is more likely a case of permanent disequilibrium. High hospital reimbursement rates have induced a large quantity supplied; at given out-of-pocket prices, there has not been enough quantity demanded to clear the market.

8.3.8 Multimarket Analyses

The competitive model is well suited to making predictions about the effect of supply and/or demand changes in one market on price and quantity in a related market. Let us take an example of two substitute services, inpatient and outpatient surgical care. Because of the development of quicker acting anesthetics, outpatient surgery has become more feasible. Further, the total cost of outpatient surgery is much less than inpatient surgery for most cases, and outpatient surgery for many procedures is now covered.

Analytically, the impact of moving from no outpatient coverage for a procedure (e.g., tonsillectomy) to outpatient coverage is shown in Figure 8–6. The pre-outpatient-coverage market for inpatient procedures is characterized in Graph A. Here S is the inpatient supply curve and D_i is the inpatient demand curve. In Graph B, D_n is the demand curve for outpatient tonsillectomies (without insurance) and S is the supply curve. Note that the demand function for *inpatient* care is dependent on the out-of-pocket price for *outpatient* surgery because the two are substitutes.

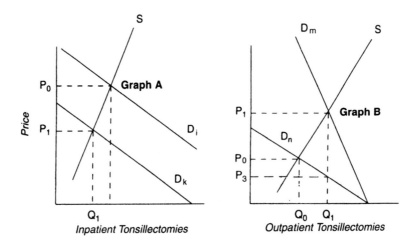

Figure 8–6 Representation of multimarket analysis. Demand curves in inpatient and outpatient markets are related (the services are substitutes). When the out-of-pocket price in the outpatient market falls (because of an increase in insurance coverage), the demand curve in the inpatient market shifts inward and price and quantity fall.

Initially, there is no insurance coverage for outpatient tonsillectomies and P_0 is the prevailing price. An increase in outpatient coverage will shift the market curve for outpatient care outward (to D_m in Graph B) and simultaneously lower the out-of-pocket price of outpatient care from P_0 to a point such as P_3. This will result in an inward shift in the D_i curve for inpatient care to D_k. The inpatient price will fall and the quantity of inpatient procedures will be reduced. Note also that the outpatient procedures will be increased.

Similar types of analyses can be conducted for other types of substitute procedures. It can also be conducted for complements, such as film and radiologist services. In some cases, it is not clear whether two services are substitutes or complements. For example, it is not clear whether nursing home care replaces hospital care or is used in conjunction with it. The same holds for home health care and hospital care. In these instances, the model cannot provide unambiguous conclusions.

8.4 EVIDENCE FOR AND AGAINST THE COMPETITIVE MODEL

8.4.1 Overview

There has been some use of the competitive model in explaining resource allocation trends in medical care markets. In the physician services market, the phenomenon of rapidly rising physician fees, both before and after the watershed year of 1966, when Medicare and Medicaid were instituted (see Chapter 14), was explained using the competitive model by hypothesizing that the rapid increase in medical care insurance caused demand shifts and consequent rising prices. In this market, the length of time required to train new physicians means a slow supply response, even in a competitive market, and prices would be expected to rise

(Garbarino 1959; Newhouse et al. 1977). In the hospital care market, the same type of explanation can be made for rising hospital costs, with one modification. Although insurance was increasing during this time period, hospital input prices, notably employee wages, were also rapidly rising. This latter phenomenon would shift the supply curve inward. Couple this with a rapidly outward shifting demand curve for hospital care, and the net effect would be a larger price increase. Whether utilization would increase or decrease would depend on the magnitude of both shifts. As seen in Chapter 2, hospital utilization increased. Our "after the fact" explanation would state that the supply and demand shifts were such that the increase in utilization was likely to occur. (An application of the competitive model to the hospital field is found in Ro [1977].)

The competitive model has also been used to explain the persisting queues and unmet demands that have resulted from the institution of the National Health Service (NHS) in Great Britain in 1946. The NHS is characterized by a zero money price paid by consumers, per capita remuneration for general practitioners, and salaried remuneration for surgeons. The competitive model applied to this type of health care system would predict large increases in quantity demanded following the lowering of the price to zero. Supply decisions passed into the hands of the central government, and large increases in supply did not materialize. As a result, persistent shortages occurred, particularly in hospital care (Culyer and Cullis 1976).

Although the competitive model is a useful device for explaining price and quantity movements and uncovering the causes of shortages of medical care, much attention has focused on the shortcomings of the model. Evidence of the existence of shortcomings might be gotten in three ways. First, we might examine data on market outcomes, such as profits and prices. If such outcomes are not what we would expect in a competitive market (i.e., not what the competitive model predicts would happen), we could infer that the model does not explain what we have observed and seek alternative models to better explain the data. Secondly, we might observe some conditions and characteristics of a market, such as consumer ignorance or product quality level differences. If the observed characteristics are at odds with the competitive model's assumptions, we should consider seeking a different model that incorporates realistic assumptions. Third, we might observe direct actions on the part of providers that suggest the prevalence of noncompetitive practices. These might include constraints on certain activities usually thought of as competitive, such as entry into the market. We now turn to some of the evidence that the competitive model has serious flaws as a model of the health care market.

8.4.2 Excessive Profits

Studies made of the profits accruing from medical practice have shown these profits to be persistent and considerable. These profits, which are the net incomes of the physicians operating the practices, must be adjusted for the costs incurred in medical training, including fees paid and earnings forgone while practicing medicine or during internship and residency. Even after adjusting for these costs, the net present value of medical practice indicates the existence of persistently high profits (i.e., earnings in excess of normal returns) (Lindsay 1976; Sloan 1976). Generally, the competitive model predicts that such excess profits would eventually be bid away by new providers entering the industry to take advantage of the high returns. This has not occurred in medical practice.

8.4.3 Fee Differences among Patients

The competitive model predicts that one price will prevail in the market for all suppliers and demanders. Before the spread of health insurance, physician pricing was characterized by a sliding scale of fees, with high-income patients paying higher prices than low-income patients. This phenomenon has led economists to reject the competitive model as inappropriate for the physician services market and to substitute a monopoly model (Kessell 1958; Newhouse 1970; Ruffin and Leigh 1973; Wu and Masson 1974; see Chapter 9).

8.4.5 Quality of Care

The competitive model assumes that a homogeneous service is being bought and sold and that competition is based on price. Yet product quality is a major element of a hospital's output, and health insurance companies often offer different types of policies in terms of coverage (viewed as differences in the quality of the policy as well as differences in service).

When a supplier can vary its quality, it can attract consumers on the basis of its quality. It follows that some "brand loyalty" may ensue, and buyers will not switch brands easily (because of a slight increase in price, for example). This phenomenon is called *product differentiation*, and it implies that each supplier then faces a downward-sloping demand curve, not a horizontal one (as is the case in perfect competition), and can choose to compete with other providers on the basis of price or product quality. The competitive model is not equipped to handle this feature of the health care market, which requires a somewhat more complex model.

8.4.6 Restricting Competitive Behavior

Additional evidence of anticompetitive control mechanisms is found by examining the behavior of physicians when confronted with potentially competitive colleagues. Two practices have been restricted by physician associations: the advertising of physician fees and the participation by physicians in prepayment group practices. In an ideal world, such as that set out in the model in Section 8.2, advertising is unnecessary because consumers know all about physician fees. But in the real world considerable consumer ignorance exists, and advertising would reduce ignorance about alternative physician prices (and perhaps qualifications). Coupled with fee cutting (price reductions), advertising would result in more business for the fee-cutting advertiser but in generally lower prices and profits in the industry.

Advertising bans have been enforced by state medical societies (Kessell 1958), and although such bans are no longer legally enforceable, their existence in the past was evidence that physicians were able to intervene in the market on behalf of themselves and eliminate some degree of competition in the market. Bans on advertising (and other competitive practices) have been used as evidence of the availability of mechanisms to restrict competition.

8.4.7 Consumer Ignorance and Supplier-Induced Demand

The competitive model operates under the assumption that consumers possess a considerable degree of information about their condition, the products they need, and the outcomes of using the products. In fact, consumers appear to operate under a considerable degree of ignorance in this area, which has led some commentators to view physicians as essentially agents acting on behalf of consumers (Feldstein 1974). If physicians do behave as agents for their patients, the implicit assumption that suppliers and demanders are acting independently must be rejected. Demand is subject to direct supplier influence.

Nor can we assume that, if they do act as agents for their patients, physicians always behave in the patients' best interests. Because of information asymmetry, the possibility exists that physicians can use their influence to further their own interests. Consumer demands can be shifted by the suppliers through the provision of biased information.

Demand shifting can be detected in market outcome statistics in some circumstances. According to the competitive theory, an increase in the per capita supply of physicians results in an increase in market supply. With everything else held constant, this should bring down the price of health care. Yet it has been alleged that the relationship between physician per capita supply and price is exactly opposite to that predicted by the model; that is, the more physicians per capita in an area, the higher the observed price (Evans 1974; Fuchs and Kramer 1972). The reason why this phenomenon is not considered proven is that a number of intervening factors exist that may cause demand to rise at the same time as physician supply increases.

Let us make a simple comparison of two hypothetical medical markets, one in a small town and one in a large metropolitan center with several medical schools. The large city may have more physicians per capita than the small town, and yet the price for a visit to a physician may be greater. This "raw" relationship by itself does not mean that the higher supply has caused the higher price. Many other intervening variables must also be taken into account, among them insurance, the health status of the two populations, and the quality of care provided. The third factor, the quality of care, is especially important in making comparisons, mainly because it is such a difficult variable to measure and thus may be ignored. It may well be that the quality of care in the city is higher than in the town. If all factors other than the quality of care were adjusted for, we might still observe a positive relationship between physician density and price. Until quality has been adjusted for, however, we cannot be certain that the higher price is not due to the fact that better quality service is being provided.

This type of confounding relationship has caused controversy regarding the observed relationship between price and physician density (Sloan and Feldman 1978). Some commentators have proceeded as if it were true and have constructed alternative supplier-induced demand models.

8.5 COMPETITIVE BIDDING

The competitive market has often been held up as an ideal, a standard in the light of which other allocative arrangements might be judged. One mechanism that has been put forward as potentially providing a competitive-style outcome for public programs is competitive bidding. Competitive bidding occurs when a purchaser (e.g., a government agency) requests bids from alternative competing providers and allocates the right to treat patients based on the bids. The object of this practice is to have the patients treated for the least cost.

One approach to developing a model of the competitive bidding process is to examine the behavior of an individual supplier who is facing a single paying agency and who is competing with other providers for the right to provide the services. In constructing such a model, it is essential to recognize that the bids are made under conditions of risk. When they submit their bids, the bidders do not know for certain whether or not they will be selected as providers. Their behavior can be modeled in a manner similar to that of consumers who are faced with risky medical expenses.

The bidder faces two possible outcomes: (1) the bid is accepted, or (2) the bid is rejected. To simplify matters, let us assume that no losses are associated with an unsuccessful bid (i.e., the bidder is no worse off than if he or she did not bid). What the bidder must do is compare the outcomes of the various bids to assess which will prove the most satisfactory.

Our simplified model is presented in numerical form in Table 8–1. We make the following assumptions. First, a request is put out calling for providers to bid for the right to serve a given number of patients in a public program. The bids are to be expressed in per capita terms for a certain set of services (physician care, hospital care, and drugs). Second, five options (labeled A through E) are open to the bidder: bids of $100, $95, $90, $85, and $80. Third, as the bidder lowers his or her bid, the probability of having the bid accepted increases. At a bid of $100, there is a 20-percent chance of the bid being accepted. This rises to 90 percent with a bid of $80. Fourth, the bidder's profits, if the bid is accepted, are equal to the revenues less the costs of serving the designated number of patients. Given the number of patients (Q) and the costs per patient (C), the higher the accepted bid, the higher will be the profits [equal to $(B \times Q) - (C \times Q)$]. Fifth, we translate the profitability situation of the bidder into a wealth level. We assume that, without a contract, the bidder's wealth would be $200. A successful bid thus adds to the successful bidder's wealth level by the level of the bidder's profits.

The bidder is thus faced with a trade-off between profits (and hence wealth) and the probability of a successful bid. The individual bidder can increase the likelihood of success but only by lowering the bid and thus lowering the profits. Given the range of alternatives, which option will the bidder choose? As set up now, our model is incomplete; it does not incorporate the objectives of the bidders or the bidding rules set up by the contracting agency.

With regard to bidder's objectives, let us assume first that the bidder is extremely risk averse. He or she puts a high personal value on small gains and successively lower additional values on larger gains (i.e., wealth, for the bidder, has a diminishing marginal utility). Under this assumption, reflected in Column 6 of

Table 8–1 Hypothetical Bidding Data

					Utility Levels	
Option	Bid Price	Probability of Acceptance	Profits (if bid accepted)	Wealth Level (if bid accepted)	Risk Averter	Risk Taker
A	$100	.2	$800	$1,000	126	2,000
B	95	.4	400	600	122	800
C	90	.6	200	400	118	400
D	85	.8	100	300	110	200
E	80	.9	50	250	100	100

Table 8–1, the bidder will choose the option that maximizes his or her *expected* utility, measured as the product of the probability of success (P_s) and the utility associated with the wealth level of that option. In our example, the risk averse bidder will choose Option E, which yields an expected utility of 100. Option D, for example, would yield an expected utility of 88. Although the profits for this option are greater, the bidder prefers to select a very safe but relatively unprofitable option.

A risk taker, whose tastes might be like those summarized in Column 7, considers high levels of wealth to be of the utmost importance, which is shown by the sharply increasing utilities of wealth. To this bidder, substantial profits are so important that they overshadow the very small chances of attaining them. To the risk taker, Option E has an expected utility of 100, whereas Option A has an expected utility of 2000. Option A is the one to be selected by the risk-taking bidder.

Competitive bidding does not automatically lead to a low-price bid. Much of the outcome depends on the bidders' costs and goals. But there are several other factors as well. First, an increase in the number of bidders will reduce the probability of any single bidder being successful. Depending on the bidders' utility schedules, a larger number of competitive bidders may cause each bidder to reduce his or her bid. Second, there are a number of selection and reimbursement methods that a contracting agency can resort to. These may influence the bidding strategies of the bidders (Christianson et al. 1984). One method is to reimburse each winning bidder (more than one provider in an area may be chosen as a winner) at the level of the bid he or she submitted. Thus, if Bidder 1 submitted a bid of $95, Bidder 2, $90, and Bidder 3, $85, and if Bidders 2 and 3 are selected as providers, then Bidder 2 would be reimbursed at $90 and Bidder 3 at $85. This method tends to encourage bidding providers to gamble and seek a higher price, since there is a potential reward to them for doing so (they are reimbursed at the price they bid if their bid is accepted). An alternative method will check this tendency to gamble. If the set of rules entailed that all winning bidders would be reimbursed at the rate bid by the lowest winning bidder, there would be no benefit to a winner making a higher bid if he or she deems that some other winner will bid lower. Indeed, raising the bid merely reduces the chances of being successful.

Competitive bidding rules may lead to a competitive market–type outcome. Whether it does will depend on a number of factors, including the number of bidders, their attitudes toward risk, and the bidding rules set up by the agency. In 1982 the California legislative assembly passed a law allowing selective contracting by third-party payers with hospitals and physicians. Previously, third-party payers in California could not exclude any providers from the group they were obligated to reimburse for services provided.

8.6 SUPPLIER-INDUCED DEMAND

8.6.1 A Pedagogic Model

In Chapter 4 we focused on the asymmetry of information between consumers and providers in the medical care market. We raised the possibility that consumers may not have good information about their health status or the probable effect of medical care on their health. Although consumers are not likely to be completely ignorant, they often rely on physicians to act as agents and inform them about these variables. Physicians can, in many instances, provide information that will allow patients to form a demand curve. But this information may not be fully correct. Physicians can affect the demand curve for medical care by providing information that is inaccurate. If physicians do induce demand unnecessarily, perhaps in response to the excess capacities of their practices, then where the ratio of physicians to population is high, demand will be shifted out more. Ultimately, the extent of unnecessary inducement of demand is an empirical question—and a difficult one to answer.

A large number of studies have been developed that attempt to incorporate supplier-induced demand into the framework of medical markets. Many of these models focus on the provider (physician) and assume implicitly that the ability to shift demand is unlimited. Because consumers have access to information about the quality of advice they receive from their physicians, it is more realistic to recognize that limitations to demand generation may exist. We present a simple model of medical care markets that brings out some of their more important features (Pauly 1980).

We assume that consumers' "taste" for medical care depends on information about initial health status (H_0); the effect of medical care on health ($\Delta H/\Delta M$, where M stands for medical care); and the impact of health on utility, incomes, and prices. It also depends on the number of physicians in the market. In particular, a lower physician (M.D.) to population ratio (shortened to *MDPOP*) will lead to a higher demand for each physician in the market.

For each patient, we suppose there is a "true" level of H and $\Delta H/\Delta M$ that can be determined by the patient's physician. If the physician is fully truthful with the patient, a demand curve for the patient can be derived (D_{true} in Figure 8–7). This demand curve is downward sloping, which means that, for any given level of belief about H and $\Delta H/\Delta M$, the quantity demanded will be responsive to out-of-pocket price.

Of course, the physician can tell the patient that H and $\Delta H/\Delta M$ have values other than the actual ones. If the patient believes the physician, the patient's demand curve will shift outward (i.e., at any price the quantity demanded will be greater). But the physician is only one source of information, and the patient can get information elsewhere if he or she questions the physician's assessment. It is therefore likely that there is an upper limit to the physician's ability to generate demand that is not grounded in reality. We will call the demand curve at this upper limit D_{limit}.

8.6.2 Supply

Having specified the demand characteristics of the model, we now turn to the supply side of the market. With regard to physician behavior, the following assumptions are made:

- Each physician has an upward-sloping marginal cost (*MC*) curve (i.e., as more services are provided, marginal costs increase).
- The price of services is fixed by a fee schedule, and so fees are beyond physician control.

8.6.3 Objectives

A number of studies have identified many possible physician objectives, ranging from healing patients to maximizing profits. We will assume each physician's

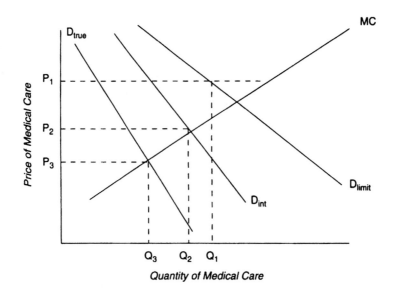

Figure 8–7 Representation of supplier-induced demand. The three demand curves, D_{true}, D_{int}, and D_{limit}, represent the demand of three successive levels of supplier inducement; no unnecessary inducement (D_{true}), an intermediate level of inducement (D_{int}), and the maximum level of inducement possible (D_{limit}). The physician's marginal cost is MC. Three alternative fee levels, P_1, P_2, and P_3, are shown. The quantity of medical care "induced" will depend on the fee level, the degree of inducement, and the physician's MC. However, at high fee levels, patient-influenced limitations may be a factor in determining utilization.

goal is profit maximization for the sake of convenience, not because it is the most realistic assumption. It also elucidates the "worst case" scenario and shows how the most selfish physicians will behave under specified conditions.

The model has been designed to predict the quantity of medical care provided. We will now show that this quantity will depend on the specific price received by the physician. Let us start with a high price, such as P_1 in Figure 8–7. At this price, the physician will generate demand to the limit and provide services at level Q_1. At this point, marginal revenue (MR) is greater than MC, and the physician would be able to earn additional profits if demand could be generated beyond D_{limit}. But the patient cannot be pushed further, and so this is the best the physician can do.

If the price were lower, at P_2, the physician would generate demand up to some intermediate point D_{int} and would provide Q_2 units of service. Beyond this point, MC would exceed MR, and the physician would reduce profits by inducing further demand. At an even lower price, P_3, the physician would not generate any unnecessary demand and would provide Q_3 units of service. The conclusions of even this simple model are that, with the most selfish of physicians, the quantity demanded—and the degree of demand generation—will depend on the given price.

What about an increase in the supply of physicians (i.e., an increase in the *MDPOP*)? From the viewpoint of the individual physician, such an increase would lead to a reduction in each demand curve (D_{true}, D_{int}, and D_{limit}) because these curves are the individual physician's demand curves and each physician will have a smaller market. In these circumstances, each physician's quantity of services supplied will be reduced. Overall demand cannot be generated beyond the maximum, and, at a price such as P_3, there is not likely to be any change in overall services.

As pointed out above, there are a number of reasons why consumers might not be totally gullible and vulnerable to demand-generating tactics. First, consumers can obtain information from sources other than their physicians. Second, a number of studies have suggested that there is a limit to the willingness of physicians to generate demand (Rossiter and Wilensky 1984; Stano 1987a, 1987b), although the nature of this reticence has not been spelled out. Analysts have alternatively modeled the generation of ungrounded demand as a cost to physicians and as a cause of disutility (perhaps as a result of feelings of guilt). In either case, generating too much unnecessary demand will make the physicians (as well as the patients) worse off.

As has been hypothesized, the generation of ungrounded demand will result in higher marginal costs to the physician and, depending on revenues, may yield more profits. But what if the physician's objectives included patient well-being? The impact of this goal will be to reduce the degree to which the physician would be willing to generate demand.

The above model has dealt with demand generation and patient utilization at given prices. It presents a pedagogic treatment of the issue of demand generation and its likely degree of restriction. But it ignores the fact that, contrary to what might be expected, higher physician fees have been associated with an increase in *MDPOP*. We turn now to possible explanations of this surprising relationship between fees and supply.

8.6.4 MDPOP and Physician Fees: A Positive Relationship?

One hypothesis concerning price formation in the physician services market is that when supply shifts out, price increases (Evans 1974). This prediction is contrary to that of the competitive model, which predicts that price will fall when supply increases. The standard competitive model discussed in this chapter is represented geometrically in Figure 8–8. In this figure, D_1 represents an initial demand level and S_1 an initial supply level. The initial supply level corresponds to an initial supply of physicians (an initial level of *MDPOP*). Let us now increase the level of *MDPOP* to the point where the supply shifts out to S_2. Physicians, according to this theory, will offer more services, and, as supply shifts out, prices will fall and utilization will increase. This prediction does not square with the alleged empirical fact that increases in price accompany increases in physician supply (*MDPOP*). In order to fit the theory to the facts, a number of observers have contended that suppliers can shift out demand. For example, suppose the suppliers in our example could push the demand curve out to D_2. Even if the supply was to increase from S_1 to S_2, the equilibrium price would increase to P_3. Of course, supplier-induced demand can also occur when prices *fall* after an outward shift in supply. If, following an increase in supply to S_2, suppliers were only successful in shifting the demand to D_3, the price would fall even though suppliers had been successful in shifting the demand. Thus, a fall in price when supply increases is consistent with both the competitive and the supplier-induced demand theories! This makes it impossible to distinguish between them. Only when prices are observed to rise following an increase in *MDPOP* and all

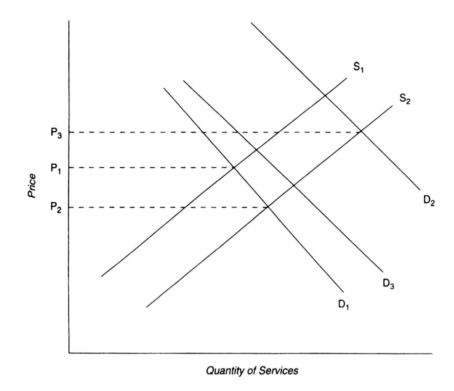

Figure 8–8 Diagram showing the difficulties in identifying the supplier-induced demand based on actual market data. An increase in the physician population will result in an increase in supply from S_1 to S_2. Absence of supplier-induced demand will cause a fall in price from P_3 to P_1, a result of a movement along demand curve D_1. However, supplier-induced demand is consistent with both an increase in price (if demand shifts to D_2) and a reduction in price (if demand shifts, but only to D_3).

else stays the same can we be sure that the supplier-induced demand model is the appropriate model.

The major problem in verifying the existence of supplier-induced demand lies in the fact that other demand- and supply-influencing variables are changing along with *MDPOP*. Let us say that supply shifts from S_1 to S_2 and we observe a price increase from P_1 to P_3. In order to be sure that we are actually observing supplier-induced demand, we must be sure that we have controlled for all other variables that could affect demand and supply. If, for example, S_1 represents supply conditions in Salt Lake City and S_2 conditions in San Antonio, the demand differences between the two markets may have occurred because of supplier-induced demand or myriad other demand-influencing factors, such as health status, quality of care, insurance coverage, and so on. Further, even if we have controlled for differences in *MDPOP* between the two markets, we must be sure that other intervening supply variables have not resulted in greater increases (or decreases).

A number of statistical studies have been undertaken to estimate the extent of supplier-induced demand. The majority of these have focused their attention on *utilization* of medical care and how it has been influenced by *MDPOP*. For example, Rossiter and Wilensky (1984) studied data obtained from a national sample survey of families (known as the National Medical Care Cost and Expenditure Survey) to determine the effect of a number of variables, such as direct price, travel time, health status, and the physician to population ratio, on the number of physician-initiated visits. Physician-initiated visits, although suggested by physicians, are not the same as physician-induced visits, since the term *inducement* connotes lack of necessity. There is no way of telling from a data set such as that used by the authors the degree to which physician-initiated visits were unnecessary and induced by physicians for their own benefit. The results of the study indicated a very small effect of *MDPOP* on ambulatory care utilization: An increase in the ratio by one physician per 100,000 population resulted in an increase in expenditures on physician-initiated visits of only seven cents. However, the authors did not directly test the supplier-induced demand hypothesis.

Cromwell and Mitchell (1986) and Fuchs (1978), on the other hand, did directly test for the effect of supplier-induced demand in the market for surgery by examining the effect of surgeon population ratios on surgery utilization and surgeons' fees. The data set in the Cromwell-Mitchell study consisted of metropolitan area statistics on families' characteristics and surgical utilization obtained from the Health Interview Survey of the National Center for Health Statistics coupled with Medicare surgical fee data. The authors studied how both surgical fees and surgery utilization rates differed among markets (metropolitan areas) when variables such as age distribution, education level, average coinsurance rate, the number of general practitioners per 1,000 population, and the number of surgeons per 1,000 population varied. They also controlled for the supply effect of higher fees causing more surgeons to locate in the area.

Their results indicated a price elasticity for surgical operations of –0.15 when all identified demand-shifting variables were held constant. With regard to the variable *MDPOP* for surgeons, they identified a considerable effect of this variable on surgical utilization and on surgical fees. In the case of utilization, the magnitude of the relationship was such that a 10-percent increase in surgeons in the population resulted in a 9-percent increase in surgical operations. With regard to fee increases, a 1-percent increase in surgeons in the population resulted in a .9-percent increase in surgeons' fees. The authors presented these results as indicative of a significant supplier-induced demand effect in the market for surgery. However, because of the many variables influencing supply and demand and the difficulty of controlling for these in statistical tests, there is controversy surrounding any results in this area (Dranove and Wehner 1994; Feldman and Sloan 1988).

EXERCISES

1. Predict the effect of the following changes on the market price and quantity utilized of eye examinations conducted by ophthalmologists:
   a. an increase in the degree of insurance coverage for eye exams (i.e., lower insurance copayments by the patients)
   b. an increase in the number of ophthalmologists
   c. an increase in the average age of the population
   d. a reduction in the price of optometry services (which are substitute services)
   e. an increase in the price of eyeglasses, which are complementary goods

2. Given the initial demand and supply curves for prescription drugs and an equilibrium price and quantity, predict the direction of change of the equilibrium price and quantity if the following occur:
   a. More consumers enter the market.
   b. The price of nonprescription drugs, which are substitutes, falls.
   c. The price of bottled water, a complement, falls.
   d. Consumers become more enamoured with the wonders of modern drugs.
   e. Consumers become better educated about the dangers of taking excess drugs.

3. Given an initial equilibrium in the market for clinical care, predict the effect of the following changes on equilibrium price and quantity:
   a. an increase in nurses' wages in the clinic market
   b. an increase in the number of clinics
   c. an increase in clinic productivity
   d. a reduction in supply costs for clinics

4. Beginning with an initial equilibrium in the market for private, noninsured dermatology services, predict the effect on price and quantity for the following changes:
   a. an increase in consumer tastes for cosmetic dermatological services
   b. an increase in nurses' wages
   c. an increase in the severity of patient illness
   d. a reduced quality of care offered by dermatologists

5. For-Profit Labs, Inc. (FPL) is a private laboratory that does only routine blood counts. With total assets of $8,000,000 last year, FPL took in $3 million in revenues and had expenses of $200,000. The average firms in other industries make a return of 10 percent on their assets. The market for lab services is potentially competitive, but right now there are only a few firms in the industry. However, lab technicians are free to enter the industry if they wish. Firms in the industry charge $300 for blood counts, and their costs are $20. What do you expect will happen in the long run?

6. The market for physiotherapists is competitive. Chiropractic services and physiotherapy services are substitutes. Currently the price per visit is $40 and the quantity utilized is 30,000 visits annually. Physiotherapists face stiff competition from chiropractors. Currently, chiropractors charge $35 per visit and there are 15,000 visits annually in the region. The chiropractic association has decided to license another 20 practitioners in the region. This will lower the price to $25 per visit. There is no change in the supply of physiotherapists. What will be the direction of the effect of the change in chiropractors on the price and quantity utilized for physiotherapy services?

7. The market for physiotherapist visits is shown in the accompanying diagram. The current equilibrium price is $30 and the equilibrium quantity is 150 visits. The health care authorities are concerned that the price is too high and so have proposed lowering the price to $10 per visit. They contend that at a lower price more people will get to use these services. Predict the effect on quantities demanded and supplied and on quantity of services actually utilized as a result of such an intervention.

8. The equilibrium price for physiotherapy visits is $30 and the quantity utilized is 150 visits as a result of the demand and supply conditions in this diagram. The state legislature is concerned that the current price does not

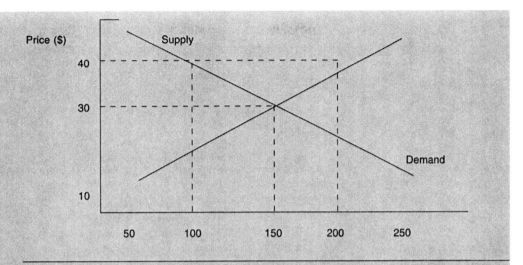

give the physiotherapists enough incentive to produce a high volume of services. A proposal has been made to increase the price paid by the consumers to the suppliers to $40. What will the resulting quantities demanded and supplied and the resulting utilization be?

9. The demand and supply for hospital care in the Garden State is given in the following diagram. Currently, the state legislature has mandated that all hospital care must be free and that providers will be reimbursed at a rate of $450 per day. The Hospital Association has expressed its concern that at this reimbursement rate there will not be enough hospital care to "go around" and meet all the demands. It is proposed that the reimbursement rate be increased to $600 a day. What is the quantity demanded and supplied and the quantity utilized at the two rates? What is the total amount funded at the two rates?

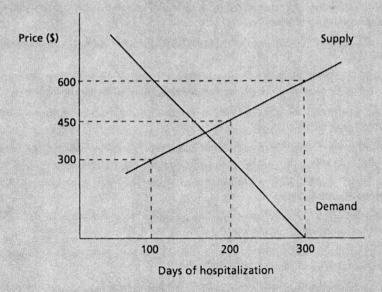

10. The state health care commission is planning to put out bids for hospital care. Key Hospital is considering making a bid but is unsure how much to

bid. The hospital's actuary has developed four options: bid a price per case of $1,000, $800, $600, or $400. The hospital currently has a wealth level of $1,000. Added profits associated with each level are provided in the accompanying table. Also provided in this table are the estimated probabilities of each of the four bids being accepted and the hospital board's utility of each wealth level. Given that the hospital is a risk averse, utility-maximizing entity, what bid should it make?

Option	Bid Price	Probability of Bid Being Accepted	Added Profits If Bid Accepted	Wealth Level If Bid Is Accepted	Utility of a Given Level of Wealth
A	$1,000	.2	$4,000	$5,000	380
B	800	.4	3,000	4,000	340
C	600	.6	2,000	3,000	280
D	400	.8	1,000	2,000	200
No bid				1,000	100

BIBLIOGRAPHY

On the Competitive Market Model

Buchanan, J.M. 1965. *The inconsistencies of the National Health Service.* Occasional paper 7. London: Institute of Economic Affairs.

Christianson, J.B., and W. McClure. 1979. Competition in the delivery of medical care. *New England Journal of Medicine* 301:812–818.

Culyer, A.J., and J.G. Cullis. 1976. Some economics of hospital waiting lists in the NHS. *Social Policy* 5:239–264.

Evans, R.G. 1974. Supplier induced demand. In *The economics of health and medical care,* ed. M. Pearlman. London: MacMillan.

Feldstein, M.S. 1970. The rising price of physicians' services. *Review of Economics and Statistics* 52:121–133.

———. 1974. Econometric studies in health economics. In *Frontiers in quantitative economics,* ed. M. Intriligator and S. Kendrick. Amsterdam, The Netherlands: North-Holland.

Frank, R.G., and W.P. Welch. 1985. The competitive effects of HMOs: A review of the evidence. *Inquiry* 22:148–161.

Friedman, M. 1962. *Capitalism and freedom.* Chicago: University of Chicago Press.

Fuchs, V.R., and M. Kramer. 1972. *Determinants of expenditures for physicians' services in the United States, 1948–1968.* Publication no. HSM 73–3013. Washington, DC: National Center for Health Services Research.

Garbarino, J.W. 1959. Price behavior and productivity in the medical market. *Industrial and Labor Relations Review* 13:3–15.

Greene, V.L., et al. 1993. Do community-based long-term care services reduce nursing home use? *Journal of Human Resources* 28:297–317.

Hay, J.W., and M.J. Leahy. 1984. Competition among health plans. *Southern Economic Journal* 50:831–846.

Kessell, R. 1958. Price discrimination in medicine. *Journal of Law and Economics* 1:20–53.

Lindsay, C.M. 1976. More real returns to medical education. *Journal of Human Resources* 11:127–129.

Mwabu, G., et al. 1993. Quality of medical care and choice of treatment in Kenya. *Journal of Human Resources* 28:838–862.

Newhouse, J.P. 1970. A model of physician pricing. *Southern Economic Journal* 37:147–183.

Newhouse, J.P. et al. 1977. Policy options and the impact of national health insurance revisited. *International Journal of Health Services* 7:503–509.

Pauly, M.V., and K.M. Langwell. 1983. Research on competition in the market for health services. *Inquiry* 20:142–161.

Rizzo, J.A., and R.J. Zeckhauser. 1992. Advertising and the price, quantity, and quality of primary care physicians' services. *Journal of Human Resources* 28:387–421.

Ro, K.K. 1977. Anatomy of hospital cost inflation. *Hospitals and Health Services Administration* 22:78–88.

Salkever,D. 1978. Competition among hospitals. In *Competition in the health care sector*, ed. W. Greenberg. Washington, DC: Federal Trade Commission, Bureau of Economics.

Schwartz, W.B., and D.N. Mendelson. 1990. No evidence of an emerging physician surplus. *JAMA* 263:557–560.

Sloan, F.A. 1976. Real returns to medical education. *Journal of Human Resources*. 11:118–126.

Sloan, F.A., and R. Feldman. 1978. Competition among physicians. In *Competition in the health care sector*, ed. W. Greenberg. Washington, DC: Federal Trade Commission, Bureau of Economics.

Sloan, F.A., and J.H. Lorant. J.H. 1976. The allocation of physicians' services. *Quarterly Review of Economics and Business* 16:86–103.

Wu, W.S., and R. Masson. 1974. Price discrimination for physicians' services. *Journal of Human Resources* 9:63–79.

Zwanzinger, J., et al. 1990. Measures of hospital market structure: A review of the alternatives and a proposed approach. *Socio-Economic Planning Sciences* 24:81–95.

Zwanzinger, J., et al. 2000. Can cost shifting continue in a price competitive environment? *Health Economics* 9:211–226.

Competitive Bidding

Brown, E.R., et al. 1985. Competing for medical business. *Inquiry* 22:237–250.

Christianson, J.B. 1984. Provider participation in competitive bidding for indigent patients. *Inquiry* 21:161–177.

———. 1985. The challenge of competitive bidding. *Health Care Management Review* 10, no. 2:39–54.

Christianson, J.B., et al. 1983. The Arizona experiment: Competitive bidding for indigent medical care. *Health Affairs* 2:87–103.

Christianson, J.B., et al. 1984. A comparison of existing and alternative competitive bidding systems for indigent medical care. *Social Science and Medicine* 18:599–604.

Dranove, D., et al. 1992. Is hospital competition wasteful? *Rand Journal of Economics* 23:247–262.

Freeland, M.S., et al. 1987. Selective contracting for hospital care based on volume, quality, and price. *Journal of Health Politics, Policy and Law* 12:409–426.

Hoerger, T.J., and A. Meadow. 1997. Developing Medicare competitive bidding: A study of clinical laboratories. *Health Care Financing Review* 19:59–85.

Johns, L. 1989. Selective contracting in California: An update. *Inquiry* 26:345–353.

Johns, L., et al. 1985. Selective contracting in California: Early effects and policy implications. *Inquiry* 22:24–32.

Keijser, G.M., and B.L. Kirkman-Liff. 1992. Competitive bidding for health insurance contracts. *Health Policy* 21:35–46.

Kirkman-Liff, B.L., et al. 1985. An analysis of competitive bidding by providers for indigent medical care contracts. *Health Services Research* 20:549–577.

McCall, N., et al. 1985. Evaluating the Arizona health care cost containment system. *Health Care Financing Review* 7:77–88.

Melia, E.P., et al. 1983. Competition in the health care marketplace. *New England Journal of Medicine* 308:788–792.

Melnick, G.A., and J. Zwanzinger. 1988. Hospital behavior under competition and cost containment policies. *JAMA* 260:2669–2681.

Melnick, G.A., et al. 1992. The effects of market structure and bargaining position on hospital prices. *Journal of Health Economics* 11:217–233.

Mobley, L.R. 1998. Effects of selective contracting on hospital efficiency, costs and accessibility. *Health Economics* 7:247–262.

Robinson, J.C., and H.S. Luft. 1988. Competition, regulation, and hospital costs, 1982 to 1986. *JAMA* 260:2676–2681.

Robinson, J.C., and C.S. Phibbs. 1989. An evaluation of selective contracting in California. *Journal of Health Economics* 8:437–455.

Zwanzinger, J., and G.A. Melnyck. 1988. The effects of hospital competition and the Medicare PPS program on hospital cost behavior in Ontario. *Journal of Health Economics* 7:301–320.

Supplier-Induced Demand

Auster, R.D., and Oxaca, R.L. 1981. The identification of supplier-induced demand in the health care sector. *Journal of Human Resources* 16:327–342.

Blackstone, E.A. 1980. Market power and resource misallocation in neurosurgery. *Journal of Health Politics, Policy and Law* 3:345–360.

Carlsen, F., and J. Grytten. 1998. More physicians: Improved availability or induced demand? *Health Economics* 7:495–508.

Cromwell, J., and J.B. Mitchell. 1986. Physician induced demand for surgery. *Journal of Health Economics* 5:293–313.

Dranove, D. 1988. Demand inducement and the physician–patient relationship. *Economic Inquiry* 26:281–298.

Dranove, D., and P. Wehner. 1994. Physician-induced demand for childbirths. *Journal of Health Economics* 13:61–73.

Evans, R.G. 1974. Supplier induced demand. In *The economics of health and medical care*, ed. M. Perlman. London: Macmillan.

Feldman, R., and F. Sloan. 1988. Competition among physicians. *Journal of Health Politics, Policy, and Law* 13:239–264.

Fuchs, V. 1978. The supply of surgeons and the demand for operations. *Journal of Human Resources* 13 (suppl.): 35–55.

Hay, J.L., and M.J. Leahy. 1982. Physician induced demand. *Journal of Health Economics* 1:231–244.

Hemenway, D., and D. Fallon. 1985. Testing for physician induced demand with hypothetical cases. *Medical Care* 23:344–349.

Labelle, R., et al. 1994. A re-examination of the meaning and importance of supplier induced demand. *Journal of Health Economics* 13:347–368.

Pauly, M.V. 1979. What is unnecessary surgery? *Milbank Quarterly* 57:95–117.

———. 1980. *Doctors and their workshops*. Chicago: University of Chicago Press.

Pauly, M.V., and M.A. Satterthwaite. 1980. The pricing of primary care physicians' services. *Bell Journal of Economics* 12:488–506.

Reinhardt, U. 1978. Comment. In *Competition in the health care sector*, ed. W. Greenberg. Washington, DC: Federal Trade Commission.

———. 1983. The theory of physician-induced demand and its implications for public policy. *Beitrage zur Gesundheitsökonomie* 4:153–172.

Rice, T.H. 1983. The impact of changing Medicare reimbursement rates on physician induced demand. *Medical Care* 21:803–815.

Rizzo, J.A., and D. Blumenthal. 1996. Is the target income hypothesis an economic heresy? *Medical Care Research and Review* 53:243–266.

Rossiter, L.F., and G.R. Wilensky. 1983. A reexamination of the use of physician services. *Inquiry* 20:162–172.

———. 1984. Identification of physician-induced demand. *Journal of Human Resources* 19:231–244.

———. 1987. Health economist-induced demand for theories of physician-induced demand. *Journal of Human Resources* 12:624–626.

Market Power in
Health Care

1. Use the monopoly model to predict the price charged or quantity of services utilized.
2. Use the monopoly model to explain how providers are able to charge different groups of patients different prices.
3. Describe the functioning of a market where the buyers have market power.
4. Describe a measure of market power and demonstrate how it can be applied in a market situation.
5. Describe the determinants of market power.
6. Explain the concept of nonprice competition and describe a model with market power and nonprice competition.
7. Demonstrate how the monopoly model can be used to predict resource allocation in markets with preferred provider organizations.

9.1 INTRODUCTION

Market power refers to the ability of one participant in a market to influence the terms on which he or she makes an exchange. Market power can be wielded by both buyers and sellers. For example, a heart surgeon can be in a position to influence the fee that patients or insurers pay. Similarly, an insurance company or government health insurance program can be in a position to influence the rate at which it reimburses providers for supplying services to its members.

Essential ingredients of market power are the limited availability of viable substitutes for the service and the ease with which buyers and sellers can weigh these alternatives. A hospital may be the only hospital for hundreds of miles, in which case it possesses some degree of market power (i.e., it has some leeway in setting prices and other terms for the services it provides). On the other hand, a large number of HMOs may be vying to become providers for a firm's employees; in this case, the HMOs have little or no market power, although the firm may possess some.

Market power is important because, if possessed by buyers or sellers, it might allow them to wield influence over the use of resources to their benefit and to the

202

detriment of the other bargaining parties. In this chapter we develop an analysis of how market power influences market outcomes (i.e., prices, quantities, and quality). Our analysis is "explanatory" in the sense that we are asking how one set of factors (related to market power) influences specific phenomena. Discussion of the desirability (or undesirability) of market power must wait until we discuss yardsticks with which to gauge actual market conduct.

We will examine several models that explain resource allocation when either buyers or sellers possess some degree of market power. In Section 9.2 we look at two models of the behavior of the ultimate wielder of market power—the monopolist—that offer predictions about how monopolistic suppliers and demanders set price and quantity. All suppliers and demanders would benefit if they possessed market power, and so a pertinent question is, how does one obtain it? In Section 9.3 we consider the determinants of market power. This section includes a general discussion of market power as well as an account of how providers in one market possessing many of the preconditions of a competitive market, the physician services market, were nevertheless able to develop and maintain a considerable degree of market power and use it to bolster their incomes.

The monopoly model and the competitive model are two polar extremes of models of market power. In many (perhaps most) markets, market power and competition are mixed to varying degrees. In Section 9.4 we discuss several models of incomplete market power that elucidate how product quality can be an important outcome in provider competition.

9.2 MONOPOLISTIC MARKETS

9.2.1 Simple Monopoly

A supplier has a monopoly in a market when it is the sole source of supply in that market. In a monopolistic market, the demanders do not have any close substitutes for the service and there are barriers to the entry of new sellers. Of course, some substitutability usually exists. For example, in health care an alternative to treatment usually exists, even if that alternative is to do nothing.

We will develop the monopoly model in the context of a supposed monopolistic market, the market for pediatric ambulatory services. We assume that in this market there is a single group practice. The product is defined as quality-constant pediatric visits. The simple monopoly model consists of demand, cost, and behavioral assumptions.

9.2.2 Demand

With regard to demand, we assume that the pediatric group faces a single market demand curve (see Table 9–1 and Figure 9–1). Note that there is a price ($10) at which patients will abstain from making any visits. As discussed in Section 3.5, as one moves down the demand curve, one moves through elastic, unit elastic, and inelastic portions of the demand curve, and the total revenue (*TR*) will increase, level off, and decrease. The marginal revenue (*MR*) is falling throughout, although it is positive when it is associated with the elastic portion of the demand curve and zero at the unit elastic point on the demand curve. For the provider, the *MR*

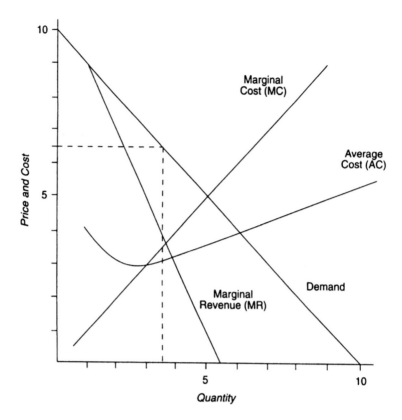

Figure 9–1 Equilibrium price and output in a monopolistic (single-seller) market. The monopolist faces a given demand curve for the service, and from this curve is derived its marginal revenue curve. The monopolist's cost conditions are presented in marginal (*MC*) and average (*AC*) terms. The profit-maximizing monopolist will set price and quantity such that its *MR* = *MC*. Equilibrium price is between 6 and 7, and equilibrium quantity is between 3 and 4. (This graph is based on data in Table 9–1.)

represents the additional *TR* that it will receive by lowering the price enough to sell one more visit. Note that as the provider lowers its price, it sells more units, but all of them are sold at the new, lower price. The *MR* is the net change in *TR* and is equal to the difference in the two *TRs* at the two quantity levels.

The monopolist has the ability to set price at any level it wishes. This ability represents the ultimate degree in market power. (Of course, the price it sets will influence the quantity demanded, something the monopolist will want to keep in mind when setting the price.)

9.2.3 Cost

Our cost assumptions are that the total fixed cost (*TFC*) is $3 and that the total variable cost (*TVC*) is increasing in such a way that marginal cost (*MC*) increases as output expands (see Table 9–1, Column 6). The total cost (*TC*) is the sum of *TVC* and *TFC*.

Table 9–1 Revenue and Cost in a Hypothetical Monopolistic Market

Price	Units of Output	Total Revenue (TR)	Marginal Revenue (MR)	Total Cost (TC)	Marginal Cost (MC)	Profits (TR – TC)
$10	0	0		3		–3
9	1	9	9	4	1	5
8	2	16	7	6	2	10
7	3	21	5	9	3	12
6	4	24	3	13	4	11
5	5	25	1	18	5	7
4	6	24	–1	24	6	0
3	7	21	–3	31	7	–10

9.2.4 Objectives

Profits (Column 7) are equal to *TR* – *TC*, and they initially increase and then decrease as output expands. But we cannot tell what price will be charged and what output (and profit) levels will be attained until we know what objectives the provider is pursuing. We will initially assume that the provider's objective is to maximize profits.

Our analysis of the model is as follows. First, the price will be set at that point on the demand curve at which *MR* comes closest to (or equals) *MC* (without *MC* exceeding *MR*). Let us assume that the monopolist initially set its price at $10 per visit. It would have no buyers at such a price (see Table 9–1), and its losses would be confined to its fixed costs, since it would have no variable costs at zero output. If price was lowered to $9, one visit would be sold and the *MR* would be $9. One additional visit would cost only $1 extra (*MC* = $1) and would add $8 to the previous output level's profits. Total profit would therefore be $5. This is certainly better than not operating at all but not as good as lowering the price to $8, selling two units in total, and deriving an additional $7 in revenue in the process (*MR* = $7). For then it would cost the pediatricians only $2 more to provide this added visit, and they would be adding another $5 (*MR* – *MC*) to the previous profit level, making the profits $10 in total. Indeed, the practice would lower its price to $7, selling three visits. It would stop there, because beyond this level of output *TC* increases more than *TR* increases, and as a result *MR* – *MC* becomes negative. Any further increase in output would detract from total profits.

The above analysis is shown graphically in Figure 9–1, which has smoothed-out revenue and cost functions. Here we see that the *MR* and *MC* curves intersect (meaning *MR* = *MC*) at a quantity of between 3 and 4 (because of our smoothed-out values). This corresponds to a price on the demand curve of between $6 and $7. Profitability cannot be increased by raising or lowering the price.

Let us now see what the model implies. First, the provider will set the price at that point on the demand curve above which the *MR* and *MC* curves intersect. Because *MC* is positive, *MR* must also be positive (since *MR* = *MC*) at the profit-maximizing point. It should be noted that *MR* is positive only at those quantities that correspond to the *elastic* portion of the demand curve. Therefore, a monopolist will set the price only on the elastic portion of its demand curve. Indeed, if the price was set on the inelastic portion of the curve, say at $3, *MR* would be negative, meaning that a reduction in output coming from a price increase would raise total revenues. At the same time a reduction in output would reduce *TC*. Profits would therefore always be greater at a higher price (one on the elastic portion of the demand curve).

In addition, since the most profitable level of output is determined by *MR* and *MC* alone, and since *MC* is unaffected by fixed costs, the profit-maximizing price will similarly be unaffected by changes in fixed costs. Let us say that fixed costs in our example increase to $5. Profits would be lower by $2 at every level of output. But the maximum profit level of output would still be the same (at $Q = 3$), only now the provider would be earning less profit. This important result implies that if the provider's fixed costs increase (e.g., because of an increase in mortgage rates), it cannot do anything about it. If it tries to pass on these added fixed costs to the consumer by raising the price, it will only be moving away from the profit-maximizing position; in raising price it will sell less, and total revenue will decrease more than total cost. This, of course, is not true for an increase in variable costs (i.e., *MC*).

In a similar vein, if the profit-maximizing monopolist received a fixed subsidy (i.e., one unrelated to output) of $2 to treat poor patients, *TR* would be increased at every level of output by $2, but *MR* would not be affected. The monopolist's profit-maximizing price will not change. That is, the profit-maximizing monopolist will not lower the price to induce people to demand more.

One outcome of the monopoly model is that the firm could be persistently earning excess profits. Since the *AC* curve incorporates all the monopolist's costs, including opportunity costs, the monopolist's profits in this analysis are equal to *TR* – *TC* or, using average terms, the product of the unit margin ($P – AC$) and output (Q). These profits are true economic profits. That is, they are profits over and above all the costs required to operate the enterprise, including a normal return for the owner's efforts and capital. Furthermore, nothing in the model will allow the monopolist's profits to be bid away. There are no potential entrants into the market who can charge a lower price. As a result, the monopolist can earn above-normal profits that persist over time. Note the contrast with the competitive market model, in which entry is inexpensive and any excess profits will attract new entrants, who will expand supply and lower price and profits.

9.2.5 Price Discrimination

Under some conditions a monopolist can further increase its profits by charging different prices to different buyers. This is called *price discrimination*. Price discrimination can be practiced only when the product or service in the lower price market cannot be resold in the higher price market. In addition, the demand elasticities in the two markets have to be different to make the practice worthwhile.

Let us assume that a pediatric practice can separate its patients into two distinct markets according to patient income. Assume further that demand elasticity is influenced by income so that each market will have a different demand curve. Thus, one of the preconditions for price discrimination is met. The product sold is patient visits. These can hardly be sold in one market and resold in the other, so the other precondition is met as well. The demand curves for the two separate markets, "rich" and "poor," are shown in Figure 9–2, Graphs A and B. Our cost assumption is that the *MC* eventually rises, as shown in Graph C. Note that there is one *MC* for the

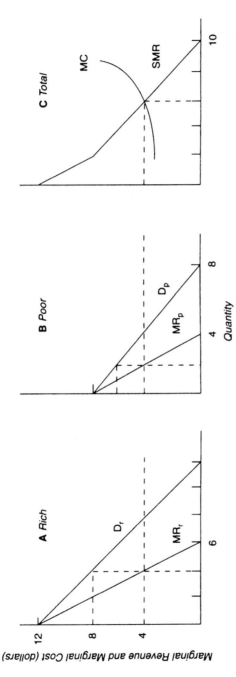

Figure 9–2 Price setting by a discriminating monopolist. If the monopolist can separate its markets into two submarkets, "rich" and "poor," the price charged in each submarket will be derived from firm-level conditions and will occur where the marginal revenue in that submarket equals the overall marginal cost to the firm. The curve *SMR* in Graph C shows the total quantity in all submarkets at each level of *MR*. Note that the equilibrium occurs in each market at the same value of *MR*.

entire operation; production is not separated. Our behavioral assumption is that the pediatric practice seeks to maximize its profits.

Given these assumptions, we can use the monopolistic model to elucidate the monopolist's pricing policy. In doing so, we must rely on the equimarginal principle of maximization. To maximize profits, the provider will set the price (and therefore the quantity) in each market so that (1) the MR earned by lowering (raising) the price in all markets is the same and (2) overall the MR in each market is equal to the MC of producing that total level of output.

The derivation of the profit-maximizing prices is shown in Figure 9–2. The curve MC shows the provider's marginal cost for all units provided (it does not have a separate cost for each market), and the curve SMR shows the quantity that would be supplied overall when the firm allocated output to each market according to the specific level of MR. SMR is thus the sum of quantities in both markets at a given level of MR. Given the MR curves for the poor and the rich markets (MR_p and MR_r) at an MR level in both markets of $ 4, the corresponding quantities in the markets are 4 and 2, respectively. The SMR curve for those quantities will be at a quantity of 6, where $Q_m = Q_p + Q_r$.

The firm's maximum profit position will be determined by equating MC with the MR in each market. Overall, this occurs where $MC = SMR$ (at quantity 6). The corresponding outputs in each market are 4 and 2, and the prices in the two markets that equate the MRs are $8 and $6, respectively. Profits, which are equal to the sum of TR in each market less TC, will be greater than if the same price was set in all markets.

Price discrimination such as this cannot exist in a competitive market, and this is one reason why physician pricing has been characterized as monopolistic. In a competitive market, if two submarkets had different prices, "traders" would buy goods in the low price market and resell them (at a higher price but below the market price) in the second market. For many years, physicians, particularly specialists, resorted to a sliding scale of fees when setting prices, charging the richer patients more than the poorer ones (Kessell 1958). By the 1970s, physician services became more highly insured, and the sliding scale all but disappeared by that time (Newhouse 1970).

9.2.6 Physician Pricing and Supply in Public Programs

A variant of the two-payer monopoly model outlined in Section 9.2.5 has been used to explain physician pricing and supply in relation to the reimbursement policies of Blue Shield (Sloan and Steinwald 1978), Medicare (Paringer 1980; Rice 1984), and Medicaid (Cromwell and Mitchell 1984; Hadley 1979; Kushman 1977) and the 1972–1975 price limitations set by the Economic Stabilization Program (Hadley and Lee 1978–1979).

The Medicare studies examined the effect of Medicare reimbursement levels (80 percent of the reasonable charges) on the assignment decision—the decision of physicians to accept the Medicare-determined fee as full payment for their services. On an individual-case basis, physicians can accept Medicare assignment of their patients. A physician who accepts the reasonable fee in full (i.e., who accepts assignment) for a specific patient receives 80 percent of the fee direct from Medicare and can bill the patient for the copayment. If the physician does not accept assignment, he or she can bill the patient whatever fee he or she chooses. In this case Medicare will reimburse the patient directly for 80 percent of its reasonable fee, and the physician must collect the entire charge from the patient. The acceptance by physicians of assignment relieves patients from the financial risks associated with higher physician fees.

The analysis is set out graphically in Figure 9–3. The physician is assumed to be a monopolist facing two submarkets: one with private patients and one with patients in a public program. (We ignore the extra billing in this analysis.) The output is defined as patients served. D_p is the demand curve for private patients, and MR_p is the related *MR* curve. The public agency reimburses the physicians for its patients at a fee level F_m; since the fee level is fixed, F_m is also the physician's *MR* for public patients. Assume that the physician's *MC* curve is at MC_1. Finally, assume that the physician is a profit maximizer.

According to the equimarginal principle, the physician will supply services to Q_1 private and $(Q_3 - Q_1)$ public patients, since at this output $MR_p = F_m$ and both are equal to MC_1. The private patients will be charged a price of P_m. To attract any additional private patients, the physician would have to lower the price to private patients below P_m, which would imply an *MR* for private patients below that for public patients. A profit-maximizing physician will thus prefer to serve additional public patients where the *MR* is constant at a level F_m rather than lower his or her price and have a marginal revenue below F_m.

A lower public fee would lower the supply to the public patients (it would also cause the physician to lower his or her private fee, since the physician will now

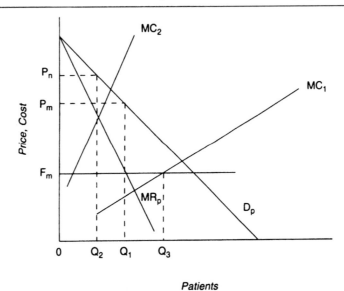

Figure 9–3 Representation of price setting by a monopolist facing a private market (with demand represented by D_p and marginal revenue by MR_p) and a publicly financed market (with a set fee and therefore a marginal revenue of F_m). With a marginal cost of MC_1, the monopolist will set the price to equate the *MR* in both markets. In this case, the price in the private market is set at P_m. The marginal revenue for public and private patients will be the same, MC_1. Total output supplied is Q_3, with $Q_3 - Q_1$ going to public patients. With an *MC* such as MC_2, the monopolist would not supply any output to the public patients; the price and output levels in the private market would be P_n and Q_2.

move down the MR_p curve). A physician facing the same demand curve but with a higher MC (say, MC_2) will not supply any services to public patients and will set a private fee of P_n. This analysis demonstrates that the public and private sectors are interdependent. A public program that lowers fees will reduce the supply to the public market and will also affect the private market.

A model similar to the one discussed in the previous section has been used to explain hospital cost shifting, a tactic purportedly used by hospitals to raise fees on self-pay and commercially insured patients in response to low reimbursement levels by Medicare, Medicaid, and, in some instances, Blue Cross (Danzon 1982; Sloan and Becker 1984; Sloan and Ginsburg 1984).

9.2.7 Nursing Home Markets and Public Rates

The two-payer monopoly model is also suited to analyzing economic behavior in the nursing home market. Generally, in this market, there are two major groups of payers: self-pay (relatively uninsured) patients and state Medicaid agencies. Many Medicaid agencies pay nursing homes a flat rate, whereas self-pay patients are charged according to market conditions. With Medicaid agencies being economy minded and having the power to set rates, one option they have in pursuing the goal of budget containment is to set low rates.

Because the nursing homes can differentiate their products, they can develop some form of "brand loyalty" on the part of patients and prospective patients. When they have patients with some degree of preference, nursing homes will face demand curves that have some elasticity (i.e., are downward sloping). The more loyal their patients are, the more inelastic their demand curves will be.

Figure 9–3 can therefore be interpreted as pertaining to nursing home markets. In this diagram, assume that F_m is the rate that Medicaid pays to nursing homes, D_p is the demand of private pay patients, and MC_1 is a nursing home's marginal cost. At the fee level (and marginal revenue) of F_m, the nursing home will equate its marginal cost so that it is equal to the MR for each class of patients. It will therefore serve Q_3 patients, with Q_1 of these being private and $Q_3 - Q_1$ being Medicaid. If the Medicaid agency lowered its rates below F_m, fewer Medicaid patients (and more private pay patients) would be served. Shortages of Medicaid patient nursing home beds would therefore appear (Paringer 1980).

9.3 MONOPSONY—BUYERS' MARKET POWER

A large buyer that faces many small sellers may be in a position to exert market power. Market power possessed by buyers is referred to as *monopsony*. In the health care sector, the monopsony model has been applied to situations as diverse as the labor market for nurses, the purchase of hospital services by big insurers such as Blue Cross plans (Foreman et al. 1996; Staten et al. 1987), the purchase of specialized medical services by managed care plans (Pauly 1998), and the procurement of organs for transplant (Barnett et al. 1993).

The basic monopsony model can be illustrated by the example of a large hospital chain that is a purchaser of aspirin. The supply curve faced by the monopsonist is the result of many small sellers' willingness to produce and sell aspirin at any given price. Higher prices result in a greater quantity supplied, so the supply curve looks like S in Figure 9–4.

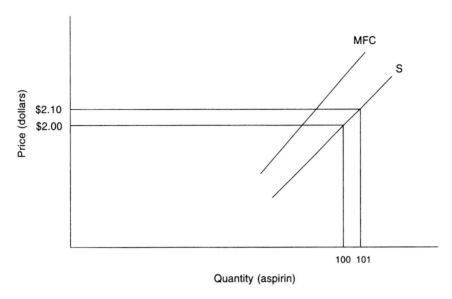

Figure 9–4 Supply and marginal factor costs (MFC) for a buyer with market power. The MFC curve is derived from the supply curve(s).

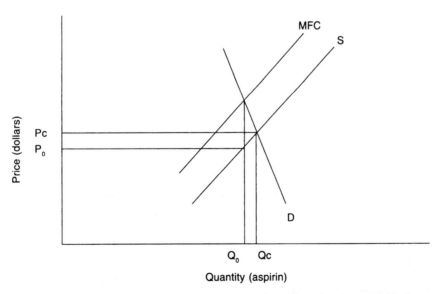

Figure 9–5 Price setting with buying power. D is the monopsonist's demand curve and indicates marginal benefit to the monopsonist of an additional unit purchased. To maximize profit, the monopsonist would purchase the quantity mat which marginal benefit equals MFC (Q_0). The price paid for this amount is P_0. Under monopsony, price and quantity (P_0, Q_0) are lower than they would be under perfect competition (P_c, Q_c).

For the monopsonist, however, the supply price associated with any quantity of aspirin does not give a true indication of the cost to it of expanding its purchases. In order to induce suppliers to sell added quantities, it must offer a higher price. Of course, it must pay this higher price not just on the added purchases but on all its purchases. This means that for the monopsonist the marginal cost of an additional unit of aspirin is higher than its price. This is illustrated in Figure 9–4. Initially the buyer is purchasing 100 units at a price of $2, spending a total of $200. To induce sellers to supply 101 units, the price offered must rise to $2.10. The new total spending on aspirin is thus $2.10 x 101 = $212.10. So the added expense is not just the $2.10 price for the 101st unit but also the additional .10 paid on the initial 100 units. The expense of adding another unit of an input for a monopsonist is called the *marginal factor cost (MFC)*, and it will be higher than the supply price, as shown by the *MFC* curve.

Since there are many substitutes for aspirin, the hospital chain will have a somewhat elastic demand curve indicating its marginal benefit for any quantity (based on increased revenue the input will enable it to earn). In making a purchase decision, it will weigh this marginal benefit against the *MFC* and buy the quantity at which these two are equal. At any quantity less than this, there would be increased profit as a result of expanding purchases. At any higher quantity, profit would be enhanced by a reduction in quantity purchased.

The result is shown in Figure 9–5. Q_0 units will be purchased at a price of P_0 per unit. The contrast of this result with the result that would occur in perfect competition is noteworthy. If the demand curve had represented the total demand of many small buyers, equilibrium would have been at $P_c Q_c$. So the effect of monopsony is to decrease price and quantity compared to what which would occur in perfect competition.

9.4 MARKET STRUCTURE AND ITS DETERMINANTS

9.4.1 Measuring Market Concentration

Market structure has a major influence on market power. Structure is usually presented in terms of an index or percentage, representing the size of the largest firm (or four firms or eight firms) relative to the overall market's output or else measuring the distribution of firm size in the market. A four-firm concentration ratio shows the percentage of the total market (in terms of sales, assets, or some other indicator of firm size) represented by the largest four firms. For example, a completely monopolized market has a concentration ratio of 100 percent; a market with 20 firms, total sales of $1 billion, and combined sales for the largest four firms of $500 million would have a four-firm concentration ratio of 50 percent. The choice of four or eight firms is arbitrary and does not indicate the concentration of the remainder of the market. A more general measure of concentration, which incorporates all firms in the market, is the Herfindahl (*H*) index. According to this index, concentration is measured as

$$H = \Sigma(S/M)^2 \times 10,000$$

where *S* is the size of each firm and *M* is the size of the total market. The figure 10,000 is used as a multiplier because *H* is usually presented as a sum of percentages expressed in absolute terms. The summation sign (Σ) indicates summation over all firms. Thus, if a monopolist with sales of $200 is the only firm in the market, its H index is (200/200) × 10,000, or 10,000. If there were three hospitals, each with sales of $100, the H index for that market would be 3,300 [$\Sigma(100/300)^2 \times 10,000$].

There is no true cutoff point for a concentrated versus a nonconcentrated market, although a figure of about 1,800 is sometimes used (Wilder and Jacobs 1986). Generally, it is thought that the greater the degree of concentration, the greater will be the ability of the leading firms to influence price, quantity, and other characteristics of output.

9.4.2 Determinants of Market Structure

Market structure can be thought of as having market and governmentally imposed (regulatory) determinants. Let us examine these in the context of the health insurance market. In the United States, the health insurance market is largely a localized market, in part because each state requires operating licenses for any insurance company operating within the state and also because of unique relations between local providers and some insurers (primarily the Blues). Aside from government insurance, health insurance has been broken down into two categories of operators, the Blues and the commercial insurance companies. The Blues comprise Blue Cross (for hospitalization insurance) and Blue Shield (for medical and other insurance). In some states the two plans are combined. The Blues are nonprofit in terms of organization. Commercial insurers include a large number of mutual (member-owned) and commercial (for-profit) firms, none of which has a substantial share of the health care market. Blue Cross and Blue Shield collect about one-quarter of the total health insurance premiums nationally, although their share of the private insurance market varies considerably by state.

9.4.3 Economies of Scale

Among the most important market determinants of market power are economies of scale. Let us assume that the market demand for private health insurance is D_m in Figure 9–6 and that the long-run average cost curve for a state-of-the-art insurance company is LAC. Two things should be noted in our example. First, the long-run average cost incorporates capital and other fixed setup costs as well as current operating costs; if there are high start-up costs for the industry, the LAC at low output levels will be quite high. Second, the LAC in our example includes insurance administration costs and the amount the insurance company reimburses the providers. The shape of the LAC curve in our example is such that the minimum cost is reached at a large scale of output (about 12 million subscribers).

9.4.4 Pricing Policies

Given certain cost conditions, one firm could capture a considerable portion of the market. To do so, however, it must resort to a second, and related, market share determinant: pricing policy. If the insurance company sets a very low price relative to costs of other insurers (represented by the curve LAC_2), say, $80 per subscriber, market demand would be quite large (20 million subscribers). In this case, the insurance company would have considerable discretion in choosing its own output level; the level chosen would depend, of course, on its objectives. If it provided

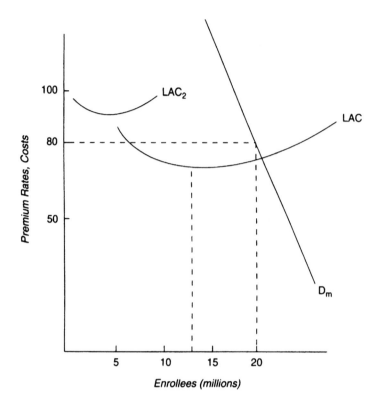

Figure 9–6 Output in an insurance market with alternative cost conditions. D_m represents market demand for insurance coverage. If the cost conditions are represented by cost curve *LAC*, one firm can capture a substantial portion of the market by virtue of its economies of scale and pricing policies. A producer with the cost conditions represented by *LAC* could set a price of, say, $80; if it did so and chose to supply 13 million policies (as shown by the dashed line), another producer with the same cost conditions could not reach a large enough scale of output to match the first producer's cost (and price). If the cost conditions were represented by LAC_2, no producer could dominate the market in this way.

services for 13 million subscribers at this price, there would be an excess demand of 7 million potential subscribers. If the technology of insurance provision was known to other potential entrants, a second firm could provide insurance on a cost basis like that represented by the *LAC* curve. However, to reach a unit cost of $80, it would need to operate at a scale of 8 million subscribers. Since the potential entrant could not obtain such a volume, it might simply produce at a higher cost, charge a higher price, and obtain a smaller share of the residual market.

The final distribution of market shares will thus depend on the size of potential economies of scale relative to the potential market and also on the pricing policies of the larger firms. As seen in Figure 9–6, if the initial insurance company charged a higher price, say, $90 or $100, potential entrants would have less problem gaining an entry to the market.

If, on the other hand, the state-of-the-art cost curve was like LAC_2 (with no substantial economies of scale), no firm could obtain a substantial share of the market, and a concentration of firms would be unlikely. There is some evidence economies of scale exist in health insurance operations, but these economies are not of the magnitude that would permit a single firm to dominate the health insurance market (Blair et al. 1975).

9.4.5 Input Prices and Taxes

A third cause of market concentration relates not to the cost-scale relation but to the potentially different levels of cost curves for different providers. If, for example, one provider could obtain its inputs (workers, materials, etc.) at a lower cost than a second provider, its cost curve would be lower at all scales of output than the cost curve of the second provider. The first firm could capture a larger share of the market by turning its cost advantage into a price differential. One such input price differential is the discount that many Blue Cross plans receive from hospitals (Feldman and Greenberg 1981a, 1981b; Goldberg and Greenberg 1985), which is perhaps partly due to the special traditional relationship between Blue Cross and hospitals (Blue Cross was founded by hospitals). Whereas commercial insurance companies typically have reimbursed hospitals for close to full charges, about half of the Blue Cross plans have received discounts ranging from 2 to 30 percent and averaging from 8 to 15 percent. These discounts have the effect of lowering the LAC curves of the Blue Cross plans relative to the commercial ones, allowing Blue Cross to gain an increased market share by charging lower premium rates. One recent estimate attributed 7 percent of Blue Cross's market share to this cost differential.

9.4.6 Regulation

There might also be regulatory causes of market concentration. Like the Blue Cross discount, discriminatory regulations can give one firm or type of firm a cost advantage that allows it to lower price and increase market share. One such regulation is the tax on health insurance premiums, which is imposed on commercial insurance companies in all states; in some states the Blue plans are exempt from such a tax, which is about 2 percent of premiums. In addition, the Blue plans, being nonprofit, are exempt from income taxes and, in some states, from property taxes. Such exemptions lower the Blues' total costs, giving them a cost advantage.

However, these advantages need not always result in a larger market share. As shown in Section 6.6, firms can incur costs providing on-the-job benefits for the managers. This is particularly true for nonprofit firms, whose profits cannot be directly shared by the managers. Thus any cost advantage possessed by a nonprofit firm can be appropriated by the managers rather than be passed on to consumers in the form of lower premiums. On-the-job amenities have been hypothesized to be a factor in the behavior of Blue Shield plans that were not "controlled" by physicians. Blue Shield plans deemed to be physician controlled were found to have lower operating costs. One possible explanation is that the physician-controlled plans passed on surpluses to the physicians in the form of reimbursements. Non-physician-controlled plans could appropriate potential surpluses and in the process generate higher operating costs (Eisenstadt and Kennedy 1981).

9.4.7 Market Power in the Market for Physicians' Services

Market structure and market power are not always equivalent. In the physician services market, there are a number of manifestations of market power, and yet the market structure does not have a high degree of provider concentration. For instance, for many years physicians were able to maintain a sliding scale of fees, indicating price discrimination. Also, their incomes have been well above normal, even allowing for the high cost of medical training. Yet significant economies of scale in medical practice are not present, and there is a very low degree of market concentration, conditions that normally accompany monopolistic pricing and profit levels.

The explanation of this paradox is that the medical profession developed a mechanism of control to police its members and prevent them from engaging in competitive practices such as price cutting (Kessell 1958; Rayack 1970). This control mechanism was basically in the hands of organized medical associations at the county, state, and national levels.

The key players were the teaching hospitals, the American Medical Association, the local medical associations, and practicing physicians, especially specialists (see Figure 9–7). The operation of the mechanism depended on the fact that it benefited

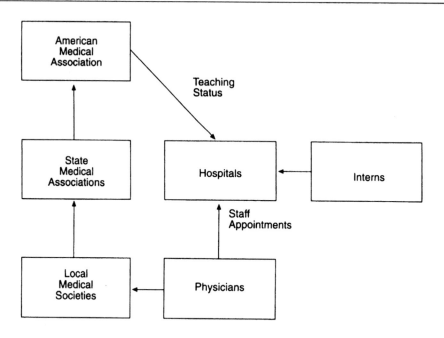

Figure 9–7 Representation of the control mechanism that existed in the medical profession. Key players included hospitals with teaching programs that required accreditation from the Council on Teaching Hospitals (AMA associated) and physicians (who benefited from staff appointments in hospitals). Membership in local medical societies was required for a staff appointment to a hospital, a regulation enforced by the AMA through its control over hospital accreditation. Local medical societies could enforce regulations (regarding pricing policies, for example) through their control over membership.

several of the key groups: (1) interns were an important (and low-cost) input in the operation of teaching hospitals, and (2) physicians, especially specialists, needed membership on hospital medical staffs to make a good, secure living.

The basis of the mechanism was a convention developed by the American Medical Association (AMA) regarding the certification of teaching hospitals. According to this convention, known as the Mundt Resolution, hospitals that were certified as teaching hospitals were advised that their medical staffs should be composed only of physicians who were members of local medical societies. Since the AMA certified teaching hospitals, the resolution carried great weight.

Here is an example of how the resolution helped to limit competitive behavior on the part of physicians. County medical association members generally disapproved of price cutting and other competitive practices. One target of disapprobation was prepaid group medicine. Prepaid group practices (proto-HMOs) charged a single fee for all members, thus undermining the price discrimination system that had become prevalent. The expulsion of physicians who joined prepaid group practice staffs from county medical societies occurred in several instances (Kessell 1958), and the threat of expulsion was sufficient to make physician recruitment difficult for these practices. In addition, other competitive activities, such as advertising, were also discouraged by the organized medical profession.

The control of competitive practices by the medical profession at large has not relied solely on such formal mechanisms. With the growth of specialization, physicians have become increasingly dependent on referrals from colleagues. Physicians who engaged in competitive practices could be "controlled" to some degree if they lost referrals from colleagues (Havighurst 1978).

In recent years there has been a considerable amount of regulatory activity, especially on the part of the federal government, to contain anticompetitive practices on the part of physicians and other health care providers.

9.5 NONPRICE COMPETITION AND MARKET POWER

9.5.1 Overview

The vast majority of health care markets are neither perfectly competitive nor completely monopolistic. Consumers develop some loyalty or attachment to specific providers, but this loyalty is not total. Furthermore, product quality or attributes other than price play a key role in the output of most health care providers; therefore, quality has a key role to play in the competitive process as well. In this section, we discuss market power and the role of nonprice competition.

In addition to price, there are many product attributes that have the potential to attract patients. Providers can increase convenience by adding office hours in order to reduce their patients' waiting time. They can build satellite facilities and clinics to cut down on their patients' travel time. Pharmacists can initiate delivery services, emergency services, family prescription monitoring records, and prescription waiting areas. Insurance companies and HMOs have a wide variety of services that might be covered, and they can also vary the degree to which these services can be covered (e.g., through the use of copayments, deductibles, and treatment limitations). Note, however, that in all such instances additional quality is expensive to provide.

There are three relevant varieties of price-quality competition: (1) price competition alone, (2) quality competition alone, and (3) joint price and quality competition.

9.5.2 Monopolistic Competition

Competition in both price and quality is called *monopolistic competition*. In a monopolistic competition model, we assume that there are many competitors and potential competitors (i.e., there is low-cost entry). Each firm can vary its product quality (e.g., location of facilities, operating hours, etc.) and in the process will develop some consumer loyalty (and hence market power). That is, consumers will not be as willing to change suppliers at the drop of a price as in the quality-constant perfect competition case.

Let us develop our model using the example of an HMO. We will assume that Palmedico HMO is one among a number of alternative providers (some of whom might offer more traditional insurance and fee-for-service options). Palmedico, we will suppose, is a provider of average efficiency, and we can characterize the partial loyalty of its subscribers by means of a downward-sloping demand curve (*D* in Figure 9–8, Graph A). Associated with this demand curve is an *MR* curve. Palmedico's cost curve will depend on the characteristics of its product: the extent of coverage,

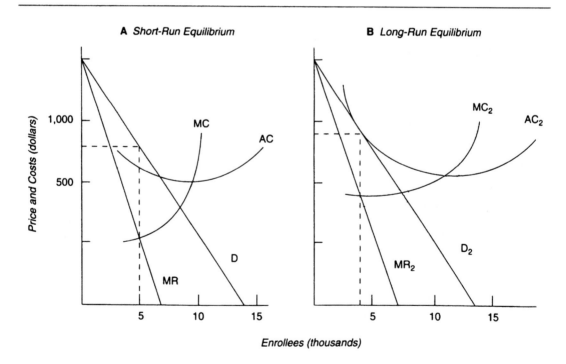

Figure 9–8 Representation of equilibrium in monopolistic competition. In the short run (Graph A), the provider's equilibrium price and quantity are set where $MR = MC$ (at 5,000 enrollees and a price around $750). In the long run (Graph B), competitive responses, including increases in quality, lead to an equilibrium where no excess profits are made (price equals average cost).

the credentials of its staff, its operating hours, the number of satellite clinics it operates, and so on. Initially, let us assume that Palmedico is a profit-maximizing institution. Given these conditions, it will set its price at the quantity where $MR = MC$. Hence, the price will be around \$750 per subscriber and the enrollment will be 5,000.

At this price Palmedico is earning excess profits, and since it is a representative firm in the industry, presumably others are earning excess profits as well. Since entry is inexpensive, other potential entrants will be attracted by the prospect of high profits. To gain enrollees, they may reduce price, and they may also offer potential enrollees a higher quality product (longer clinic hours or more clinic sites, for example). Palmedico's demand curve will shift to the left unless it responds with an increase in quality and a decrease in price, which we assume it does. As a consequence, its costs increase (because of the higher quality). The same forces will affect all firms in the market.

As long as there are any excess profits to be made, this process will continue and the quality of each firm's product will continue to rise. For each firm, demand will first shift outward in response to its higher quality and then inward in response to the quality and price changes instituted by its competitors. Profit margins (the excess of price over average cost) will continually be lowered as a result of the competition. For any firm, we cannot predict whether price will ultimately increase or decrease (i.e., we cannot predict the net result of the competitive process) because demand has shifted in both directions and costs have changed as well. For the same reason, we cannot predict the direction of enrollment. However, the final equilibrium will appear as in Figure 9–8, Graph B, where AC_2 just touches the firm's demand curve D_2. The equilibrium quantity is at the point where $MC = MR$ (i.e., it is the most profitable position Palmedico can have); in this case, Palmedico is just breaking even. All that we can say for certain about this equilibrium is that AC_2 represents a higher quality level; we cannot say for certain whether price and enrollment are higher or lower. For this reason, the monopolistic competition model has been criticized as being incomplete: It fails to make predictions about the direction of some key variables—price and quantity.

Competition between nonprofit firms would have a similar outcome. If our behavioral assumption was that the firm wants to maximize enrollees, for example, quality and price competition would still prevail and the final result would be that each provider breaks even. Models similar to the monopolistic competition model in this section have been used to explain resource allocation decisions in markets containing numerous HMOs (Christianson and McClure 1979; Goldberg and Greenberg 1980) and numerous retail drugstores (Cady 1976). The importance of nonprice factors (including quality) in these markets has been stressed. Similar models have also been used to explain the diffusion of (high-quality) technological developments in the hospital industry, such as the use of radioisotopes and intensive-care units (Lee and Waldman 1985; Rapoport 1978).

9.5.3 Monopolistic Competition and Preferred Provider Organizations

The monopolistic competition model has been used to analyze how PPOs affect hospital price and quality behavior (Dranove et al. 1986). The basic model is applied to interhospital competition, and the impact of PPOs on each individual hospital's demand curve is predicted.

A PPO is an organization that has been formed to contract with providers in order to obtain discounted prices. The PPO shops around among providers (hospitals and physicians) for lower prices and then contracts with the providers who offer better terms on behalf of insurers and/or employers. (The PPO might also institute utilization review.) The discounts are passed on in the form of lower copayments for insureds who choose the preferred providers. Consumers, in effect, are given incentives to choose providers on the basis of price. This increases the elasticity of demand facing any individual hospital because consumers lose some of their loyalty to "their" hospital.

Using the monopolistic competition model to analyze this phenomenon, we begin with the assumption that there are many differentiated firms, each facing a downward-sloping demand curve (D_1 in Figure 9–9). We will assume that each firm has the same demand conditions and that each firm's demand curve is elastic (though the market curve can be inelastic). The implications of this will be seen below. Also, each firm has the cost conditions shown in Figure 9–9: marginal cost is constant up to a point, then it starts to increase. The corresponding ATC curve is U-shaped. Initially, we will assume that short-run equilibrium is at point A with a price P_0 and quantity Q_0. This is based on the firm's cost conditions, demand conditions, and profit-maximizing objectives.

The change in demand conditions is the crux of this model. The introduction of a PPO will have the effect of increasing the elasticity of each individual hospital's demand (to D_2). That is, the effect of the PPO is to make each hospital more

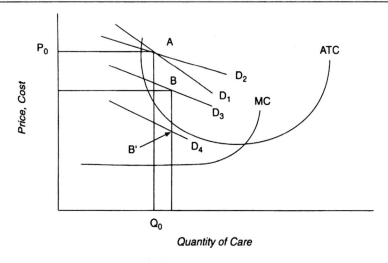

Figure 9–9 Representation of the effect of a PPO on a "typical" hospital's behavior. The initial demand curve facing the hospital (prior to the introduction of the PPO) is D_1, and the cost conditions of the hospital are represented by ATC and MC. The introduction of the PPO will initially increase the elasticity of the hospital's demand curve (to D_2). In response, the hospital will lower its price. All other hospitals are facing the same situation and will do the same. As they do so, each hospital's demand curve will shift inwards. The result of these cuts is uncertain, but the demand curve could wind up at D_3 (in which case each hospital will still make a profit) or at D_4 (in which case each would operate at a loss). In the latter case, some hospitals would have to cut costs or shut down operations entirely.

vulnerable to price changes instituted by other hospitals. With its demand elasticity increased, each hospital, assuming it acts as if all else is held constant, will lower its price to increase revenues and profits (this would be a profit-maximizing response of a firm facing an elastic demand curve). However, if all hospitals do the same, each hospital's demand curve will shift down (to D_3), and the new equilibrium will be at a point such as B (where each hospital shares in the larger market demand, which has expanded because of the lower price charged by all hospitals). Initially, price will fall, but hospitals in such a market may respond further. If B (on a curve such as D_3) is above the ATC curve, then the hospitals will still be making a profit after the price cut and no further change will result. On the other hand, if the collective price cuts drive the new demand curve down to D_4 (so that the equilibrium point is at B'), the hospitals will all be suffering a loss, and they will have to cut costs (by reducing services, downsizing, etc.) or some will have to leave the market. Cost cutting will shift the cost curves downward, while abandonment of the market by a few hospitals will result in a greater market share for the remaining ones. The final result will be the same: The PPO will have had an impact on hospital services ("quality") and market share.

Note that if the hospitals are operating on the constant portion of their marginal cost curves and no hospitals exit (each hospital's demand thereby remaining the same), then "downsizing" (a reduction in services and thus "quality") will be the outcome.

9.5.4 Increased Concentration

When concentration increases and providers are fewer in number, the probability of price collusion increases. Price collusion involves an explicit agreement or implicit understanding among competitors in a market to limit price competition. If there are only a few suppliers in a market and each understands that the ultimate outcome of price competition is lower prices and profits for all, the likelihood of suppliers refraining from price competition increases.

Explicit agreements to restrict price competition are illegal, but cautious pricing behavior directed at avoiding conflicts in pricing policies among competitors is not. Such cautious behavior is more likely to be found when a market contains a small number of competitors, because as the number of competitors increases, "cheating" is more likely. With fewer suppliers, the cost of detecting cheating is lower. Also, the impact of one supplier's price cuts is less dispersed; that is, each supplier's demand curve is shifted inward more when there are only a few suppliers.

Markets with a small number of suppliers and a significant degree of provider interdependence are called *oligopolistic*. Although vigorous price competition is not usually a characteristic of an oligopolistic market, quality competition is. In providing higher quality to attract and retain patients, the costs of oligopolistic competitors increase and profits are reduced.

Oligopolistic competition might occur when there are a few HMOs and traditional insurers in a market competing for the business of a large number of enrollees. In this case, we would expect to see rising quality but not much price competition (Hay and Leahy 1984). However, for an oligopolistic market to persist, entry by new competitors must be difficult, and the startup costs for an HMO may be low enough to make entry easy and attractive. The eventual result might be price competition. Also, buying power may discourage providers from engaging in oligopolistic behavior. In many markets, businesses play a considerable role in selecting which insurers (including HMOs) will insure their employees. If the buyer's side of the market is dominated by a few large businesses, price competition may become important despite the low number of providers.

9.5.5 Nonprice Competition

Price competition is sometimes not relevant. When patients are fully or substantially insured for a service and have a free choice among suppliers, they will choose suppliers based strictly on nonprice or quality considerations. Quality competition then becomes the only form of competition, and if the supply side of the market is competitive, costs will increase in response to quality improvements until the suppliers reach the break-even point or the limits placed by third-party reimbursers are reached. Analyses of this type of competitive process have been done for hospital markets (Farley 1985; Joskow 1980) and dialysis markets (Held and Pauly 1983). Studies across hospital markets have shown that, in market areas with greater degrees of competition (measured by the number of hospitals), hospitals are more likely to offer specialized heart surgery (Robinson et al. 1987) and specialized clinical services (Luft et al. 1986). Although these studies focused strictly on quality measures of output, there is some evidence that quality competition among hospitals is more prevalent than price competition (Noether 1988).

EXERCISES

1. Given the following demand and cost conditions for a monopolistic medical practice, predict the profit maximizing price and quantity of services utilized.

Price	Quantity of visits demanded
$10	0
9	1
8	2
7	3
6	4
5	5
4	6

   Cost conditions: fixed costs are $5 and marginal cost is $3.50 per visit.

2. The state Medicaid agency has set a rate of $5.50 per visit for all Medicaid enrollees who visit a physician. Each physician also has private paying patients. The demand curve for each physician can be characterized as follows, and physicians can be regarded as individual monopolists.

Out of pocket price	Quantity of visits demanded
$8	0
7	1
6	2
5	3
4	4
3	5
2	6
1	7

Each physician also has a cost schedule that can be characterized as follows:

Quantity of visits provided	Total cost
0	$5
1	7
2	11
3	17
4	25
5	35
6	47

a. If each physician is a profit maximizing provider, how many visits will he/she provide to public and private patients?

b. What will the number of visits provided be if the Medicaid Agency lowers its rate to $3 per visit, but the demand remains the same?

3. A physician practice serves two groups of patients. One group, with limited insurance, has demand represented by Demand Schedule A; the other, with extensive insurance, has demand represented by Demand Schedule B. The cost to produce a visit is $7.50. The practice wishes to price discriminate in order to maximize revenue. What price should it charge each patient group?

Demand Schedule A		Demand Schedule B	
Price ($)	No. of visits	Price ($)	No. of visits
10	1	10	5
9	2	9	6
8	3	8	7
7	4	7	8
6	5	6	9

4. The following tables show the hospitals operating in two cities and their annual patient days:

City 1		City 2	
Hospital	Patient days (000)	Hospital	Patient days (000)
A	15	H	60
B	85	I	60
C	110	J	54
D	45	K	48
E	70	L	39
F	25	M	39

Compare the concentration of the markets in the two cities using the four-firm concentration ratio and the Herfindahl (H) index.

5. Following is the supply schedule faced by a monopsonist and its demand schedule for the goods. Determine how much will be bought and what price will be paid by the monopsonist.

Price ($)	Units supplied	Price ($)	Units demanded (nurse)
1	1	$10	1
2	2	9	2
3	3	8	3
4	4	7	4
5	5	6	5
6	6	5	6
		4	7
		3	8

6. What characteristics of market structure make quality competition more likely than price competition? Which type of competition is more desirable from the viewpoint of the consumer? Discuss.

7. Explain why the market for physician services might exhibit some of the behavior of a monopoly market despite an apparently competitive structure.

BIBLIOGRAPHY

Monopoly and Physicians

Havighurst, C.C. 1978. Professional restraints on innovation in health care financing. *Duke Law Journal* 1978:303–388.

Kessell, R. 1958. Price discrimination in medicine. *Journal of Law and Economics* 1:20–53.

Leffler, K.B. 1978. Physician licensure: Competition and monopoly in American medicine. *Journal of Law and Economics* 21:165–186.

Newhouse, J.P. 1970. A model of physician pricing. *Southern Economic Journal* 37:147–183.

Rayack, E. 1964. The supply of physicians' services. *Industrial and Labor Relations Review* 17:221–237.

———. 1970. *Professional power and American medicine.* Cleveland, OH: World Publishing Co.

Profits in Medicine

Lindsay, C.M. 1973. Real returns to medical education. *Journal of Human Resources* 8:331–348.

———. 1976. More real returns to medical education. *Journal of Human Resources* 11:127–129.

Sloan, F.A. 1976. Real returns to medical education. *Journal of Human Resources* 11:118–126.

Price Discrimination and Physician Reimbursement

Cromwell, J., and J. Mitchell. 1984. An economic model of large Medicaid practices. *Health Services Research* 19:197–218.

Gabel, J.R., and T.H. Rice. 1985. Reducing public expenditures for physician services. *Journal of Health Politics, Policy, and Law* 9:595–609.

Hadley, J. 1979. Physician participation in Medicaid: Evidence from California. *Health Services Research* 14:266–280.

Hadley, J., and R. Lee. 1978–1979. Toward a physician payment policy: Evidence from the economic stabilization program. *Policy Sciences* 10:105–120.

Kushman, J.E. 1977. Physician participation in Medicaid. *Western Journal of Agricultural Economics* 2:22–33.

Muller, C., and J. Ostelberg. 1979. Carrier discretionary practices and physician payment under Medicare Part B. *Medical Care* 17:650–666.

Paringer, L. 1980. Medicare assignment rates of physicians: Their responses to changes in reimbursement policy. *Health Care Financing Review* 1 (summer): 75–89.

Rice, T. 1984. Determinants of physician assignment rates by type of service. *Health Care Financing Review* 5 (summer): 33–42.

Seldon, B.J., et al.1998. Market power among physicians in the U.S., 1983–1991. *Quarterly Review of Economics and Finance* 38:799–824.

Sloan, F.A., and B. Steinwald. 1978. Physician participation in health insurance plans. *Journal of Human Resources* 13:237–263.

Hospital and Nonprofit Agency Pricing

Barnett, A.H., et al. 1993. Inefficient pricing can kill. *Southern Economic Journal* 60:393–404.

Bauerschmidt, A.D., and P. Jacobs. 1985. Pricing objectives in non-profit hospitals. *Health Services Research* 20:153–161.

Bishop, C.E. 1988. Competition in the market for nursing home care. *Journal of Health Politics, Policy, and Law* 13:341–360.

Brooke, J.M., et al.1997. Hospital-insurer bargaining: An empirical investigation of appendectomy pricing. *Journal of Health Economics* 16:417–434.

Danzon, P.M. 1982. Hospital "profits." *Journal of Health Economics* 1:29–52.

Hay, J.W. 1983. The impact of public health care financing policies on private sector hospital costs. *Journal of Health Politics, Policy, and Law* 7:945–952.

Jacobs, P., and R.P. Wilder. 1984. Pricing behavior of non-profit agencies. *Journal of Health Economics* 3:49–61.

Johnston, W.P., et al. 1985. Interhospital variations in hospital pharmacy mark-ups. *American Journal of Hospital Pharmacy* 42:2492–2495.

Keeler, E.B., et al. 1999. The changing effects of competition on non-profit and for-profit hospital pricing behavior. *Health Economics* 18:69–86.

Sloan, F.A., and E. Becker. 1984. Cross subsidies and payment for hospital care. *Journal of Health Politics, Policy, and Law* 8:660–685.

Sloan, F.A., and P.B. Ginsburg. 1984. Hospital cost shifting. *New England Journal of Medicine* 310:893–898.

Wilder, R.P., and P. Jacobs. 1986. Antitrust considerations for hospital mergers: Market definition and market concentration. *Advances in Health Economics* 7:245–262.

Market Power and Health Insurance

Adamache, K.W., and F.A. Sloan. 1983. Competition between non-profit and for-profit health insurers. *Journal of Health Economics* 2:225–244.

Beazoglou, T., and D. Heffley. 1994. Reevaluating the "procompetitive" effects of HMOs: A spatial equilibrium approach. *Journal of Regional Science* 34:39–55.

Blair, R.D., et al. 1975. Economies of scale in the administration of health insurance. *Review of Economic Statistics* 57:185–189.

Dranove, D. et al. 1986. The effect of injecting price competition into the hospital market: the case of Preferred Provider Organizations. *Inquiry* 23:419–431.

Eisenstadt, D., and T.E. Kennedy. 1981. Control and behavior of nonprofit firms: The case of Blue Shield. *Southern Economic Journal* 48:26–36.

Feldman, R., and W. Greenberg. 1981a. Blue Cross market share, economies of scale and cost containment efforts. *Health Services Research* 16:175–183.

————. 1981b. The relation between Blue Cross market share and the Blue Cross "discount" on hospital charges. *Journal of Risk and Insurance* 48:235–246.

Frank, R.G., and W.P. Welch. 1985. The competitive effects of HMOs: A review of the evidence. *Inquiry* 22:148–161.

Frech, H.E. 1988. Competition among health insurers revisited. *Journal of Health Politics, Policy, and Law* 13:279–291.

Frech, H.E., and P.B. Ginsburg. 1978. Competition among health insurers. In *Competition in the health care sector*, ed. W. Greenberg. Washington, DC: Federal Trade Commission.

Goldberg, L.G., and W. Greenberg. 1977. The effect of physician-controlled health insurance. *Journal of Health Politics, Policy, and Law* 2:48–78.

————. 1985. The dominant firm in health insurance. *Social Science and Medicine* 20:719–724.

Lynk, W.L. 1981. Regulatory control of the membership of corporate boards of directors: The Blue Shield case. *Journal of Law and Economics* 24:159–174.

Wholey, D.R., and J.B. Christianson. 1994. Price differentiation among health maintenance organizations: Causes and consequences of open-ended products. *Inquiry* 31:25–39.

Monopsony

Barnett, A.H., et al. 1993. The medical community's opposition to organ markets: Ethics or economics? *Review of Industrial Organization* 8:669–678.

Foreman, S.E., et al. 1996 . Monopoly, monopsony and contestability in health insurance: A study of Blue Cross plans. *Economic Inquiry* 34:662–677.

Pauly, M.V. 1987. Monopsony power in health insurance: Thinking straight while standing on your head. *Journal of Health Economics* 6:73–81.

————. 1988. Market power, monopsony, and health insurance markets. *Journal of Health Economics* 7:111–128.

————. 1998 . Managed care, market power and monopsony. *Health Services Research* 33:1439–1460.

Staten, M. et al. 1987. Market share and the illusion of power: Can Blue Cross force hospitals to discount? *Journal of Health Economics* 6:43–58.

Monopoly and Monopolistic Competition

Bamezai, A., et.al. 1999. Price competition and hospital cost growth in the United States. *Health Economics* 8:233–244.

Cady, J.F. 1976. *Restricted advertising and competition*. Washington, DC: American Enterprise Institute.

Christianson, J.B., and W. McClure. 1979. Competition in the delivery of medical care. *New England Journal of Medicine* 301:812–818.

Farley, D.E. 1985. *Competition among hospitals: Market structure and its relation to utilization, costs and financial position*. Hospital Studies Program, Research Note 7. DHHS publication no. PHS 85–3353. Washington, DC: U.S. Department of Health and Human Services, National Center for Health Services Research and Health Care Technology Assessment.

Getzen, T.E. 1983. The market and evaluation in quality assurance. *Evaluation and the Health Professions* 6:299–310.

————. 1984. A "brand name" theory of medical group practice. *Journal of Industrial Economics* 33:199–217.

Goldberg, L.G., and W. Greenberg. 1979. The competitive response of Blue Cross and Blue Shield to the health maintenance organization in Northern California and Hawaii. *Medical Care* 17:1019–1028.

———. 1980. The competitive response of Blue Cross to the health maintenance organization. *Economic Inquiry* 18:55–68.

Hay, J.W., and M.J. Leahy. 1984. Competition among health plans: Some preliminary evidence. *Southern Economic Journal* 50:831–846.

Held, P.J., and M.V. Pauly. 1983. Competition and efficiency in the end stage renal disease program. *Journal of Health Economics* 2:95–118.

Joskow, P.L. 1980. The effects of competition and regulation on hospital bed supply and the reservation quality of the hospital. *Bell Journal of Economics* 11:421–447.

Kelly, E.T., et al. 1975. An examination of the effect of market demographic and competitive characteristics on gross margins of prescription drugs. *Medical Care* 12:956–965.

Lee, R.H., and D.M. Waldman. 1985. The diffusion of innovations in hospitals. *Journal of Health Economics* 12:371–380.

Luft, H.S., et al. 1986. The role of specialized clinical services in competition among hospitals. *Inquiry* 23:83–94.

Mobley, L.R. 1996. Tacit collusion among hospitals in price competitive markets. *Health Economics* 5:183–194.

———. 1997. Multiple hospital chain acquisitions and competition in local health care markets. *Review of Industrial Organization* 12:185–202.

Morrisey, M.A., and C.S. Ashby. 1982. An empirical analysis of HMO market share. *Inquiry* 19:136–149.

Noether, M. 1988. Competition among hospitals. *Journal of Health Economics* 7:259–284.

Nyman, J. 1987. Prospective and "cost-plus" Medicaid reimbursement, excess Medicaid demand, and the quality of nursing home care. *Journal of Health Economics* 6:129–146.

Rapoport, J. 1978. Diffusion of technological innovations among non-profit firms. *Journal of Economics and Business* 30:108–118.

Robinson, J.C. 1988. Hospital competition and hospital nursing. *Nursing Economics* 6:116–124.

Robinson, J.C., and H.S. Luft. 1987. Competition and the cost of hospital care, 1972 to 1982. *JAMA* 257:3241–3245.

Robinson, J.C., et al. 1987. Market and regulatory influences on the availability of coronary angioplasty and bypass surgery in U.S. hospitals. *New England Journal of Medicine* 317:85–90.

Robinson, J.C., et al. 1988. Hospital competition and surgical length of stay. *JAMA* 259:696–700.

Chapter 10

Health Insurance

1. Explain the utility-maximizing model of an individual's demand for health insurance.
2. Explain how the insurer's loading fee and the government's allowance of health insurance as a tax-free benefit will influence the demand for insurance.
3. Explain the influence of moral hazard on the demand for medical care and health insurance.
4. Explain why an individual may prefer insurance with a copayment rather than insurance without any copayment.
5. Calculate the elasticity of demand for health insurance and explain its importance.
6. Explain the concept of adverse selection.
7. Explain the role of the insurer in shifting risks.
8. Describe the supply function for insurers.
9. Explain the meaning of *community rating* and *experience rating*.
10. Explain the implications of adverse selection in insurance markets with information asymmetry and community rating.
11. Explain what tools insurers have at their disposal to avoid information asymmetry.
12. Explain the working of the insurance market with experience rating.

10.1 INTRODUCTION

As has been noted in earlier chapters, health insurance has a significant influence on markets for medical care. In this chapter we focus on the market for health insurance itself. The analytical basis for the discussion is a theory of decision making in the presence of risk. First, a model of demand for health insurance is developed. Then we consider the supply behavior of insurance providers. Finally, a model of a competitive market for health insurance is presented. While much of the chapter applies the basic supply-demand framework to a new context, it also introduces some concepts that are unique to insurance markets, specifically moral hazard and adverse selection.

10.2 DEMAND FOR HEALTH INSURANCE

10.2.1 Individual Demand for Insurance

The simple analysis of demand for medical care in Chapter 3 was based on the condition that the consumer knows with certainty what his or her state of health will be during the relevant time period. This underlying assumption is not plausible for many medical problems. In these cases, a consumer cannot be certain whether a problem will occur. The consumer does know, however, that he or she *might* be sick during a particular period and might have to visit a physician and even be hospitalized.

In this type of situation, a consumer faces the choice of whether to prepare financially for medical contingencies. He or she can prepare by purchasing insurance. This action entails an increased outlay (the premium) at the outset, followed by reduced outlays should an illness occur. The basic theory of the demand for insurance presents a systematic view of how certain underlying variables—tastes, wealth, price, the likelihood of an illness, and the loss resulting from the illness—can influence the decision to buy insurance. Following is a presentation of the basic assumptions of the model:

- *Consumer tastes.* To characterize consumer tastes with regard to the alternative situations resulting from an illness, let us assume that, when an illness occurs, it leads to medical care expenses that constitute a loss of wealth. To specify what this loss means to the individual, we must introduce a concept to characterize the individual's well-being at alternative levels of wealth—the concept of *utility*. One hypothetical individual's taste for wealth is presented in the form of an index of utility in Table10–1. This index shows what level of utility is associated with each specific level of wealth. Thus, a level of wealth of $1,000 is associated with a level of utility of 100, a level of wealth of $990 is associated with a level of utility of 99.8, and so on. The size of the specific numbers in the utility index are arbitrary. What is important is that higher wealth gives higher utility (i.e., increased wealth makes the individual "better off"). We further assume that the function is characterized by diminishing marginal utility. That is, each additional $10 of wealth results in less additional utility than the previous $10. For example, at $850, an extra $10 will yield 3 extra units of utility; at $860, an extra $10 will yield 2.8 extra units; and so on.

  If wealth has diminishing marginal utility for an individual, that individual is said to be *risk averse*. The basic idea is that, for a given wealth level, a loss of a given amount is of greater subjective importance (utility) to the person than would be a gain of an equal amount. Utility is the subjective index of the relative importance of wealth.

  In this model a utility function is unique to an individual. Thus it does not imply that additional wealth means less to a rich person than it does to a poor person. This kind of comparison, called *interpersonal comparison*, would involve specifying different people's utilities on the same scale.
- *Level of wealth.* Our second assumption is that the individual initially has a level of wealth of $1,000.
- *Medical expenses in the event of illness.* Our third assumption is that, if the individual becomes sick, he or she will face medical expenses of $100. This expenditure is assumed to fully restore the loss in health.

Table 10-1 Relationship between Wealth and Utility

Wealth	Total Utility	Marginal Utility
$800	57.0	4.2
810	61.2	4.0
820	65.2	3.8
830	69.0	3.6
840	72.6	3.4
850	76.0	3.2
860	79.0	3.0
870	81.8	2.8
880	84.4	2.6
890	86.8	2.4
900	89.0	2.2
910	91.0	2.0
920	92.8	1.8
930	94.4	1.6
940	95.8	1.4
950	97.0	1.2
960	98.0	1.0
970	98.8	0.8
980	99.4	0.6
990	99.8	0.4
1000	100.0	0.2

- *Likelihood of illness.* A fourth assumption concerns the element of uncertainty. We will assume that we can assign probabilities to the various possible health states the individual may experience. Let us say there is a .1 probability of illness (i.e., of 10 people in similar circumstances, 1 will become ill) and a .9 probability the individual will remain well and will not incur any medical costs. These are the only two possibilities, so the sum of the probabilities equals 1.
- *Price of insurance.* The individual can shift the risk of loss on to an insurer but will have to pay a premium to do so. In exchange for this premium, the insurer assumes the risk (i.e., the insurer will fully pay the $100 if the person should get sick).
- *Behavioral assumption.* The sixth assumption is that the individual wants to maximize the expected value of his or her utility. Thus the individual will choose that course of action from which he or she can expect to receive the highest level of utility.

The model's conclusions are obtained by determining how, under these assumed conditions, the individual will behave so as to maximize expected utility (i.e., which of the two options, buy insurance or do not buy insurance, the individual will chose). The model predicts that if health insurance is available on the right terms, the individual will buy it to reduce risk (and hence increase expected utility). To see how this conclusion is derived, let us examine how much wealth and utility the individual would expect to have with and without insurance.

The decision problem is summarized in Table 10–2. Without insurance, the individual has a 90-percent chance of having $1,000 in wealth and a 10-percent chance of having only $900 because of the payout for medical care. The expected value of wealth will be 90 percent of $1,000 plus 10 percent of 900, or $990. This is the sum of the amounts the individual expects to receive under various conditions

Table 10–2 Comparison of "Buy Insurance" and "Do Not Buy" Insurance Options

Price of Insurance	Wealth after Insurance Purchase	Utility after Insurance Purchase	Expected Utility with No Insurance	Decision
$10	$990	99.8	98.9	Buy
20	980	99.4	98.9	Buy
30	970	98.8	98.9	Do not buy
40	960	98.0	98.9	Do not buy

adjusted for the probabilities that those conditions will arise. If $1,000 is the level of wealth, the utility is 100 units. If $900 is available, the utility is 89 units. But the individual has only a 90-percent chance of having 100 units of utility and a 10-percent chance of having 89 units. The expected value of the utility achieved will be 90 percent of 100 plus 10 percent of 89, or 98.9.

So without insurance, the expected value of income is $990 and the expected value of utility is 98.9 units. The utility associated with a *certain* wealth of $990 is 99.8. So a certain wealth of $990 would be more desirable to the individual than the risky situation (because 99.8 > 98.9). A certain wealth of $990 could be obtained by buying an insurance policy costing $10. Payment of the $10 premium would reduce the initial $1,000 wealth to $990, but there is then no risk of further loss because even if illness occurs the insurance would cover the costs. Thus the individual in our model would have a demand for insurance at a premium of $10. Note that the premium of $10 here is called the actuarially fare premium or pure premium. It is the amount an insurer would have to charge to break even when insuring a large number of people assuming no administrative costs of operation.

In fact, the person in our example would be willing to pay considerably more than $10 for insurance. Suppose that for $20 he or she could buy insurance coverage against the $100 loss. By buying the insurance, the individual would be certain of having $980. This is because the individual's wealth would be reduced by the amount of the premium ($20), and if he or she became ill, the insurer would pay the cost. Certainty of having $980 would yield 99.4 units of utility, which is a higher expected utility than that in the "no insurance" situation. Being a utility maximizer, the individual would buy the insurance on these terms. Indeed, he or she would pay up to roughly $30 to avoid the risk of losing wealth due to illness, because at that price the expected utility with no insurance is approximately equal to the utility of the certain wealth after the purchase of insurance.

Of course, he or she would not buy insurance "at any price." For example if the premium were $40, the expected utility in the risky situation (98.9) is greater than the utility associated with a certain wealth of $960 (98.0), and the "do not buy insurance" option would be the more attractive one. Insurance demand also depends, of course, on the size of the possible loss. Suppose, for example, that the possible medical expense is not $100 but rather $150, either because the illness is more serious or because the price of medical care is higher. In this situation, the individual faces an expected loss of $150 if he or she becomes sick. The individual would have an expected utility of 97.6 units (10 percent of 76 plus 90 percent of 100) in the "no insurance" situation. If the individual was certain of having $960, he or she would be certain of receiving 98 units of utility. Therefore, in this case the individual would be willing to pay something over $40 for insurance.

The conclusion is that, as the possible loss increases, the amount of money the individual is willing to pay to avert the possible loss increases as well, and the individual will be willing to buy additional insurance coverage if the terms are right. The size of the financial loss in relation to the individual's wealth and the associated utilities is called the *financial vulnerability factor*. A second factor, which is related to the probability of illness, is referred to as the *risk perception factor* (Berki and Ashcraft 1980). In our example, if the probability of becoming sick increased from 10 to 20 percent, the expected utility in the "no insurance" situation would fall to 97.8 (80 percent of 100 plus 20 percent of 89). This is associated with a wealth level of close to $960, indicating that the individual would be willing to pay up to about $40 to avoid the risk of a $100 loss.

The amount an individual is willing to pay for insurance depends on the specific extent of his or her risk aversion. This is represented by the rate at which marginal utility diminishes with increasing wealth. An individual with constant marginal utility would be risk neutral. For such a person, insurance at the actuarially fair premium would be no more desirable than the "no insurance" option. The greater the rate of decrease of marginal utility for a person, the more risk averse he or she is and the more willing to pay premiums above the actuarially fair premium.

10.2.2 Limitations of the Theory

The theory of insurance demand has the virtue of explicitly organizing some of the variables that are central to the decision to purchase insurance. As presented, however, it has important limitations. The following observations may be of help in understanding what these limitations are.

First, the reader may find it strange that the utility function, which is supposed to measure satisfaction, does not include medical care. This is indeed a shortcoming of the model, because well-being can depend on appropriate care. The model looks only at financial aspects of the situation, in effect assuming that the care fully and instantly restores health, with no utility implications of either the illness or the process of getting care. Clearly this is an unrealistic assumption. Including medical care, however, creates a model that is much more complicated and more difficult to apply, and while it is important to understand that we have abstracted from reality, this should not detract from the value of the model. The present model has the virtue of focusing on the benefits of risk shifting, which is an economic good distinct from medical care.

Second, insurance has the effect of lowering the direct price of medical care. One would expect the demand for medical care to increase under these circumstances, yet in the basic insurance model we have assumed that medical care demand does not change with the lower, postinsurance price. That is, the model implies that, if an individual becomes ill, he or she will demand the same amount of medical care with or without insurance. This means that the elasticity of demand for medical care is zero, an unlikely scenario for most types of medical care. Again, such an assumption was necessary to simplify the model.

Third, we have assumed that the individual pays the full amount of the premium. In fact, often a consumer's out-of-pocket premium is substantially less than the total premium. The consumer might receive insurance through his or her employer, who pays part or all of the premium. This is not to say that the consumer receives "free" insurance. The consumer, through a bargaining unit or via an employer's policy, negotiates for or receives a total compensation package that includes wages (a direct money component) and benefits (e.g., pension rights and health insurance). The individual pays taxes on the money portion of compensation and with after-tax wages directly pays his or her share of the premiums. Under the Internal Revenue Code, many nonwage benefits received through the employer, including health insurance, are not taxed. Therefore, insurance has a lower price when purchased through employment benefits than directly by the consumer.

This point is illustrated numerically in Table 10–3. In our example, the marginal tax rate of the individual or family is 20 percent, which means that, for each $100 in taxable income the employee receives, he or she pays $20 in taxes and takes home $80. Now if $625 of additional compensation is made in the form of wages and there are no deductible expenses, the individual will pay $125 (20 percent of $625) in taxes and will have $500 left over to purchase goods or services, including health insurance. If, on the other hand, the $625 in compensation is in the form of employer-provided health insurance, then this compensation is not taxed and $625 in insurance coverage can be received. A dollar's worth of coverage purchased with after-tax wages is thus worth $(1 - T)$ times the value of the coverage received via employer benefits, where T is the marginal tax rate. Thus $(1 - T) \times \$1$ is sometimes called the price of $1 of employer-provided premiums (Taylor and Wilensky 1983). In terms of our demand model, such tax benefits will lower the cost of health insurance to the individual and thus will increase its demand.

10.2.3 The Market Demand for Insurance

Insurance availability requires the existence of at least one organization willing to accept the risks and pay the costs when they arise. To determine under which market conditions this will occur, let us assume an insurance company is being formed to cover the risks of 1,000 people with tastes, incomes, and health experience exactly like those of the representative individual in Section 10.2.1. We can now give a more definite meaning to the "probabilities" assigned to the alternative health states. Assume that the insurance company can be almost certain that 100 of the 1,000 consumers will become ill and require medical care during the month. Because pooling a large number of risks yields a considerable degree of certainty, it becomes possible to assign a risk to each consumer and evaluate his or her expected loss experience in terms of the group.

The insurance company knows that, in a group of 1,000 consumers, 100 will most likely become ill and will require $100 worth of medical care The expected medical expenses total $10,000 for the group. As we have seen, the actuarially fair rate, the expected loss per individual consumer, is $10. If each consumer pays a

Table 10–3 A Comparison of Health Insurance When Purchased by Employer and Employee

	Purchased by Employee	Purchased by Employer
Compensation	$625	$625
Tax	125	0
After-tax money available for purchasing premiums	500	625

premium of $10, the expected losses of the group will just be covered. According to the analysis in Section 10.2.1, every consumer would be willing to pay a premium equal to the actuarially fair rate to reduce the risk of large losses. Indeed, with diminishing marginal utility, they would be willing to pay somewhat more.

The insurance company cannot charge the actuarially fair rate, because resources are necessary to administer an insurance business and some level of profit or surplus must be earned. The insurance company must charge more to cover these administrative costs and profits. The additional fee charged by the insurance company is called the *loading fee*. The premium each individual pays is thus made up of two components: the fee for benefits received and the loading fee. In our example, let us assume that the insurer has administrative expenses of $750 in total and desires a profit of $250; the total load is thus $1,000. The insurance company must charge premiums of $11,000, of which $10,000 will be paid out in benefits. With premiums spread over 1,000 consumers, if all pay the same premium rate, the rate will be $11 per consumer.

Strictly speaking, the price of insurance is the loading fee, not the premium. In this case, the price of insurance is $1 per insurance consumer. This price can be expressed in several ways, including as a ratio of premiums to benefits ($11/$10 or 1.1), as a cost per policy ($1), or as a ratio of the loading fee to benefits (0.10). The reason the loading fee is the price of insurance is that the product is insurance, the protection from risk, not the provision of medical care. The gains the consumer receives from insurance coverage are the utility gains from the risk reduction. The price of this risk reduction is the loading fee. It is the level of this fee that will determine whether or not the individual will purchase insurance.

The overall market demand will thus depend on the various factors that influence individual demand and the number of individuals in the market. If all individuals have exactly the same tastes, incomes, sickness profiles, and so on, then they will have the same demand for insurance. In actuality, this is unlikely to be the case. Individuals will differ by illness level, wealth, and degree of risk aversion. Their gains from risk reduction will thus differ, and as the price of *insurance* (the loading fee) increases, some individuals will drop their coverage and market demand will fall off.

10.2.4 Moral Hazard

Once an individual has purchased medical insurance, the direct price he or she pays for medical care decreases. If the individual has purchased full insurance, this price is zero. However, as was shown in Chapter 3, when the direct price of medical care decreases for any reason (including as a result of buying insurance), the quantity demanded will increase (i.e., the absolute value of the elasticity of demand is greater than zero). This phenomenon—the existence of an elasticity of demand for medical care in response to insurance—is known in the insurance industry as *moral hazard*. The term suggests that individuals "shirk" their responsibilities and consume recklessly when they are insured. From the point of view of economics, they are simply behaving in accordance with the principle expressed by the downward-sloping demand curve.

The existence of moral hazard has been used to explain why individuals only partially insure against health care risks, that is, why they accept copayments and deductibles rather than full insurance coverage (Feldstein and Friedman 1977;

Friedman 1974). Such analyses are more complicated than the basic insurance models, but the essentials can be presented in a simple fashion. Let us assume that an individual has the same utility function as in the model discussed in Section 10.2.1. Other basic assumptions are as follows:

- The probability of being sick is 0.2 and of being well is 0.8. That is, out of each 100 consumers, 20 will get sick.
- If a consumer gets sick, the price of each unit of medical care is $5.
- The individual's initial level of wealth is $1,000.

We also initially ignore, as in our previous model, utility received directly from medical care and health. We now distinguish three options: in Option 1, the individual has no insurance but pays the market price ($5.00) per unit of medical care used; in Option 2, the individual is fully insured and pays a zero price for medical care; and in Option 3, there is a 10-percent copayment and thus a direct price to the individual of $.50 per unit of medical care.

Because demand varies with price, the quantity of medical care demanded will vary in the three situations. We assume that in Option 1, where the direct price is $5.00, 10 units of medical care will be demanded. In Option 2, where the price is 0, 30 units will be demanded. In Option 3, where the price is $.50, 12 units will be demanded. We now wish to focus on the demand for insurance. To simplify the analysis, let us specify a loading fee of zero (no load), which means that the premium rate will equal the expected loss to the individual. The information for this example is summarized in Table 10–4.

Let us first consider Options 1 and 2. We will compare the expected utilities ($E(U)$) to determine which provides the highest utility level (and hence which is preferred). If the expected utility in Option 1 is greater than that in Option 2, then the individual will not buy insurance, since having no insurance yields a higher expected utility than having full insurance. In fact, under Option 1 the individual faces a 20-percent chance of becoming sick, paying the full $50 in medical costs, and having $950 left over. The utility of $950 in wealth is 97 (see Table 10–1). On the other hand, the individual has an 80-percent chance of not getting sick, in which case the level of wealth remains at $1,000 and the utility is 100. The $E(U)$ for this situation is 99.4 (80 percent of 100 plus 20 percent of 97). The $E(U)$ under Option 2 is equal to the utility of the original level of wealth minus the premium (i.e., the utility of $970). This amounts to 98.8. Since "no insurance" has greater expected

Table 10–4 Example of the effects of moral hazard

	Situation 1 (No insurance)	Situation 2 (Full insurance)	Situation 3 (10% copayment)
Price paid by individual for one unit of care	$5	0	$.50
Units of care demanded	10	30	12
Amount paid by insurance company for care	0	$150	$54
Pure premium	—	$ 30	$10.80
Expected utility	99.4	98.8	99.6

utility than full insurance, the individual will demand "no insurance" under these conditions.

Let us now bring Option 3 into the picture. First note that the premium is less than under full insurance, where 30 units of medical care were demanded. Under Option 3, 12 units are demanded, but because of the 10-percent copayment, the insurance company pays only $4.50 per unit, or $54.00 in total. The individual, having a 20-percent probability of becoming sick, will pay a premium of $10.80. In addition, if the individual is sick, he or she pays a copayment of $.50 per unit, or $6.00 overall. The $E(U)$ for this situation is roughly 99.6 [20 percent of $(1,000 - 10.80 - 6.00)$ plus 80 percent of $(1,000 - 10.80)$]. This is greater than the expected utility of not buying insurance. Now the individual will buy insurance.

However, this may not be the preferred option. Other copayment rates will have other expected utilities. What is important to note is that the individual will, in some circumstances, prefer insurance with a copayment to that with full coverage (or no coverage) if the moral hazard is great enough.

One shortcoming of this model should be mentioned. Medical care has utility, as does insurance. We have ignored this fact. Indeed, the extra units of medical care consumed in Options 2 and 3 yield extra utility in their own right. It may well be that the marginal utility of these units would make the full coverage option preferable to one of lesser coverage. While this may be the case, the point of this discussion is that, if the conditions are right, insurance with a copayment may be preferred to all other options.

10.2.5 Demand Responsiveness to the Price of Health Insurance

In Chapter 3 we discussed the concept of the elasticity of demand for medical care, which is a measure of how responsive the quantity of medical care is to out-of-pocket price changes. In a similar vein, one can estimate an elasticity of demand for health insurance showing how buyers will respond to changes in the price of insurance. The formula can be written as follows:

$$E_d = \frac{(\text{PREM}_2 - \text{PREM}_1) / (P_2 - P_1)}{(\text{PREM}_2 + \text{PREM}_1) / (P_2 - P_1)}$$

where E_d is the elasticity of demand for insurance coverage, PREM is the dollar amount of premiums demanded (with subscripts 1 and 2 referring to Situations 1 and 2), and P is the price of insurance (with subscripts 1 and 2 referring to Situations 1 and 2). Note that the price of insurance is the loading fee, as discussed in the previous section. Let us say that the loading fee increases from $80 per policy to $100 and that as a result consumers reduce their premiums from $1,050 to $950. Then the elasticity of demand is

$$\frac{(1,050 - 950) / 2,000}{(100 + 80) / 180}$$

It is very important to know the magnitude of this variable for policy purposes. The exemption from income tax of health insurance benefits is equivalent to a reduction in the price of health insurance. This exemption has the effect of increasing the demand for health insurance benefits, such as reductions in the copayment. Lower copayments increase the quantity of medical care demanded. In the immediate post–World War II era, when the government was trying to encourage the consumption of medical care, this increase in demand was not regarded as a problem. In current times, with the concern over medical care costs, the issue has grown in importance.

Several studies have been undertaken to establish the responsiveness of the demand for insurance to changes in the price of insurance. Taylor and Wilensky (1983) examined how premiums increase as the variable tax rate (1 – marginal tax rate) falls. (This variable was taken to be a proxy for the after-tax price of employer-provided health insurance.) They found the elasticity to be –0.2. In other studies, the value has ranged from –0.2 to –1. There is considerable uncertainty, then, as to the value of this variable. If we accept –0.2 as the correct figure, then an individual in the 20-percent marginal tax bracket who received $1,000 in employer-provided premiums has been able to buy $1 in premiums for 80 cents. If the government eliminated this subsidy, the price would rise to $1 and the quantity of insurance demanded (premiums) would fall to about $955.

Such a reduction in benefits would mean higher copayments and would subsequently translate into less medical care demanded and, with an elastic demand for medical care, into lower medical expenditures. The reader should be aware of the interaction between insurance and medical care markets. What happens in one market influences what happens in the other.

10.2.5 Choice of Health Plan

The purchase of a particular health insurance policy through employment-based insurance requires two decisions, one by the employer and one by the employee. Many employers provide their employees with a selection of health plans and allow them to make their own decisions about the types of coverage and service they will obtain. The plans with more complete coverage will cost more, and for each of these the insurer will charge a higher premium. Often the employer will pay a fixed contribution toward the premium regardless of the plan chosen, and the employee will pay out of pocket the difference between the premium and the employer's contribution. The employee, in such cases, has a choice among alternative types of health care coverage. From an economic standpoint, we are concerned with discovering what factors influence consumer demand for alternative plans.

Which economic determinants influence the choice of health plan is a topic of considerable importance. If individuals or families with specific characteristics (e.g., sick people, young couples with families) prefer one type of plan over another on economic grounds, selection is said to be *biased*. *Biased selection* thus means that these individuals or families with certain characteristics will demand one particular plan systematically. Often the basis for the selection of a plan is economic. In such cases, the selection is a manifestation of demand behavior.

The economic significance of this lies in the fact that, as a result of these selections, different health plans will have different populations with different experiences of health care utilization. One plan (e.g., a traditional plan) may appear to be expensive relative to another (e.g., an HMO). Some of the difference in price may be due to the enrollment of families with different characteristics in the plan (e.g., older people may tend to enroll in the traditional plan). Any comparison of the cost of the two plans that *did not account for these differences* would be misleading. Thus, we must be aware of these factors and of their causes.

To demonstrate the concept of biased selection, we will apply our insurance demand model to two alternative situations. In both, there is an employer with 2,000 employees. Each employee has one chance in five (i.e., a probability of .2) of becoming sick. However, the employees can be divided into two groups of 1,000 each. Those in the "unhealthy" group will require $200 in medical care if they become sick; those in the "healthy" group will require only $100 of medical care. Individuals in both groups have an initial wealth level of $1,000 and the utility function shown in Table 10–1.

The insurance plan in Situation 1 is a "high-option" plan, in that it covers all expenses in the event of illness. We will assume, for simplicity's sake, that the insurance company has no loading fee. The premium is thus equal to the expected loss for the employee. The total payout will be $40,000 ($200 × .2 × 1,000) for the unhealthy employees and $20,000 for the healthy employees. On average, the payout is $30 per employee. We will assume that all consumers pay according to *community rating*; that is, each pays the same premium regardless of his or her experience. The full premium is $30. The employer's contribution is assumed to be $20 per employee, and the employee's contribution is $10. It should be remembered that the employer's $20 contribution is employee compensation, and normally there would be tax advantages in receiving compensation in this way. We will ignore these benefits to keep our example uncomplicated.

With our assumptions specified, we now examine the demand for the high-option plan. This is done using the utility model of insurance demand that we introduced in previous sections. According to this model, individuals will demand an insurance plan if the expected utility associated with the plan is greater than the expected utility in the absence of the plan. Consider first the unhealthy group. The expected loss for a person in this group if he or she became sick and had no insurance would be $200. The person would be left with $800 in wealth (yielding a utility of 57.1). However, 80 percent of the individuals in this group will remain healthy, and each of these individuals will be left with $1,000 and have an associated utility level of 100. The average expected utility for the entire group would be 91.4 (80 percent of 100 and 20 percent of 57.1). Similarly, the average expected utility of the healthy group would be 97.8 (20 percent of the utility of $900 plus 80 percent of the utility of $1,000), since their costs are only $100.

To determine the situation of these groups when they have insurance, we must know the premium. In this case it is $30. This amount is treated as a reduction in employee's wealth even though some of it may be employer paid, because more nonwage benefits would mean less wages (and so, in the absence of tax considerations, we can regard them as equivalent). If each employee incurs a premium cost of $30, he or she will be left with wealth of $970 and have a utility level of 98.8. Since utility with insurance for both groups is greater than utility with no insurance, both groups would demand insurance coverage.

Let us now introduce Situation 2, in which there is a low-option plan with the following characteristics. First, there is a limit on the benefits of $100. That is, if anyone becomes sick, the insurance company would cover the first $100 of expenses, but beyond that the individual would be responsible. The premium of such a plan would be lower, because the insurance company's payout would be limited to only $100 per episode of illness. In fact, it would be $20 (.2 × $100).

Our utility model can again shed light on the choice of plan. First of all, the unhealthy group members, if they joined such a plan, would pay the $20 premium plus the excess of illness expenses ($200) over covered expenses ($100), or $100 per illness. Their wealth would be $880 if they were sick and $980 if they were well, and their expected utility would be 96.4 (20 percent of 84.4 plus 80 percent of 99.4). Utility theory predicts that these individuals would be better off joining the high-option plan (where the expected utility is 98.8) and so would choose the high-option plan. The healthy group, on the other hand, would spend $20 on premiums for the low-option plan and would have no additional out-of-pocket expenses. They would retain $980 whether or not they were sick, and their expected utility would be 99.4. This is greater than under the high-option plan, and so they would choose the low-option plan.

Our model thus shows that the characteristics of a group partially dictate the choice of plan. An unhealthy group uses more care and will demand higher coverage. There are a number of reasons why one group might consist of high-cost users: the individuals might be older, have special health problems, be more likely to have children, and so on. If, for whatever reason, the group members have higher expected costs, then they will *systematically* select a plan with a higher degree of coverage.

Of course, when biased selection occurs, the rejection of the high-option plan by the healthy group would leave relatively more unhealthy people in that plan, and so the average cost of that plan would increase. This is an example of what is called *adverse selection* and has implications for the functioning of the insurance market, which are discussed below.

There is a very important issue that the model throws light on. As shown above, different benefit plans will attract different types of consumers. For example, a high-option plan will attract individuals who are less healthy and tend to use more care. In a previous section, we established that individuals with more complete coverage will demand more medical care (because of lower out-of-pocket costs) whatever their health status. If we review actual data comparing plans and notice that individuals in the higher option plan use more care than in the lower option plan, what can we conclude? In fact, it could be both the lower out-of-pocket price and the difference in health status that contributed to differences in utilization. This confounding of causal factors in health care demand has been a source of bias in many studies comparing utilization between plans. For example, a number of studies have compared utilization between enrollees in HMOs and conventional insurance plans. The general conclusion has been that hospital utilization under HMO coverage is lower than under conventional coverage (Miller and Luft 1995). But the issue has been somewhat clouded by the lack of clear evidence that the groups being compared were similar in terms of health status.

10.3 SUPPLY OF HEALTH INSURANCE

10.3.1 Supplier Behavior

The product of insurers is the assumption of risks initially borne by consumers, including the risk of heavy medical costs. An insurer has the choice of accepting or not accepting risks on behalf of consumers, and there are a number of factors that will induce any insurer not to accept certain risks. Not only consumers have preferences regarding risk; owners and managers of insurance companies react to risk as well. The insurer is in business to earn profits, which yield utility for its shareholders. Its tastes reflect those of its shareholders. The insurer's wealth (and hence utility) depends on the revenues collected by the insurer and on the insurer's costs, including its payout.

10.3.2 Risk and Size of the Insured Population

The degree of risk of most interest to the insurer is not that faced by any specific individual but rather the mean risk for the insured population. This is what determines the claims the insurer can expect to be faced with. However, because we are dealing with random events, in any given round of insuring the actual value of claims the insurer experiences will almost always differ from the mean. Thus the insurer is concerned with the variability of the insured population's risk, that is, the likelihood that in any given year it will be very far above or below the mean value. Because of such variability, insurers must hold contingency reserves (i.e., funds available for covering claims in years when claims are unusually large).

An important thing to note is that this variability is inversely related to the number of people insured. As we add additional insured consumers, the insurer is less likely to experience a loss for the insured consumer group that is very different from the expected value. In other words, the insurer's risk of large losses is reduced as the size of the insurance pool increases, assuming the loss experiences of individuals are independent. So even if all the consumers face a high degree of risk (i.e., a big spread between financial outcomes), the variability faced by the insurance company can be much smaller because of the effect of big numbers on variation. This effect is referred to in statistics as the *law of large numbers*.

The actual computation of this effect is beyond the scope of this book. However, the very powerful effect of the number of people insured can be illustrated using a simple example. Suppose each person has a risk function as follows: there is a 25-percent probability of an $800 loss, a 50-percent probability of a $700 loss, and a 25-percent probability of a $600 loss. The expected mean loss is thus $700. In any given year, the actually realized mean of a group's loss will not be exactly $700, but if the group is large, it won't be very far away from that.

The likelihood of extreme losses for the group as a whole is less than for any individual. For example, for any *one person* the probability of a loss of $800 is .25. However, for a group of 100 such people with independent loss experiences, it is very unlikely that the *mean* loss would be $800. Such a result would imply that all 100 people experienced an $800 loss! Much more likely is the result that some will experience that loss and others will lose $700 or $600. The relevant computation shows that for this group the mean loss with 25-percent probability is $704.70 or more. If the group size were 1,000, a mean loss of $704.70 or more would have probability of only .018, and for a group of 10,000 the probability of a mean loss as large as $704.70 is virtually zero.

10.3.3 Insurer Costs

The calculation of expected costs involves two components: claims paid out and the insurer's administrative expenses. The administrative expenses are incurred in the selling of insurance policies and the administration of claims. Economies of scale may play a role in determining administrative costs. If that is the case, larger insurers will have lower per member administrative costs than smaller insurers. Claims paid out are determined by the price of medical care and the quantity of medical care used by the consumers. To some extent, both of these are outside the control of the insurer. Prices of medical care are determined in the market for such care, and medical care consumed depends largely on the health status of the insured population. However, an analysis that assumed that both of these are taken as given by the insurer would be seriously flawed for two reasons. First, insurers often have some market power and play a very active role in setting the price of medical care; sophisticated bargaining arrangements (many covered in subsequent chapters) exist under ordinary insurance arrangements as well as under preferred provider and managed care arrangements. Second, utilization of care is also subject to a host of forces, including the moral hazard phenomenon and direct insurer-provider relationships under managed care.

10.3.4 Insurer Revenues

The insurer's revenues are the premiums it receives from the consumers. There are two basic ways in which premiums can be set: through experience rating or through community rating. *Experience rating* involves the setting of premiums for individuals or groups according to their risk of loss. Healthy, low-risk individuals will be charged lower premiums than unhealthy, high-risk individuals. In *community rating*, a single rate is set for the entire insured population based on the average experience of that population. High-risk individuals and low-risk individuals all pay the same rate regardless of their expected loss.

10.3.5 Predictions about Supply

A simple supply model would show a typical positive relationship between price and quantity supplied. At higher premiums, an insurer would be more willing to take on additional risks. We can also draw conclusions about the effect of changes in other variables on the supply schedule of the insurer. Increases in the supply schedule (more risks accepted at a given premium rate) will be induced by the following: a less risk averse utility function on the part of the insurer, a greater initial level of reserves, a reduction in administrative costs, and a drop in the losses that may be experienced by the consumers. Several additional aspects of supply behavior are worthy of emphasis.

First, if all consumers do not have the same risk function and the insurer can choose between experience rating and community rating, the analysis becomes more complex. Suppose there are two groups, one high risk and the other low risk. With experience rating, a premium would be set that reflected each group's loss experience. The insurer would then have to decide for each group whether to supply insurance, a decision that would be based on the premium rate, marginal costs, and so on, for that particular group. Use of community rating would create a different situation. Again, there would be two groups, each with its own marginal costs. But now there would be a single premium rate, which would fall somewhere between those of the high-risk and low-risk groups. A for-profit insurer would have an incentive to develop criteria to distinguish between high-risk and low-risk individuals and refuse to insure the former (i.e., it would engage in so-called preferred risk selection). In fact, community rating began and evolved as a method in the nonprofit sector, where firms follow different objectives. A nonprofit firm may have as an objective increasing the availability of insurance coverage for higher risk groups. If it did have this objective, its behavior would differ from the behavior of a for-profit firm.

Second, insurers can lower their costs (and increase their profits) by reducing the consumers' utilization of insured health care services and by lowering the amounts they reimburse the providers of care. Indemnity insurers have developed a number of utilization-reducing instruments, including preadmission review and rules requiring second opinions for surgery. Indeed, HMOs were developed as a means of controlling the intensity of medical care provided to patients. However, even indemnity insurers have become active in the managed care arena and have resorted to utilization-reducing mechanisms.

Third, whereas previously insurers had played a passive role in the setting of prices, they have become increasingly active in contracting with providers and pushing for favorable terms. For example, in a preferred provider arrangement, insurers seek specified prices from providers. Insurers have sought to gain a market advantage over providers so they can either pass the lower prices on to consumers or else can capture the gains for themselves.

10.4 ADVERSE SELECTION IN HEALTH INSURANCE MARKETS

In Section 10.2 the concept of self-selection in insurance coverage was introduced. Insurance plans with specific types of coverage will attract consumers who will benefit the most from the coverage. In the presence of information asymmetry, this can create a situation, called *adverse selection*, that could damage an insurance market to such a degree that it ceases to exist. Although in practice economists have questioned whether this phenomenon is an empirically important one, it has drawn considerable attention in the literature (Pauly 1986).

In our insurance model, we will assume that there are three separate groups of 100 individuals with the following demand conditions:

- In Group 1, the healthiest, each individual has a 10-percent probability of becoming ill and requiring medical care; in Group 2, the intermediate group, the probability is 40 percent; and in Group 3 it is 80 percent.
- The cost of medical treatment for an individual in any group (i.e., the total amount of the loss in the event of illness) is $100.
- Individuals have the utility function presented in Table 10–1.

Based on these assumptions, the expected utility of being uninsured for any individual will be the weighted average of the utility of $1,000 (which is 100.0, according to Table 10–1) if the individual stays healthy and the utility of $900 (which is 89.0) if he or she becomes sick. For Group 1 individuals, this is $(.9 \times 100) + (.1 \times 89.0)$, or 98.9. The expected utilities for Groups 2 and 3 are 95.6 and 91.2, respectively. Each member of Group 1 would pay at most a premium of approximately $30 (resulting in a utility of 98.9) to be insured. For any premium above this amount, the members would accept the risk and not buy insurance. For any premium lower, they would demand insurance coverage. The indifference premium is approximately $60 for Group 2 and approximately $90 for Group 3.

We turn now to the supply side of the market. The relevant assumptions are as follows:

- The insurance company's administrative costs are $2,000.
- Total insurance company expenses consist of the administrative costs plus the amount the insurer reimburses for medical care.
- The insurance company merely wants to break even, so revenues will just equal costs.

As for the pricing policy of the insurance company, which is a critical element in the model, there are a number of alternatives the company could choose. For example, it could employ an experience rating methodology, which involves dividing the total pool into subgroups and setting rates according to each subgroup's expected loss. In an experience rating pricing scheme, Groups 1, 2, and 3 would all pay different premiums because they have different levels of expected loss. The second type of pricing policy is community rating. In a community rating scheme, all individuals pay the same rate. Community rating would probably be the method chosen if the insurer were not able to distinguish between individuals in the three groups. It could not, then, charge a different premium based on expected loss.

Let us assume that an information asymmetry does exist. That is, the consumers know which group they fall into, but the insurer does not have that health status information. Under this condition, a single community rate is charged to all individuals. We will now determine how the market might operate over time. Initially, the insurance company, wanting to break even, will charge a rate high enough to cover all the reimbursements for the three groups ($13,000) plus the administrative costs ($2,000). Over the 300 individuals, this rate amounts to $50 per individual. This rate exceeds Group 1's indifference premium, and so members of Group 1 will choose not to insure. Members of Groups 2 and 3, on the other hand, will insure. With Group 1 dropping out of the market, total expenses for Groups 2 and 3 are $14,000. Again, the insurance company cannot distinguish between them, and so it must charge a single community rate, this time of $70 per individual. But this rate will be above the amount members of Group 2 are willing to pay, and they will drop out of the market, leaving only Group 3. The rate will be raised to $100, but this will exceed Group 3's indifference premium. The members of Group 3 will drop out of the market as well, causing the market to collapse. This phenomenon is a joint result of adverse selection (those with the highest risks remain in the market) and community rating (chosen as a method because of the information asymmetry).

The popularity of the above model might be attributable to its doom-and-gloom prediction of market disappearance, but there is some question as to how well it fits the present market for health insurance. There is scant empirical evidence to decide its applicability, but it has drawn attention to the phenomenon of community rating and its potential role in market failure. And, in fact, in the present model the market would perform differently if experience rating was used. To see this, assume that for each group a premium is set equal to its expected medical costs plus $666 (which is one-third of the total administrative expenses). Then each group would pay a premium that was less than what it would be willing to pay. For example, Group 1 individuals would be charged $16.66 in premiums ($1,000 + $666 divided by 100 people). This is below what they would be willing to pay for insurance coverage. Thus it is the community rating pricing policy that caused the market to disappear.

There have been questions raised as to whether community rating results from informational asymmetry or other factors. Insurance companies have or can get considerable amounts of information about potential consumers by looking at age and medical history and by conducting medical exams. In fact, insurance companies use experience rating for pricing individual policies. This being the case, it may not be informational asymmetry that leads to community rating (Feldman 1987) but other causes. For example, employers may want to be equitable to all employees and so offer a single (community) rate for all—the young, the old, the sick, and so on. Employees, including low-risk employees, may accept this in part because they are happy with the idea that when they become unhealthy later in life their premiums will be community rated as well.

EXERCISES

1. Mrs. Smith's utility function is the same as that shown in Table 10–1. Her initial level of wealth is $1,000. Her annual medical expenses if she got sick would be $120. Her probability of getting sick (and thus incurring the medical expenses) is 0.2. The price of an insurance policy is $30.
   a. If Mrs. Smith were a utility maximizer, should she purchase insurance?
   b. Should she purchase insurance if the price were $60?
   c. Would Mrs. Smith purchase insurance at $60 if her medical expenses, in case she got sick, were $200?
   d. Is Mrs. Smith risk averse, risk neutral, or a risk taker?
2. Mrs. Rosen has a utility function like that in Table 10–1. There is a 0.5 probability that she will incur medical expenses of $200. What is the most she would pay for insurance?
3. Health insurance premiums obtained through an employer are deductible from income tax. An individual health insurance policy costs $500. The personal income tax rate is 30 percent. An employer provides premiums as a benefit. What is the price to the employee of the insurance?
4. An insurance company has a payout of health benefits of $100,000. Administrative expenses on top of that are $30,000, and profits are $10,000. What is the ratio of premiums to benefits? If there are 100 insureds, what is the premium rate each would pay?
5. A survey of insured persons indicates that, when the loading charge paid by each was $80, the premium was $2,000. When the loading charge was increased to $120, each person was only willing to spend $1,600 on insurance. What is the elasticity of demand for insurance?
6. The elasticity of an individual's demand for insurance is –0.2. When the loading fee was $100, the person purchased $3,000 in insurance premiums. The loading fee is increased to $120. How much insurance will the person purchase?
7. Buffalo Systems has 1,000 employees, all of whom are insured in the company plan. There are two groups of employees, healthy and unhealthy. Half of the employees are in each category. Persons in both groups have an

equal probability of being sick of –0.2, an initial wealth level of $1,000, and the utility function shown in Table 10–1. When a healthy person gets sick, the cost of care is $100. The cost of care for an unhealthy person is $150.

   a. If the company plan is community-rated, such that each person pays $25, would both groups choose to insure?

   b. Assume that the company introduces a low-cost plan. Those in the plan pay $20. The plan only insures up to $100. Persons pay any excess out of pocket. Which group would purchase insurance? What would be the total expenditure of each group, including out-of-pocket expenses?

8. How will each of the following affect the supply for insurance:
   a. a larger pool of insured persons
   b. lower administration costs for insurance companies
   c. higher premiums (with no change in risk experience)
   d. a greater degree of risk aversion on the part of insurers

9. What is the effect of utilization management on insurance company expenses? Consider both administrative expense and claims expense.

10. What are community rating and experience rating?

11. What is information asymmetry in health insurance? How would information asymmetry result in a single rate for all persons, even if their expected losses differ?

12. What mechanisms are available to insurers to allow them to charge premiums by risk category?

BIBLIOGRAPHY

Health Insurance Market

Abraham, K.S. 1985. Efficiency and fairness in insurance risk classification. *Virginia Law Review* 71:403–451.

Altman, D., et al. 1998. Adverse selection and adverse retention. *American Economic Review* 88:122–126.

Anderson, G., and J. Knickman. 1984. Adverse selection under a voucher system: Grouping Medicare recipients by level of expenditure. *Inquiry* 21:135–143.

Baker, L.C., and K.S. Corts. 1996. HMO penetration and the cost of health care: Market discipline or market segmentation? *American Economic Review* 86:389–394.

Berki, S.E., and M. Ashcraft. 1980. HMO enrollment: Who joins what and why: A review of the literature. *Milbank Memorial Fund Quarterly* 58:588–632.

Berki, S.E., et al. 1977. Enrollment choice in a multi-HMO setting. *Medical Care* 15:95–114.

Bradford, D.B. 1996. Efficiency in employment-based health insurance: The potential for supra-marginal cost pricing. *Economic Inquiry* 34:341–356.

Buchmueller, T.C., and P.J. Feldstein. 1997. The effect of price on switching among health plans. *Journal of Health Economics* 16:231–247.

Chernick, H.A. 1987. Tax policy toward health insurance and the demand for medical services. *Journal of Health Economics* 6:1–25.

Cleeton, D. 1989. The medical uninsured: A case of market failure? *Public Finance Quarterly* 17:55–83.

Cutler, D.M., and S.J. Reber. 1998. Paying for health insurance: The trade-off between competition and adverse selection. *Quarterly Journal of Economics* 112:433–466.

Dranove, D., et al. Competition among employers offering health insurance. *Journal of Health Economics* 19:121–140.

Farber, H.S., and H. Levy. 2000. Recent trends in employer-sponsored health insurance coverage: Are bad jobs getting worse? *Journal of Health Economics* 19:93–119.

Feldman, R. 1987. Health insurance in the United States: Is market failure avoidable? *Journal of Risk and Insurance* 54:298–313.

Feldman, R., and B. Dowd. 2000. Risk segmentation: Goal or problem? *Journal of Health Economics* 19:499–512.

Feldman, R., et al. 1989. *Employer based health insurance.* Publication no. PHS-89-3434. Rockville, MD: U.S. Department of Health and Human Services, National Center for Health Services Research and Health Care Technology.

Feldstein, M., and B. Friedman. 1977. Tax subsidies, the rational demand for insurance and the health care crisis. *Journal of Public Economics* 7:155–178.

Foreman, F.E., et al. 1996. Monopoly, monopsony and contestability in health insurance: A study of Blue Cross plans. *Economic Inquiry* 34:662–677.

Frank, R.G., et al. 1997. Solutions for adverse selection in behavioral health care. *Health Care Financing Review* 18:109–122.

Friedman, B. 1974. Risk aversion and the consumer choice of health insurance option. *Review of Economics and Statistics* 56:209–214.

Heffley, D.R., and T.J. Miceli. 1998. The economics of incentive-based health care plans. *Journal of Risk and Insurance* 65:445–465.

Hemenway, D. 1990. Propitious selection. *Quarterly Journal of Economics* 104:1063–1069.

———. 1992. Propitious selection in insurance. *Journal of Risk and Uncertainty* 5:247–251.

Huang, L.F., et al. 1989. Demand for Medigap insurance by the elderly. *Applied Economics* 21:1325–1339.

Jensen, G.R., et al. 1984. Corporate-benefit policies and health insurance costs. *Journal of Health Economics* 3:275–296.

Long, S.H., et al.1998. Do people shift their use of health services over time to take advantage of insurance? *Journal of Health Economics* 17:105–115.

Marquis, M.S., and S.H. Long. 1995. Worker demand for health insurance in the non-group market. *Journal of Health Economics* 14:47–63.

Miller, R.H., and H.S. Luft. 1995. Estimating health expenditure growth under managed competition. *JAMA* 273:656–662.

Nyman, J.A. 1999. The value of health insurance. *Journal of Health Economics* 18:141–152.

Pauly, M. 1986. Taxation, health insurance, and market failure in the medical economy. *Journal of Economic Literature* 26:629–675.

Pauly, M.V. 1989. Competition in health insurance markets. *Law and Contemporary Problems* 51:237–271.

Pauly, M.V., and B.J. Herring. 2000. An efficient employer strategy for dealing with adverse selection multiple-plan offerings: An MSA example. *Journal of Health Economics* 19:513–528.

Pauly, M.V., and S.D. Ramsey. 1999. Would you like suspenders to go with that belt? An analysis of optimal combinations of cost sharing and managed care. *Journal of Health Economics* 18:443–458.

Sloan, F.A., and E.C. Norton. 1997. Adverse selection, bequests, crowding out, and private demand for insurance: Evidence from the long-term care insurance market. *Journal of Risk and Uncertainty* 15:201–219.

Taylor, A., and G.R. Wilensky. 1983. The effect of tax policies on expenditures for private health insurance. In *Market reforms in health care*, ed. J.A. Meyer. Washington, DC: American Enterprise Institute for Policy Research.

Thomas, K. 1994–1995. Are subsidies enough to encourage the uninsured to purchase health insurance? An analysis of underlying behavior. *Inquiry* 31:415–424.

Economics of Disease Prevention and Health Promotion

Jones, L., and M.R. Bakler. 1986. The application of health economics to health promotion. *Community Medicine* 8:224–229.

Kenkel, D.S. 1994. The demand for preventive medical care. *Applied Economics* 26:313–325.

Russell, L.B. 1984. The economics of prevention. *Health Policy* 4:85–100.

Scheffler, R.M., and L. Paringer. 1980. A review of the economic evidence on prevention. *Medical Care* 18:473–484.

Shepard, R.J. 1987. The economics of prevention: A critique. *Health Policy* 7:49–56.

Chapter 11

The Labor Market

1. Define the role of the market for labor and explain how this market is linked to health and health care.
2. Describe a model of the demand for labor.
3. Describe a model of labor supply.
4. Explain how health insurance benefits are related to the supply of labor.
5. Explain the factors that affect the determination of wages and total compensation.
6. Explain how a model of the labor market can be used to explain wage and employment figures for health care workers.
7. Describe how health status affects workers' compensation.
8. Explain how market power can affect labor market outcomes in the health care sector.

11.1 INTRODUCTION

The labor market is the institution by which workers and employers come together to engage in the production of output. As a result of their interactions, the amount of labor that is hired and its compensation are determined. There are a number of health-related issues related to this market. Employers hire and pay workers according to their productivity, and in some instances a healthy worker will be more productive than an unhealthy one. Productivity is a key determinant in the employer's demand for labor. A second set of issues is related to labor supply: a worker's health status may influence his or her decision to seek full-time employment, part-time employment, or no employment at all. A third issue is related to total compensation rather than just wages. In the United States, workers receive part of their compensation in the form of health insurance. The demand for health insurance is thus connected with the labor market. If we want to understand how policies that influence the purchase of health insurance work, we need to understand how labor markets work.

Another set of issues related to the labor market deal with the determination of wages and employment for health care workers. Physicians, nurses, technicians, and so on, work under the vagaries of the health care labor market. Numerous issues have arisen in this market, including shortages of nurses and other health professionals and rising wages for health care workers.

11.2 DEMAND FOR LABOR

11.2.1 Demand for Labor by the Individual Firm

In this section we develop an analysis of the demand for a specific resource by an individual provider. The provider could be a health care–producing entity, such as a hospital, laboratory, or physician's office, or it could be a non-health-care producer. We will focus on health care providers, but the analysis can be applied to either type of institution. The dependent variable of interest is the demand for labor input. The input can be expressed in time units such as hours or days. The labor demand curve or function is defined as the quantity of labor units that a firm will demand at any given price or wage.

In economic terms, this demand is a derived demand. That is, the firm does not demand labor or any other input for itself. Rather, an input is demanded because of the revenue or output it can generate for the firm. In short, the value of an input is derived from the usefulness of the input in achieving some objective. In traditional economic analysis, this objective is profits. While health care firms may indeed have other objectives than profits, the profit maximization hypothesis is a good one to start with in analyzing the demand for labor and other inputs.

To help with the analysis, we will use the example of a commercial laboratory that provides blood tests. The time frame for our analysis will be a single day. We define the firm's product (or output) as the number of blood tests produced per day. The firm has a series of inputs, which include capital equipment, materials and supplies, fixed management time, and variable labor time. Indeed, labor units, in the form of lab technician time, are assumed to be the only variable input (although in reality reagents will vary with the number of blood tests).

- *Production function.* With inputs and outputs defined, we hypothesize the relationship between them (the production function). In Table 11–1 we present a numerical example of the relationship for the range of variable inputs from one to seven lab technician days. With one lab technician, the lab can produce 50 blood tests; with two lab technicians, it can produce 110 tests; and so on. This relationship at first exhibits increasing marginal productivity, followed by decreasing marginal productivity (the third technician produces 50 extra tests, the fourth produces 40, and so on).
- *Revenue derived from worker production.* The firm's valuation of technician time rests, not on the number of lab tests per se, but on the revenue derived from these lab tests. We make the assumption that each lab test has a fixed price of $3. Therefore, for each extra lab test produced, the firm brings in $3 in extra revenue. The total revenue from all lab tests at each level of input is shown in the fourth column of Table 11–1 (one technician brings in $150 in revenues, two bring in $330, etc.). The fifth column shows the *marginal value product (MVP)* obtained when the firm adds successive technicians. The *MVP* is defined as the additional revenue obtained from hiring one more unit of input. As with marginal productivity, this variable at first increases but then decreases. (The first technician has an

Table 11–1 The Demand for Labor by a Commercial Lab

Number of Lab Technicians	Number of Lab Tests (total product)	Additional Tests per Technician (marginal product)	Total Revenue from All Units of Production (price of product × number of units)	Additional Revenue from Addition of One Lab Technician (marginal value product)	Wage Rate
1	50	50	$150	$150	$80
2	110	60	330	180	80
3	160	50	480	150	80
4	200	40	600	120	80
5	230	30	690	90	80
6	250	20	750	60	80
7	260	10	780	30	80

MVP of $150, the second has an *MVP* of $180, and the *MVP* of the third is down to $150). The *MVP* curve is shown in Figure 11–1.

- *Labor cost.* We assume that each lab technician earns $80 per week. Since each lab technician earns the same amount, the marginal cost of the input is $80.
- *Firm's objectives.* The firm is assumed to have a goal of profit maximization. Profits, as we have defined them, are equal to revenue minus cost. The point at which maximum profits are attained occurs when the revenue gained from adding an additional worker equals the additional cost.

The predictions of our model are as follows. On profitability grounds, the firm would hire the first worker, as the resulting marginal value product ($150) exceeds the marginal cost ($80). Indeed, the firm would continue to hire workers as long as it was profitable to do so. In our example, the firm would hire up to five workers for reasons of profitability. It would reduce its profits by hiring a sixth worker. Given the assumptions in our model, the firm's quantity of labor demanded equals five workers.

The demand curve was defined as the quantity of inputs a firm demands at a specific price. If the price of a unit of input changes, so will the quantity demanded. For example, a fall in the wage rate paid by the firm to $50 will increase the quantity of labor demanded to six units, and an increase in the wage rate will reduce the quantity of labor demanded. The quantity demanded will be traced out by the *MVP* curve, as this curve shows what the additional revenue will be for any given wage rate. Therefore, the *MVP* curve is the demand curve for the input.

The demand curve will shift outward if labor becomes more productive (yielding more output and revenue for given quantities of labor) or output prices increase. Labor can become more productive if the firm increases its degree of mechanization. For example, if the firm buys more capital equipment, each worker will be able to produce more. Also, if the price per lab test increases, then each worker will also yield more revenue (though not more output).

To extend the analysis, let us introduce the effects of benefits as a form of compensation. Figure 11–2 shows a firm's demand curve for labor at alternative daily wage rates. For example, at a wage rate of $40, the firm will demand 200 labor

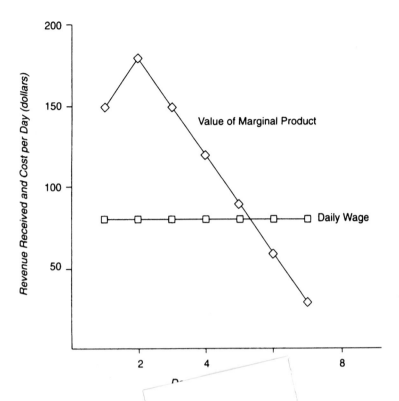

Figure 11–1 Demand curve for la or labor is based on the additional revenue generated by it (days of technician labor), called the *value of the ma* ovider profitability is determined by comparing the VMP bor.

days. The demand curve for this rate ...sed on the assumption that wages are the only form of compensa..., that is, the firm does not offer benefits such as health insurance.

Suppose, however, the firm agrees to provide $10 worth of fringe benefits per day. This adds $10 to the total labor compensation for each worker, but it does not add anything to the value of the output (the marginal value product). Therefore, the firm will still only be willing to pay $40 in total compensation for the 200th labor day—$30 in wages and $10 in fringe benefits. Thus, under the new benefits agreement, the firm would be willing to hire 200 workers at a wage rate of $30 rather than $40 ($30 in wages plus $10 in benefits is equivalent to $40 in wages with no benefits), and there is a new demand curve for labor. This curve, D_b, is the curve D_n shifted downward by exactly $10 at every quantity of labor. Any further increase in benefits would shift the demand curve down further. Furthermore, D_b, like the original demand curve, will shift in response to factors such as the price of output and the productivity of labor.

We will now introduce taxes on corporate profits as a complicating factor. Let us say that the firm pays a 10-percent profits tax. If an extra worker brings in $120 in revenues and costs the firm $100, then the before-tax profits will be $20 and the after-tax profits will be $18 [$20 × (1 − .10)]. If both wages and insurance premiums

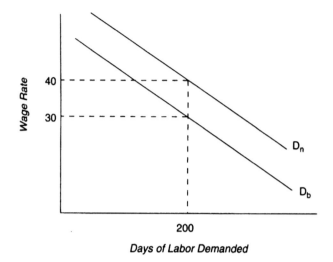

Figure 11–2 The effect of fringe benefits on the demand for labor. Curve D_n shows the demand for labor when the firm does not pay benefits. At a wage rate of $40 per day, the firm demands 200 labor days. In this case, the total wage is the same as total compensation. If health insurance benefits worth $10 per day are instituted, the demand curve relating the wage rate to the quantity of labor will fall by $10 at every quantity. This is because the firm, although still demanding 200 units at an average compensation cost of $40, is now providing each worker only $30 in wages as part of its $40 compensation package.

---

were deductible expenses, then it would not matter to the firm whether it paid out its compensation in the form of wages or insurance benefits. Under current tax law, insurance premiums are not taxed as employee income. Thus this form of compensation is preferred by the employee. This explains, in part, why benefits are so popular a form of compensation.

11.2.2 Market Demand for Labor

The market demand for labor or other inputs can be derived in the same way as other types of market demand. Assume we know the number of firms demanding labor in a certain market and the demand curve for each. We can then add together the quantities demanded for labor at each wage rate to derive a market demand curve for labor. We retain the supposition that the price of the service or product is fixed. The market demand for labor (or other inputs) is thus a downward-sloping demand curve that shifts with changes in variables such as the number of firms demanding labor and the productivity of each worker.

11.3 LABOR SUPPLY

11.3.1 Individual Labor Supply

The analysis of the supply of labor focuses on the quantity of labor individuals are willing to supply in order to earn income. The general framework used in this analysis is the consumer demand model. One main assumption of this model is that each consumer has a demand for income (usable to obtain goods) and for leisure time. The model examines how individuals alter their willingness to work in response to changes in labor compensation such as wages. The end result of the analysis is a supply-of-labor curve relating the quantity of labor supplied to the wage rate.

The unit of observation in this model is the individual consumer (although some analysts have used the household as the observation unit, because in many cases data are collected at the household rather than the individual level), and the dependent variable is the number of hours an individual is willing to work. The assumptions in our analysis are as follows.

Imagine a utility-maximizing individual who has a utility function that encompasses two distinct goods: income (usable to purchase selected goods and services) and leisure time. As more is obtained of each good, the individual moves to higher levels of utility.

The amounts of the two goods that will yield the same level of utility are shown in Table 11–2. If the individual has no income, he or she will be willing to take 60 hours in leisure. This combination of income and leisure will yield the same utility as $100 per week and 50 hours of leisure, $200 and 42 hours, and so on. Note that, whereas income increases in equal increments, leisure hours are reduced in successively smaller increments. This indicates a diminishing relative valuation placed on income. The individual will give up 10 hours of leisure to get the first $100 in income but only 8 additional hours of leisure to get the next $100.

The individual has a total of 60 available hours per week. If 50 hours are spent on leisure, then 10 hours will be spent working. Finally, the individual can work for a wage of $15 per hour for up to 60 hours. Total income equals the product of wages and hours worked.

The conclusions of the model are as follows. The individual will increase work time hours from zero as long as the value of lost leisure is less than the wage rate. For example, at the point when the individual has full-time leisure, he or she is willing to give up 10 hours of leisure (work 10 more hours) for $100 in wages, a unit value of $10 per hour. However, once the individual has achieved this new point, he or she will only be willing to give up an additional 8 hours of leisure for an extra $100 in income. This implies a marginal value of leisure of $12.50 per hour at the new point. The individual places a lower value on the next $100 increase in income and would only be willing to give up 6 more hours of leisure, implying a marginal value of $16.67 per hour of leisure. Thus the individual must be compensated at increas-

Table 11–2 Income and Leisure Time Combinations at the Same Level of Utility

Income per Week	Leisure Hours per Week (out of a total of 60 available hours)	Work Hours per Week (leisure + work = 60 hours)
$ 0	60	0
100	50	10
200	42	18
300	36	24
400	32	28
500	30	30

ingly higher wage rates to induce him or her to give up more leisure (i.e., to work more).

Let us assume a wage rate of $15 an hour. The individual is faced with a choice of whether and how much to work. The individual will work at least 10 hours, because the marginal value of the first 10 hours of work is $10. The individual would also choose to work the next 8 hours, because the value of leisure time is less than the wage. Beyond that, the value of lost leisure is greater than the wage rate. Therefore, the individual will choose to work 18 hours. If the wage rate increases, say, to $20, then the individual would be willing to give up 6 more hours of leisure and work for a total of 24 hours per week.

The positive relationship between wages and labor time measures what is called the *substitution effect of income for leisure.* Figure 11–3 shows how the quantity of labor changes as the wage rate increases (curve Supply$_1$). There is also an income effect, which may offset the substitution effect. As the wage rate increases, the total income that the individual can receive will increase, and the individual can purchase more goods and services; the individual will want to spend more leisure time consuming goods and services and hence will want to work less. It is possible that this income effect can more than offset the substitution effect, resulting in a backward-bending labor portion of the supply curve, especially at higher wage rates and income levels. However, statistical studies have shown that this is not a common event.

Supply curves for labor can have varying slopes. If an individual does not have a strong willingness to work more as wages increase, then the curve will be steeply

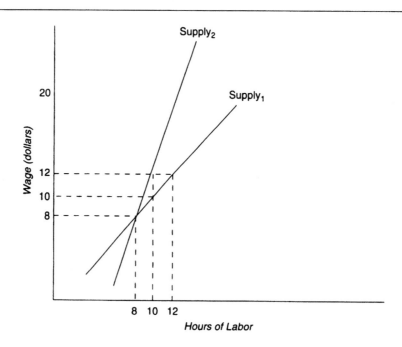

Figure 11–3 Alternative labor supply curves. Curve Supply$_1$ shows a positive relation between the wage rate and labor hours. Curve Supply$_2$ is a curve with a similar direction but a steeper slope, which means that an increase in the wage rate from $8 to $10 will induce a smaller increase in the number of labor hours supplied.

sloped (Supply$_2$ in Figure 11–3). An individual more willing to work for small increases will have a curve like Supply$_1$. In Figure 11–3, an increase in wages from $10 to $12 will, depending on the labor supply curve, increase the labor supply to 10 hours (Supply$_2$) or 12 hours (Supply$_1$).

11.3.2 Health Insurance Benefits and Labor Supply

The most common way of financing health insurance in the United States is through the payment of health insurance premiums for individuals in the workplace. Health insurance coverage is a component of total worker compensation, which consists of wages plus fringe benefits. From the viewpoint of the individual worker, the amount of total compensation is what influences labor supply. However, economists have modeled labor supply decisions using wage rates as the base price. We will follow that tradition.

In Figure 11–4 we present two labor supply curves, one for the case where fringe benefits exist and one for the case where there are none. Let us begin our analysis by

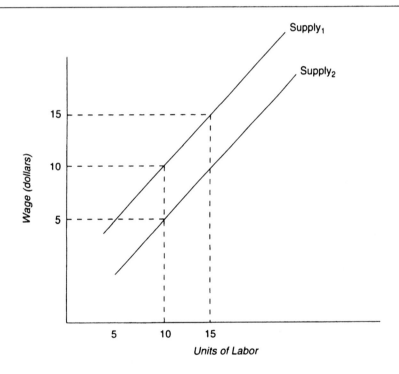

Figure 11–4 Labor supply curves with and without a benefits package. Curve Supply$_1$ shows the relation between the wage rate and units (hours) of labor supplied when there are no benefits. We make the assumption that workers place a $1 value on each dollar of benefits. If we introduce a $5 benefits package, curve Supply$_2$ indicates the new quantity supplied at each wage rate. The reason why the curve shifts is as follows. The $5 wage rate now represents $10 in compensation and will induce the same amount of labor as will a $10 wage rate with no benefits. This is true for all wage rates. If, however, $1 in benefits is worth less to the worker than $1 in wages, the shift in the curve will be less.

focusing on the situation without fringe benefits. Curve Supply$_1$ relates the quantity of labor supplied to money wages. At a wage of $10, a total of 10 units of labor are supplied, at a wage of $15, 15 units of labor are supplied, and so on.

Let us now introduce fringe benefits worth $5 per worker (an amount independent of hours worked). We will assume each worker places a value of $5 on these benefits. It is certainly possible, of course, for a worker to place a value lower than $5 on these benefits, and indeed fringe benefits may be worth very little to some workers. Under our assumption, however, the value to the worker of compensation is $10 when the wage is $5, it is $15 when the wage is $10, and so on. Put another way, the curve that relates the wage rate to the quantity of labor supplied will shift downward and to the right (Supply$_2$). At a wage of $5 (plus $5 worth of fringe benefits), the supply of labor will be the same as it would be at a wage of $10 without fringe benefits. An additional $5 increase in benefits, wages held constant, will further shift the supply curve downward and to the right. (Of course, if the workers place a lower value on these benefits than their face value, the shift will be less than $5.)

11.3.3 Market Supply of Labor

The market labor supply is composed of the sum of labor supply curves of all the individuals in the market. As with the demand curve, the labor supply curve of the market comprises the summed quantity for each individual at each wage rate. An increase in the number of individuals in the market will cause the supply curve to shift to the right.

11.4 THE COMPETITIVE LABOR MARKET

11.4.1 Assumptions

Our labor market analysis will focus on the market for lab technicians. To develop a competitive labor market model, we must make assumptions about market supply and demand factors and how they interact. The basic model is shown graphically in Figure 11–5. The original market demand curve is shown as curve D_1. At a market wage of $20 per day, the firms in the market demand 20,000 days of lab technician services. At lower wages, the quantity of days demanded increases. The market supply curve is upward sloping, as hypothesized above; this curve is shown as S_1 in Figure 11–5. At a market wage of $17.50, 17,500 days of lab technician labor will be supplied in the market. If the wage increases to $20, then 20,000 days will be supplied. In the competitive model, we must assume an equilibrium condition, that is, that the quantity supplied is equal to the quantity demanded.

11.4.2 Predictions

11.4.2.1 Supply, Demand, and Wage Rate

The first prediction of the model is that there will be a single equilibrium wage set at $20. Bargaining among demanders and suppliers of labor will result in this single equilibrium price at the equilibrium quantity of 20,000 labor days. Additionally, the equilibrium quantity and price will change with any changes in the related factors. With regard to shifts in demand, increases in the price of the product or the

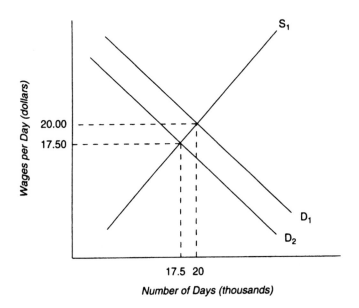

Figure 11–5 Graph of a labor market. The demand for labor is shown as curve D_1, and the supply curve is shown as curve S_1. Equilibrium occurs at a wage rate of $20 per day and a quantity of 20,000 labor days. If fringe benefits worth $5 a day are introduced, the demand curve shifts down uniformly by $5 (to D_2). The new equilibrium will be at a quantity of 17,500 days and a wage rate of $17.50.

number of firms in the market will result in increased wage rates and increased labor days. Increases in the supply of labor will result in lower wages and higher quantities of labor.

Our model can be of help in analyzing the effect of using health insurance benefits as a form of compensation. Let us say that, for each worker, the labs pay a $5 health insurance premium per labor day. The effect of this is to shift the demand curve uniformly down by $5, to curve D_2. We will assume that there is no effect on supply. The prediction in this case is that the wage rate will fall to $17.50 and the quantity of labor employed will be reduced to 17,500 days. In this case, the finance method does reduce the quantity of employment.

11.4.2.2 Health and Labor Market Outcomes

Economists have recognized the role of health in labor market outcomes. The topic that has received the most attention has been the impact of health on the supply of labor. Good health will increase the likelihood that a worker will be employed and that a worker who is employed will work longer hours (e.g., will accept full-time rather than part-time employment). In terms of the competitive labor market model, poor health will shift the labor supply curve to the left. At any given wage rate, the quantity of labor supplied will be reduced when health status is decreased. If we look at the workings of the entire market, a reduction (leftward shift) in the supply of labor will reduce the overall amount of employment and increase the wage rate of those who continue to participate in the market.

Much of the evidence of the effect of health status on earnings has come from the developing countries (Duraisamy and Sathiyavan 1998; Jack 1999). A number of such studies have shown that improved health status or factors that are associated with health status, such as nutrition and the body mass index, have a positive effect on wages. This finding is as expected, because in many developing countries there is a very low general level of health.

However, the same trends have been noted in developing countries as well. Using a national sample survey of residents in the United States, Kahn (1998) studied the comparative impact of labor market performance of persons with and without diabetes. He found that 64 percent of males who had diabetes and were between the ages of 50 and 60 were employed; the comparative figure for males without diabetes was 82 percent. The corresponding statistics for women were 40 percent and 60 percent. Thus persons with diabetes are 18 to 20 percent less likely to be employed than persons without diabetes. Kahn's statistics indicate that there is a considerable effect of diabetes on labor market behavior, especially with regard to whether persons are employed.

11.4.2.3 Occupational Risk and Labor Market Outcomes

Injury and mortality rates vary considerably between occupations and industries. In 1999 there were 6,023 work-related fatalities in the United States. The occupation with the largest number was trucking (898), followed by farming (557 deaths). On the basis of relative risks, workers in trucking had a fatality rate of 2.1 deaths per 10,000 workers. By comparison, workers in foodstores had a fatality rate of 0.4 per 10,000, roughly one-fifth that of the truckers (U.S. Department of Labor 2000). In 1998, there were 5.9 million nonfatal injuries and illnesses, or 6.7 per 100 equivalent full-time workers. Rates varied between occupations for illnesses and injuries as well. For example, there were 14.6 injuries per 100 workers in the manufacturing of transport equipment and 0.6 injuries per 100 securities brokers (U.S. Department of Labor 1999b).

If workers correctly perceive differences between risks in different occupations, then according to utility maximizing principles they will prefer low-risk to high-risk occupations (all else held constant). Indeed, starting with a very low risk occupation (e.g., restaurant work, in which there are 0.23 deaths per 10,000 workers), workers will demand risk premiums in order to induce them to accept occupations with higher risks (Viscusi 1993). There are widespread differences in wages between occupations. The factors that influence these differences include both demand variables (worker productivity, occupational characteristics, price of the final product) and supply variables (worker age, education, and skill level). The on-the-job risk of mortality is one of many factors that influences the wage rate for any occupation. If we could adjust for all factors affecting supply and demand *other than risk*, then the interoccupational differences in wages would just compensate for differences in risk.

Once we have developed measures of that component of interoccupational wage differentials that reflects differences in occupational risks of mortality, we can extrapolate these measures to obtain an estimate of the value of a statistical life. For example, let us say that there are two occupations with varying risks but that all other factors are the same. Assume that a 50-year-old male has a life expectancy of

65 in the absence of a fatal work-related injury. He has a choice of two occupations: truck driving and office work. Truck drivers experience 2.1 deaths per 10,000 workers, whereas office workers experience only 0.4 deaths. The difference is 1.7 deaths per 10,000 workers (0.00017). The adjusted wage differential (net of other factors) is $40 annually. We can make a projection of the monetary value for the remainder of the person's lifetime. If we ignore the discounting factor (i.e., the discount rate is zero percent), then the wage difference between the two occupations is $600 (15 years at $40). The value of a statistical life can then be calculated as $3.529 million ($600 ÷ 0.00017). If we want more precision, we should qualify this estimate, so it can be made more realistic: we would discount future years' wages, and we would have to account for many characteristics that are difficult to measure, such as the pleasantness of the work environment. Having made these adjustments, our estimate would be a better approximation of the valuation of risk that workers actually accept in the marketplace.

Indeed, a considerable number of studies have been conducted to measure the value of life using labor market differentials (Hirth et al. 2000). These results show a very wide variation in the value of life. For a 40-year-old male, estimates ranged from $923,000 to over $19 million. Such differences are hard to reconcile, and they have created confusion on the part of policy makers. Nevertheless, the importance of the topic for policy-making purposes, including in the health care area, ensures that a great deal of additional work will be done in this area.

11.5 MARKET POWER IN LABOR MARKETS

11.5.1 Buyer's Market Power

In the past 20 years, there have been periods of time when widespread nursing shortages were reported by hospitals. A shortage is a situation where, at the given wage rate, the quantity demanded exceeds the quantity supplied of labor. Economists have tried to explain shortages by means of economic models. The model of a hospital's buying power in the market for nurses can be used for this purpose. Let us assume that there is a single buyer of nursing services, a hospital in a small city. For this single buyer, we set out an economic model to predict pricing and output decisions.

- *Supplier costs.* With respect to the supply side of the market, we assume there are a number of nurses available to be hired by the hospital (their supply curve is drawn in Figure 11–6). At a wage of $2 weekly, two nurses will supply their services; if the wage is increased to $3, three nurses will supply their services; and so on. With respect to the demand side of the market, the successive marginal value that the single hospital places on nurses is also shown in Figure 11–6.
- *Revenues.* Let us assume (1) that additional nurses allow the hospital to treat more patients but the marginal productivity of these extra nurses diminishes and (2) that the price received for each extra patient by the hospital is constant. The hospital's value curve has been derived from the estimated additional revenue that the hospital estimates the additional nurses will bring in. The marginal revenue (equal to the price of output times the marginal output yielded by an extra nursing

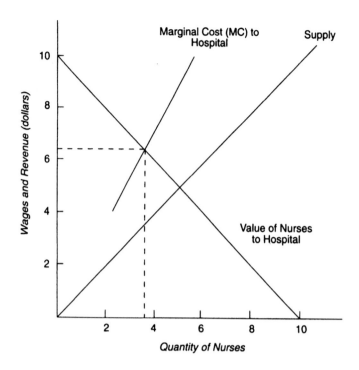

Figure 11–6 The equilibrium wage and number of nurses hired in a monopsonistic (single-buyer) market. The firm's marginal cost for hiring additional nurses is derived from the schedule of nurses in the market. The value of an additional nurse is based on the amount of output that the hospital can produce with nurses (productivity) and the price of the output (in short, the amount of revenue brought in by hiring an additional nurse). The profit-maximizing hospital will continue to hire nurses up to the point where the marginal cost equals the additional revenue from hiring another nurse.

---

unit) is $9 for the first nurse, $8 for the second, $7 for the third, and so on. Note that the total value to the hospital of three nurses is $24 ($9 + $8 + $7).

- *Behavioral assumption.* Finally, we will assume that the hospital wishes to maximize profits.

The implications of our model are that the profit-maximizing hospital will hire additional nurses as long as the marginal cost of doing so is less than the additional revenue. But the *MC* of nurses to the hospital is not the nurses' supply curve, *S*. Since *S* is sloped up, each successive nurse wants an extra dollar of pay. Assuming that the hospital must pay all nurses the same wage, by hiring the second nurse it must pay a higher wage to the first as well. As a result, the *MC* curve is more steeply sloped than the supply curve (see Figure 11–6). For example, the *MC* of the second nurse is $3 but that of the third nurse is $5 (the difference between the total cost of 3 nurses at $9 and the total cost of 2 nurses at $4). The profit-maximizing hospital will hire three nurses (between 3 and 4 in Figure 11–6), for then the hospital's added revenue will equal its *MC* for hiring nurses. At such a level of hiring, it will pay a wage of $3, since that is the wage at which three nurses will supply their services.

In a monopsonistic (single-buyer) market, fewer nurses would be hired than in a competitive market. In a competitive market, competitive forces would drive the wage up to the level where supply equals demand; more nurses would be hired and wages would be higher. However, a monopsonistic buyer can prevent more nurses from being hired, thus maintaining its profits. At the same time as it depresses wages, it creates a restriction in supply.

11.5.2 Unions as Monopoly Sellers of Labor

Feldman et al. (1982) stated that in the early 1980s unions increased nurses' wages by about 8 percent. A more recent study (Hirsch and Schumacher 1995) questioned this finding. In 1999, nurses earned $20.86 per hour, compared to $21.53 for librarians and $27.86 for high school teachers (U.S. Department of Labor 1999a), despite the fact that there was a considerable degree of unionism among nurses. In this section we present the theoretical argument that unions increase wages.

A union is an organized group of workers that allow individual workers to act as a cohesive unit when bargaining with employers. In terms of economic analysis, unions allow sellers of labor (in this case nurses) to wield monopoly power, raising their wages relative to those of nonunion workers. The monopoly model applied to the labor market is used to predict the impact of a union on wage levels. In Figure 11–7 we present a model of the labor market for nurses, with hospitals as the buyers. We assume that there are several hospitals in the market but only one unit (a union) supplying them labor. The price (wage) is measured along the vertical axis, and the quantity of nurses who are hired monthly is shown along the horizontal axis. The monthly demand for nurses is presented as curve D_L. The marginal revenue (MR) curve is derived from the demand curve. It shows the addition to total wage income of union members associated with expanded employment.

The marginal cost curve for nurses is shown as curve MCL. As the quantity of nursing time provided increases, the wage that nurses are willing to accept increases as well.

We assume that the union will maximize its "surplus," defined as the total compensation received by the workers minus any costs. Profits are defined in terms of the entire group of labor suppliers, who are behaving in unison as a labor union.

The union will bargain for a wage at that quantity of labor where the members' wage income is maximized. The profit-maximizing position is where the marginal revenue equals marginal cost, that is, at the intersection of MR and MCL. In Figure 11–7, the profit-maximizing wage is $900 a month. The union would bargain for that wage and supply 600 nurses. In contrast, the wage in a competitive market would be $700 a month and 800 nurses would be supplied at that price. The prediction of our model, then, is that unions increase wages and restrict employment.

As stated above, the question as to whether the union has raised nursing wages is an open one. Other models have been developed that incorporate both hospital and union market power. Under such conditions, the wage would be determined by the relative degree of market power of both bargaining entities, and the same conclusions would not necessarily hold.

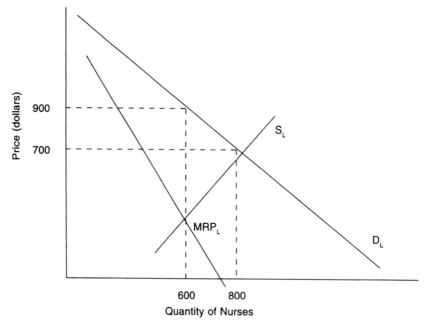

Figure 11–7 Monopolistic seller of labor. The marginal revenue product curve (MRP_L) is derived from the seller's demand for labor (D_L). The seller will select the profit maximizing position at 600 hirings, where MRP_L equals S_L (supply of labor curve).

EXERCISES

1. The Midwest Clinic is a profit maximizing organization. It has the capacity to hire up to five nursing hours. The production function for the clinic, in terms of clinic visits, is shown in the accompanying table.

Number of Nursing Hours	Number of Clinic Visits
1	12
2	22
3	30
4	36
5	40

    Midwest charges a fee of $10 for each clinic visit. It pays nurses $50 an hour. What is the quantity of labor demanded by Midwest? What will be the profit-maximizing quantity of labor demanded if the company adds $15 to the wage of each worker to pay for health insurance premiums?

2. What happens to the market supply function of public health nursing labor if:
    a. Wages increase in hospitals.
    b. Licensing requirements are made stricter for public health nurses.
    c. Nursing schools close down.
    d. There is a minimum wage imposed on nurses.
    e. The public image of public health nursing is improved.

3. What happens to the demand curve for labor of a clinic if each of the following occurs:
   a. The wage falls.
   b. The clinic purchases equipment that increases worker productivity.
   c. The price of clinic visits increases.
   d. The clinic hires more workers.
   e. The clinic hires better trained workers who are more productive.
   f. The clinic nurses provide care that is of a higher quality but takes more nursing time.
4. Explain the relationship between the wage rate and the quantity of labor supplied.
5. How does the introduction of health insurance as a benefit influence the supply curve for labor?
6. Assume a competitive model of the market for laboratory technicians in an environment of profit-maximizing laboratories. How will each of the following affect the wage rate for laboratory technicians:
   a. New equipment that increases the productivity of technicians is introduced.
   b. The local university increases the size of the graduating class of technicians.
   c. Technicians take more time in conducting tests in order to be more thorough.
   d. The government issues a generous retirement scheme for technicians over 60.
   e. The government licenses laboratories, restricting their numbers.
   f. Workers bargain for an increase in health insurance benefits; the laboratories provide insurance instead of wages.
7. Using the competitive labor market model, derive a prediction of the impact of poor health on employee wages.
8. The following is a labor supply function:

Wage per hour	Quantity of Nurse Supplied
$2	1
4	2
6	3
8	4
10	5
12	6

Nurses are used by the clinic to provide clinic visits. Each visit brings in $2 in revenue for the clinic. The relationship between nursing units and clinic visits is as follows:

Quantity of Nurses	Total Clinic Visits
1	5
2	9
3	12
4	14
5	15

The provider is assumed to maximize profits. Determine the provider's equilibrium wage and how many nursing units it will hire. The provider is a monopsonist, which means it is the sole purchaser of labor in the market.

BIBLIOGRAPHY

Labor Markets for Health Care Workers

Holtman, A.G., and T.L. Idson. 1993. Wage determination of registered nurses in proprietary and nonprofit nursing homes. *Journal of Human Resources* 28:55–79.

Lindsay, C.M. 1976. More real returns to medical education. *Journal of Human Resources* 11:127–129.

Salkever, D. 1975. Hospital wage inflation. *Quarterly Review of Economics and Business* 15:33–84.

Sloan, F.A. 1976. Real returns to medical education. *Journal of Human Resources* 11:118–126.

Thornton, J. 1998. The labor supply effects of self-employed solo practice physicians. *Applied Economics* 30:85–94.

United States Department of Labor. 1999a. National Compensation Survey: Occupational wages in the United States, 1998. Washington, DC: Bureau of Labor Statistics.

Health Insurance and Labor Markets

Gruber, J., and B.C. Madrian. 1997. Employment separation and health insurance coverage. *Journal of Public Economics* 66:349–382.

Kreuger, A.B., and U.E. Reinhardt. 1994. Economics of employer versus individual mandates. *Health Affairs* 13:34–54.

Rhine, S.L., and Y.C. Ng. 1998. The effect of employment status on private health insurance coverage: 1977 and 1987. *Health Economics* 7:63–80.

Rogowski, J., and K. Karoly. 2000. Health insurance and retirement behavior. *Journal of Health Economics* 19:529–539.

Market Power in Labor Markets

Feldman, R., and R. Scheffler. 1982. The union impact of hospital wages and fringe benefits. *Industrial and Labor Relations Review* 35:196–206.

Hirsch, B.T., and E.J. Schumacher. 1995. Monopsony power and relative wages in the labor market for nurses. *Journal of Health Economics* 14:443–476.

Link, C.R., and J.H. Landon. 1975. Monopsony and union power in the market for nurses. *Southern Economic Journal* 14:649–659.

Schumacher, E.J. 1997. Relative wages and the returns to education in the labor market for registered nurses. *Research in Labor Economics* 16:149–176.

Schumacher, E.J., and B.T. Hirsch. 1997. Compensating differentials and unmeasured ability in the labor market for nurses: Why do hospitals pay more? *Industrial and Labor Relations Review* 50:557–579.

Yett, D. 1970. The chronic "shortage" of nurses. In *Empirical studies in health economics,* ed. H. Klarman. Baltimore: Johns Hopkins University Press.

Effects of Health Status on Labor Markets

Bartel, A., and P. Taubman. 1979. Health and labor market success: The role of various diseases. *Review of Economics and Statistics* 61:1–8.

Berndt, E.R., et al. 1998. Workplace performance effects from chronic depression and its treatment. *Journal of Health Economics* 17:511–535.

Bound, J. 1989. The health and earnings of rejected disability applicants. *American Economic Review* 79:482–503.

Duraisamy, P., and D. Sathiyavan. 1998. Impact of health status on wages and labour supply of men and women. *Indian Journal of Labour Economics* 41:67–84.

Ettner, S.L., et al. 1997. The impact of psychiatric disorders on labor market outcomes. *Industrial and Labor Relations Review* 51:64–81.

Fenn, P.T., and I.G. Vlachonikolis. 1986. Male labor force participation following illness or injury. *Economics* 53:379–391.

Hamilton, B.H., and V.H. Hamilton. 1997. Down and out: Estimating the relationship between mental health and unemployment. *Health Economics* 6:397–406.

Jack, W. 1999. *Principles of health economics for developing countries.* Washington, DC: World Bank.

Kahn, M.E. 1998. Health and labor market performance: The case of diabetes. *Journal of Labor Economics* 16:878–899.

Karoly,L., and J. Rogowski.1994. The effect of access to post retirement health insurance and the decision to retire early. *Industrial and Labor Relations Review* 48:103–123.

Luft, H. 1975. The impact of poor health on earnings. *Review of Economics and Statistics.* 57:43–57.

Human Capital

Rizzo, J.A., et al. 1996. Labor productivity effects of prescribed medicines for chronically ill workers. *Health Economics* 5:249–266.

Schultz, T.P. 1997. Assessing the productive benefits of nutrition and health: An integrated human capital approach. *Journal of Econometrics* 77:141–158.

Thomas, D., and J. Strauss. 1997. Health and wages: Evidence on men and women in urban Brazil. *Journal of Econometrics* 77:159–185.

Effects of Compensation Practices on Health

McGovern, P., et al. 1997. Time off work and the postpartum health of employed women. *Medical Care* 35:507–521.

Occupational Risk and Labor Market Outcomes

Berger, M.C., et al. 1987. Valuing changes in health risks. *Southern Economic Journal* 53:867–984.

Blomquist, G. 1979. Value of life saving: Implications of life saving. *Journal of Political Economy* 87:540–558.

———. 1981. The value of human life: An empirical perspective. *Economic Inquiry* 19:157–164.

Dillingham, A.E. 1985. The influence of risk variable definition on value-of-life estimates. *Economic Inquiry* 24:277–294.

Fisher, A., et al. 1989. The value of reducing risks of death: A note on new evidence. *Journal of Policy Analysis and Management* 8:88–100.

Hirth, R.A., et al. 2000. Willingness to pay for a quality-adjusted life year. *Medical Decision Making* 20:332–342.

Linneroth, J. 1979. The value of human life: A review of the models. *Economic Inquiry* 17:52–74.

Robinson, J.C. 1986. Hazard pay in unsafe jobs. *Milbank Quarterly* 64:650–677.

Rosen, S. 1981. Valuing health risk. *American Economic Review* 71:241–245.

Thaler, R., and S. Rosen. 1975. The value of saving a life: Evidence from the labor market. In *Household production and consumption,* ed. N.E. Terleckyj. New York: National Bureau of Economic Research.

United States Department of Labor. 1999b. *Workplace injuries and illnesses in 1998.* Washington, DC: Bureau of Labor Statistics.

United States Department of Labor. 2000. *National census of fatal occupational injuries, 1999.* Washington, DC: Bureau of Labor Statistics.

Viscusi, W.K. 1978. Wealth effects and earnings premiums for job hazards. *Review of Economics and Statistics* 60:408–416.

———. 1978. Labor market valuations of life and limb. *Public Policy* 26: 360–386.

———. 1993. The value of risks to life and health. *Journal of Economic Literature* 31:1912–1946.

Part III

Evaluative Economics

Value Judgements and Economic Evaluation

1. Describe the type of question that evaluative economics is intended to answer.
2. Describe what a value judgment is and how it can be used in evaluative economics.
3. Using assumed valuations by individuals for services and costs, identify an efficient level of output in any market.
4. Compare alternative delivery arrangements in terms of their efficiency.
5. Describe how a market for health insurance can be efficient when there is less than complete insurance coverage.
6. Describe the extra-welfarist approach to identifying optimal economic arrangements.
7. Define the concept of equity.
8. Identify several alternative measures of equity and explain how these can be applied to evaluate alternative modes of finance and care delivery.

12.1 INTRODUCTION

In this chapter we begin a different level of inquiry. In previous chapters we focused on the actual allocation of resources devoted to medical care. We were interested in explaining only the various allocations that might occur in different circumstances. We did not concern ourselves with whether any particular allocation was "good" or "acceptable" or "equitable," to mention only a few of the terms we might use to label an allocation. In this chapter we begin the task of evaluating alternative possible allocations of resources. This task will lead us to such questions as whether totally free care can be judged "better" than the provision of medical care in a simple market. Or whether and in what sense a regulated system is preferable to an unregulated one. Many of these questions, it should be pointed out, are policy issues. Indeed, evaluative analysis forms the cornerstone of policy analysis, since the ultimate goal of policy is to bring about improvements in the use of resources.

Before undertaking evaluative analysis, we must lay the ground rules for conducting an evaluation. That is the mission of this chapter. In Section 12.2, the importance of having a recognizable and unvarying standard for gauging alternative allocations is discussed. The values that individual persons place on specific services can be used as the basis of a social evaluation. One procedure for building a social evaluation is discussed in Section 12.3. The standard that results from this procedure, which is used frequently by economists, is referred to as an *efficiency criterion*. Such a yardstick takes individuals' starting situations as given and therefore bypasses questions relating to equity and need as determined by clinical criteria.. The application of efficiency criteria to evaluate the performance of the health insurance market is discussed in Section 12.4, and policy goals emanating from this efficiency analysis are presented in Section 12.5. The relevance of the efficiency criteria as the sole benchmark of resource allocation has been questioned by many observers. An alternative approach, called *extra-welfarism*, is presented in Section 12.6. Finally, alternative measures of equity are considered in Section 12.7.

12.2 VALUES AND STANDARDS IN ECONOMIC EVALUATION

Suppose we are faced with a situation in which A has a curable cancer but is receiving no medical care and B is healthy but is spending $4,000 on surgical services for a facial lift. Would this be an acceptable allocation of our medical resources? Many would say it is unfair, but scarcely anybody would take the trouble to set forth the basic standard being used to judge the situation. Suppose, instead, that it was necessary heart surgery B was receiving. Would this change one's evaluation of the situation? Would a different standard be used to gauge its fairness?

In our example, the resources are being allocated differently in the two situations. However, unless we had a standard that did not itself vary from situation to situation, we really could not compare the two situations. That is, without an independent scale of fairness or acceptability, we would not have a measure capable of assessing alternative allocations. This section presents a classification of available systems of standards, focusing on the bases on which standards may be formed.

For the purposes of economic evaluation, there are two ways of deriving a system of values and then developing a ranking of alternative uses of resources. In the first method, called *delegatory* or *top-down*, a value system is imposed on the members of society. For example, it might be imposed by a higher being, such as a deity; by an interpreter of the ultimate word, such as Moses or Mohammed; or by a dictator, who settles on some value system based on his or her values. Alternatively, someone can assume the mantle of spokesperson for society, proclaiming "society wants a decent standard of health for all" or some such alleged truth. Despite the nod toward democracy, any would-be ethical authority who chooses to speak for society without a mandate based on the views of individuals within the society is really imposing his or her own views on society.

The second method for deriving a system of values is called *participatory* or *bottom-up*. In this method, the views of all members of the community play a role. One assumption underlying this method is that *everyone's* values must be taken into account in ranking alternative ways of using resources. Another assumption is that each individual is the best judge of his or her own welfare.

We now turn our focus to the value systems themselves. They vary tremendously, ranging from the very specific to the very vague. They can take the form of specific laws handed down by a deity or can be formulated in terms of general concepts such as *fairness*, *liberty*, and *equality*.

The field of health services analysis contains many examples of writers proposing value systems based on their own view of what seems desirable. For instance, some have posited a "right" to health or health care. One commentator used the principle of *agape* to derive this right (Outka 1974), whereas another appealed to a "strong sense in the population" that this right exists (Mechanic 1976).

Even assuming we could settle on a single value system, we would still face the problem of translating the chosen value system into a gauge or ranking scheme to assess alternative ways of using resources. This translation step can be controversial itself. Because any value system will be somewhat vague, different ranking schemes with very different implications can be derived from it. We would then run into the problem of which ranking scheme to choose. For example, the goal of "equality" can be interpreted in many ways—as equality of *health status* or equality of *medical care utilization*. We might decide it entails equal use of medical care for equal health status, with individuals who have poor health receiving more care than individuals who are basically healthy. This may seem plausible, but how do we decide how much more care people with poor health should get? Also, if the medical care given to those in poor health is not effective, should they still receive it?

The last step, after having decided on a ranking scheme, is to apply it to actual or proposed states of resource use (e.g., distributions of health care or levels of health) to determine their desirability from a policy standpoint.

It should be stressed that value systems imposed from above are not necessarily evil. The source of such a system may be a highly respected and beloved authority, and the system may contain laudatory ideals and translate into ranking schemes that seem reasonable and compassionate. Nevertheless, an imposed scheme is not built up from the values of the members of the society and therefore retains some degree of nonrepresentativeness.

In Section 12.3 and 12.4, a participatory system of evaluation is developed. This system, well known in economic circles as the *Paretean system* (named after the famous nineteenth-century sociologist Vilfredo Pareto), allows us to arrive at an optimum position through examining changes that could be made in resource allocations if we start from an initial position. This optimum holds only with reference to the initial starting point (i.e., the initial endowments each member of society possesses). We do not judge the starting point, which may or may not be fair, a consideration discussed in Section 12.5.

12.3 EFFICIENT OUTPUT LEVELS

12.3.1 Individual Valuations of Commodities or Activities

If we accept individuals' own valuations as the best indicators of their own welfare, we must then determine, at least in principle, what these valuations might be. Since our analysis is concerned with specific commodities, our task is simplified somewhat. We need only determine individuals' valuations with respect to those commodities with which we are concerned.

Economists have developed a hypothesis regarding an individual's valuation of units of a specific commodity. The hypothesis, which is based on our demand analysis, is that the more of any commodity the individual has, the less successive units of the commodity will be worth to him or her (as compared with other commodities). The analysis can be recast using money as the basic unit of value. To do this, we must assume that money is itself of constant value. That is, if an individual gives up $2, that $2 will always represent the same loss to the individual however much income he or she has. This assumption will hold, at least partially, if the outlay for the commodity in question is a reasonably small portion of the individual's total budget.

If an individual has an income of $10,000, spending $100 or $150 on a commodity is unlikely to cause the valuation of each dollar to change for the individual. However, as the amount that must be given up to obtain a commodity becomes very large relative to income, the utility of or the subjective valuation placed on the marginal dollar will change. We are making the assumption in this section that it does not. We should note that this is a different assumption from that made earlier in the discussion of health insurance demand (Chapter 10).

Given the assumption that money income has a constant value for individuals for all relevant ranges of expenditures, we can specify individual valuations of successive units of a commodity in terms of money. These valuations, it must be stressed, are the individuals' own evaluations of specific units of the commodity, and they qualify on participatory grounds for inclusion into our overall participatory social evaluation.

12.3.2 Values in a Selfish Market

To simplify our analysis, let us assume initially that there are two individuals in our market, A and B. Each has a specific schedule of valuations for his or her own consumption of medical care. Let us refer to these valuations as *marginal valuations* (*MVs*). A marginal valuation is defined as the extra amount of money an individual would be willing to pay for an additional unit of a commodity. Thus, an *MV* is a measure of what an extra unit of the commodity is worth to the individual in money terms.

In our initial analysis, both A and B derive satisfaction or value from their own consumption of medical services, and theirs is the only satisfaction that anyone in society gets from their consumption. A places a marginal value of $80 on his first unit consumed, $70 on his second, and so on, as seen in Columns 1 and 2 in Table 12–1. Note that the marginal values placed by each individual on successive units of medical care consumed diminish. Recall from Chapter 3 that all other factors, such as health status, income, and wealth, are held constant (i.e., the initial values of these variables are held constant). For purposes of social evaluation, then, we have a measure of the social worth of A's consumption of medical care (since no one else values this care other than A himself).

The assumed relation between marginal value and quantity consumed can be presented geometrically. In Figure 12–1, the curve MV_a represents A's marginal valuation of successive units of medical care. It is assumed, for ease of geometric exposition, that the units of medical care can be made very small so that the *MV* curve becomes smooth. A's valuation of his own consumption is referred to as the *private* (or *internal*) valuation of his consumption. On the assumption that no one else cares about A's consumption, his private valuation is the same as the social valuation (the total value placed on A's consumption by all of society).

Similarly, we present the private valuations of B in Table 12–1 and geometrically as MV_b in Figure 12–1. For whatever reason (she is poorer, more healthy, or less well educated), B places a lower value on each unit of health care than does A.

Table 12-1 Values and Costs of Medical Care

Quantity Consumed by A (Q_a)	A's Marginal Valuation (MV_a)	Quantity Consumed by B (Q_b)	B's Marginal Valuation (MV_b)	Quantity Consumed by A and B	Social Marginal Value of Consumption	Marginal Cost of Output at Consumption Level $Q_a + Q_b$
1	$80	0	$0	1	$80	$35
2	70	0	0	2	70	$35
3	60	0	0	3	60	$35
4	50	1	50	5	50	$35
5	40	2	40	7	40	$35
6	30	3	30	9	30	$35
7	20	4	20	11	20	$35
8	10	5	10	13	10	$35
9	0	6	0	15	0	$35

Indeed, her first unit has an *MV* of $50, her second has an *MV* of $40, and so on. These valuations might seem low to us, but since B is the ultimate judge of her own welfare, we cannot question these valuations: they are simply part of the data.

According to our assumption, A and B are the only members of society who participate in the medical care market. The marginal social valuations of medical care coincide with the marginal private valuations. Column 5 of Table 12–1 lists the

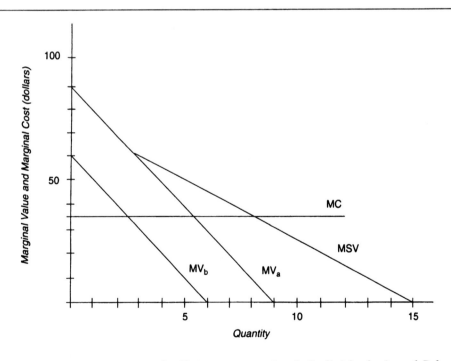

Figure 12-1 Representation of efficient output level. Individuals A and B have private marginal valuations for medical care (MV_a and MV_b respectively). Using these, we calculate the marginal social value (*MSV*) curve, which relates aggregate quantity to each individual's valuation. *MC* is the marginal social cost of medical care. The efficient level of output is that quantity at which *MSV* euqals the *MC*.

aggregated quantities that correspond to each level of *MV*. For example, at an aggregate quantity of five units of medical care (four used by A and one by B), each consumer's marginal value will be $50. If seven units were consumed (five by A and two by B), each individual's *MV* would be $40. We now have hypothesized how much each additional unit of medical care is worth to each participant. Furthermore, we have derived an aggregate-level relationship between the quantity of medical care and the marginal value to each individual if he or she was consuming at the level of consumption indicated by the *MV* curve (Figure 12–1). This aggregate curve, called the *MSV* (marginal social value) curve, shows the value to each member of the market if all individuals are consuming at the levels indicated by the curve. Because B does not have an *MV* above $60, for values above $60 the *MSV* curve coincides with A's *MV* curve.

An implicit assumption of our analysis is that consumer valuations are expressed in terms of a commodity, medical care. But medical care may not be valued for its own sake (except, perhaps, by a hypochondriac); it is usually *health* that is valued. In fact, each consumer's *MV* is made up of two components: an *MV* for health (termed *H*) and the marginal productivity of an additional unit of medical care (*M*) in producing health ($\Delta H/\Delta M$). Thus, the valuation of medical care is derivative, stemming from the two components.

We come next to the cost of producing medical care. Our initial assumption here is that each level of output is being produced at the minimum cost. This assumption is sometimes referred to as the *technical efficiency* assumption. It implies that, given production conditions and input prices, the lowest cost combination of inputs is used at any output level. In Column 7 of Table 12–1 and in Figure 12–1, we show the minimum marginal cost at which providers can produce medical care. We assume that this minimum marginal cost remains constant at $35 per unit as output increases. Note that the *MC* is the additional cost per unit of care; each extra unit costs $35 to produce.

One interpretation of *MC* is that it is the amount of money that must be paid to the inputs to hire them away from the next highest valued use. If medical care was not produced, something else of value to consumers would be. We can assume, then, that the *MC* is the amount we would have to pay the resources to induce them not to produce that something else. This approach allows us to put a value on unpaid resources that otherwise would appear to be "valueless" or "free." Thus the *MC* is marginally above (and approximates) the value that someone else would have placed on these resources in an alternative use. Viewing the *MC* in this way means that it is essentially the opportunity cost of the resources used (the value that users of other commodities would have placed on them).

12.3.3 The Socially Optimum Quantity of Medical Care

The next step in our analysis involves the definition and identification of desirable or optimum resource allocations. Since our method of evaluation is participatory, we need to identify allocations of resources that would be considered better than alternatives by all members of the community. As will be seen presently, it is possible using a participatory method to rank some allocations as superior to others, although we cannot compare every conceivable situation. Our criterion is this: the resources must be used in a way that maximizes social value. That is, if the resources are distributed in such a way that consumers are willing to pay the most for them, then output will be at the "right" or economically efficient level.

Using the valuations of A and B and the MC of medical care, we will be at a socially optimal (or economically efficient) level of output if the MVs of A and B equal the MC (i.e., $MV_a = MV_b = MC$). If output is at a level where the MVs are greater than MC, say, at an aggregate quantity of 3 in Table 12–1, then an expansion of output to 5 (an increase of 1 for A and B each) would have an MC per unit of output of $35 but would yield $50 extra in value to A and B each. Similarly, if the MC is greater than the MSV, this indicates that resources are worth more elsewhere, and so output should fall. In Figure 12–1, the optimal level of medical care is 7 units. Given our assumptions, this is how much medical care should be produced. This measure of efficiency—the distribution of output based on utility—is called *allocative efficiency*.

In reality, in a medical care market too much or too little as well as just enough medical care could be produced. Too much could be produced if the government had a policy of financing medical care and giving it away for free. At a zero price, demand will be at 15 units (where the MVs are zero); the MC of additional units will be well above this if the government is willing to ensure that all that is demanded is provided. The financing of the program could be through taxes. However, by meeting all demands, the government is clearly providing too much.

On the other hand, the market may provide too little. If medical care was in the hands of a monopolist, the monopolist would set a price well above that where $MV = MC$. If the price was $55, then three units in total would be demanded (all by A). Here the market would be producing too little care.

In addition, the optimum level of resource use could result in little or even no use of medical care by some individuals. The height of the MV curve, which is in effect a demand curve, will depend on health status, wealth, income, and so on. Poor people (e.g., B) may have low MVs. Indeed, if the MC was higher than in our example, a socially optimal quantity of output would be perfectly consistent with no consumption of medical care by B. (This is true, even though B may have poor health.) One might argue that this is unfair, and, indeed, depending on one's definition of fairness, it might well be. It should be recognized, however, that the root cause of the inequitable distribution of medical care is the inequitable distribution of wealth. A higher income for B would mean higher demand and MV curves for medical care. Of course, as far as the notion of economic efficiency is concerned, initial wealth and income levels for each individual are given. A redistribution of income or wealth among individuals might seem fair to many observers, but it would not be evaluated within the bounds of the present notion of economic efficiency.

12.3.4 Optimal Output with Altruism

To preserve the present notion of economic efficiency and to extend it to cover some distributional issues, an analysis has been developed to allow for the concern of some individuals for the low medical care consumption levels of others. Let us extend the previous example to allow for A's external demand for B's consumption of medical care. From A's viewpoint, it may well be that B has a level of consumption of medical care that is too low. If this is the case, we must find some representation of the value to A of B's medical care consumption. It is likely, of course, that A's concern for B's medical care consumption is not unlimited. A is concerned, but only up to a point, for A has other private and public concerns as well. In fact, as seen in Section 4.3, A's valuation of B's medical care consumption can be treated as any other commodity; the more B consumes, the less the marginal value to A of an additional unit. In Table 12–2, A's MV for B's consumption is $30 for the first unit, $20 for the second, and so on. In Figure 12–2, this external MV curve is shown as MV_a^b.

It may seem strange that A's altruistic concern for B's welfare can be translated into mercenary terms and be given a money measure. Our ability to do this rests on the assumption that commodities are scarce and A must make some choices at the margin. Even if A decided to give all his money away and use none of it for his family or own personal use, there would still be hard decisions to make. Should the money be donated to the cancer society or heart association? Should the money go toward the preservation of Newfoundland seals or bald eagles? Depending on their tastes, even the most altruistic of people must make choices regarding scarcity, and our analysis is merely a formalization of this fact. Of course, most people will engage in private consumption as well as altruistic consumption; their values can be presented by marginal valuation curves for both types of activities. The benefits to be obtained from others' consumption will be termed *external benefits,* and the values that people place on these benefits will be termed *external values.*

We can now arrive at a measure of the value that society places on B's medical care. This value can be called a *social value,* and it is made up of all individuals' private and external values for the specific commodity. Thus the marginal social value for B's consumption of medical care can be obtained by adding up the values both individuals place on each successive unit of medical care that B might consume. In Table 12–2, society has a marginal valuation of $80 for the first unit of B's medical care (equal to the sum of MV_b and MV_a^b), $60 for the second, and so on. These valuations are shown in Figure 12–2 as MSV_b, which is the vertical sum of MV_b and MV_a^b. By *vertical sum* we mean that each unit of B's consumption has a value to society (A and B) greater than the value placed on it by B alone. Because of this "public" dimension, we sum all values placed on each unit of B's consumption. Since each member's valuation of the commodity is measured along the vertical, or cost, axis, the summation of all members' valuations of this commodity is therefore a vertical sum.

The marginal valuation curve facing the market for medical care for A and B is MSV, which shows the quantity for all individuals at alternative MSVs for each

Table 12–2 Private and Social Values of B's Consumption of Medical Care

Quantity Consumed by B	Marginal Value to B of Own Consumption (MV_b)	Marginal Value to A of B's Consumption (MV_a^b)	Marginal Social Value of B's Consumption ($MV_b + MV_a^b$)
1	50	30	80
2	40	20	60
3	30	10	40
4	20	0	20
5	10	0	10

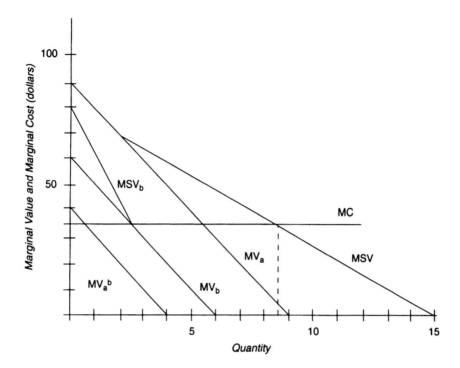

Figure 12–2 Representation of efficient output level. Individuals A and B have private marginal valuations for medical care (MV_a and MV_b, respectively); in addition, individual A places an external value on B's consumption. The marginal social value of B's consumption is the sum of the values placed on B's consumption by both A and B. The *MSV* of all medical care also reflects this externality. The *MC* is the marginal social cost of medical care. The efficient level of output is where *MSV* = *MC* (at approximately eight units).

individual. This curve is much like the *MSV* curve in Figure 12–1, except it incorporates A's valuation of B's consumption along with the private *MVs*.

The socially optimum level of output is similarly interpreted; the output is optimal at the quantity where the *MSV* for all individuals equals the *MC*. In Figure 12–2, the optimum level of output is eight units of medical care. This optimum quantity incorporates each individual's private valuations as well as any external valuations for the poor, the needy, the sick, and so on. The optimum quantity that incorporates the external concerns of A is greater than the optimum quantity if only selfish concerns exist (see Figure 12–1). However, these outcomes are results of the data, and it may well be that B's optimal consumption is still at a low level.

The results of our extended analysis are consistent with some kind of transfer of funds from A to B for the purposes of increasing B's consumption of medical care. However, the analysis does not say what kind of transfer should take place. It may be voluntary (e.g., charitable donations given by A directly to B or to some providing agency) or tax based (e.g., taxes levied on A might be used to reimburse providers). Although if taxation is used to raise funds, our analysis implies that it is voluntarily accepted by A. In either case, the optimal solution allows for some transfer, but it should be stressed that a transfer can be too much or too little. The government can over- or underprovide, based on A's criteria. All that our analysis shows is that *some* transfer is consistent with economic efficiency.

12.3.5 Alternative Delivery Arrangements

Now that we have identified an ideal or efficient output level, we can look at alternative delivery arrangements to see how they compare to the ideal. That is, we can determine whether expected output under the alternatives is too little, just enough, or too much.

12.3.5.1 "Free" and Unlimited Care

First, assume that B is given all the medical care for free that she can consume. As column three of Table 12–1 indicates, she would choose to consume six units of output. The social optimum is eight units for A and B, and the MC at this quantity is \$35. Optimally, B should consume three (i.e., where $MSV_b = MC$). For every unit B consumes beyond three, the value of B's consumption is less than the cost to society (everyone). Since someone must bear the burden of this care, and since MC exceeds MSV for all units beyond three, there is a net social loss for these units. B gains handsomely (i.e., her private benefits exceed her private costs), but overall this type of arrangement may lead to a great deal of medical care being consumed with very little value attached to it.

12.3.5.2 Competitive Market, No Philanthropy

Let us look at another arrangement, that of a competitive market with no philanthropy or government programs. Recall from Chapter 8 that equilibrium in a competitive market will occur where marginal private cost equals price. In the example here, A will consume the right amount for himself, but B will not. B's consumption will be less than the socially efficient amount because all society would have been willing to pay more for the first four units of B's consumption than the marginal cost. The competitive market does not provide a mechanism to express A's external demand for B's care. A freely operating competitive market with no philanthropy will yield less than the optimal level of output when externalities would have justified a larger output. As for a monopolistic market, the output of such a market will be less than the output of a competitive market, which means it will be even further below the optimal amount.

12.3.5.3 Competitive Market with Philanthropy

It has been contended that a competitive market even with philanthropy will not produce the optimal amount of output. To understand why, consider a situation in which there are many donors of medical care, each of whom places a value on the consumption of medical care by the needy. In this case, some social arrangement must be found for ensuring that the values of these donors will be expressed in the market. If each of these potential donors offers to give what the output is worth to him or her, the social value will equal the sum of the private values. However, if each donor feels that the others will also give, he or she might give less, hoping to get a "free ride," that is, gain the benefit of the others' donations while giving less. It is in the interests of each private donor to initially offer less than the value he or she places on the output in the hope that someone else will pay the tab. If everyone behaves in this way, the total amount given in philanthropy will be less than the socially optimal amount. Analysts who accept the efficiency criterion frequently justify compulsory government programs on the basis that they make everyone pay what the programs are worth. Of course, it is difficult to decide how much a program would be worth to each taxpayer, since the individual still has an incentive to understate the value of the program to him- or herself.

Even accepting this justification for government programs, we still must discover whether there exists an arrangement that will lead to the correct amount of medical care being utilized. As can be seen in Figure 12–2, if B was offered subsidized medical care, the efficient amount of medical care would be utilized. In this case, a charge of $30 per unit of medical care to B would lead to B's consumption of the optimal quantity—three units. The rest of society must now pick up the remainder of the tab. Since the total cost to all members of society of medical care consumed by B is $105 and since B will pay $90 of this, some arrangements must be made to collect the remaining $15 from the rest of society. This can be done in the form of taxes. Various arrangements are discussed in the next paragraphs.

We can conclude from our analysis that some form of cost-sharing arrangement can lead to the provision of an optimal or efficient amount of the product. However, other arrangements can also be efficient. One is to have needy individuals pay nothing and to impose some form of rationing. In practice, this type of arrangement requires that the rationing system used must produce the efficient outcome, and such systems are difficult to design and operate. Our analysis can also be extended to a case in which the needy individuals have different levels of income. If their demands differ because of these income levels, a system of variable subsidies tailored to income levels could be designed to have each member consume the right level of output (Pauly 1972).

What is critical in translating the preceding analysis into a policy prescription is a clear conception of what the external demands might be in actuality. Assuming that external demands for the medical care of some groups do exist and are significant, it is essential that we pin down exactly what services these external demands are for. If they are for good health, for example, then the external demanders (the A's in our analysis) may demand preventive care for consumption by the potential recipients of aid (the B's). The demands may be much more specific than that, however. The demanders might show concern only for individuals who have catastrophic illnesses requiring large financial outlays. In this case, they will not want to pay for the medical care of needy individuals who have sore throats, ingrown toenails, or acne. We know very little about the nature of medical care externalities (external demands). From an efficiency point of view, however, it is necessary to know what the external demanders are concerned about before we design a delivery system that will incorporate these externalities.

Assuming that we have identified the nature of the external demands, we can then use the preceding analysis to answer our questions, as long as we have the goal of efficiency in mind. Once the demands have been pinpointed, the types of health care that might improve the situation and the potential recipients can be identified. The consumer's portion of cost sharing should be designed to ensure that there is no overuse, which is defined as any quantity beyond which marginal social benefits are less than marginal social costs. The reimbursement mechanism chosen should lead to the least cost output.

12.4 OPTIMAL HEALTH INSURANCE

The provision of health insurance requires resources and incurs costs. In the same way that there is an optimal quantity of medical care, there is an optimal degree of insurance coverage (see Section 10.2.1). We will assume that all individuals are the same in all respects except one—the amount they must pay to obtain insurance.

Let us assume that there are 900 individuals (the number is not important) who are members of a large group and 100 individuals who are members of a small group. All individuals have an initial level of wealth of $1,000. There is a likelihood of 10 percent that each individual will get sick (i.e., 10 percent of the group will get sick). For those individuals who do get sick, the medical costs are $200 per patient. The utility function for each member (all have the same tastes) is as shown in Table 10–1. This utility function can be interpreted as a measure of "consumer welfare." With regard to the supply side of the market, we assume that there is one insurer who provides insurance at cost. The loading cost to the insurer of a large group policy is $30 whereas the cost for a small group policy is $60. Our objective is to maximize the overall utility of all members without detracting from that of any single member. This is the Paretean criterion.

The framework we will use focuses on consumer welfare (utility). In general, we can assume that consumer welfare is maximized by shifting the risk onto the insurer whenever the expected utility with insurance is greater than the utility in the absence of insurance. The postinsurance utility is the net of the economic cost of accepting the risk. Therefore, utility (welfare) is maximized whenever the risk is appropriately shifted.

In our analysis, there are two groups of individuals. Each individual faces an expected loss of $20 (i.e., 10 percent of $200), and each can obtain insurance at a cost that includes the expected loss ($20) plus the appropriate loading cost. For members of the large group, the full premium, including the loading charge, is $50. For members of the smaller group, the premium is $80. For members of the large group, there is a utility or welfare gain by shifting the risk: at a cost of $50, the utility will be 97.0 units, which exceeds the expected utility of not insuring, which is 95.8 units. There is a social gain from shifting the risk. The same is not true for the members of the smaller group. Since the cost of insurance for them is $80, they would be better off to remain uninsured. This would be true even if the cost of insurance for the smaller group was subsidized (i.e., if someone else paid part or all of the premiums). This is because we are using the criterion of social efficiency rather than individual efficiency. When we recognize that there is a *social* cost of insuring, then we must also recognize that there is an *optimal* degree of insurance coverage. This optimal degree may be zero if the arrangements for providing insurance are too costly.

We must also acknowledge that consumers may vary in many respects, including the following: risk of illness, income or wealth level, degree of risk aversion, and circumstances affecting the cost of illness. As each varies, the utility gain from shifting the risk of incurring medical expenses will also change. For example, individuals with a high risk of illness will gain more in utility terms from shifting their risk than individuals with a low risk of illness. Thus, a situation in which individuals who are less healthy have greater insurance coverage could be an optimal situation. That is, variations in insurance coverage between individuals can be economically efficient.

There is a confounding factor in this analysis—moral hazard. There can be a net welfare gain resulting from the shifting of risk. Once the risk is shifted, the out-of-pocket price of medical care to the consumer falls. If there is any elasticity of demand for medical care, then moral hazard will come into play and the quantity demanded of health care will increase. If the out-of-pocket price of medical care is low enough, the individual might consume care up to the point where $MC > MV$. There is a net welfare loss in the medical care market that occurs when the individual is ill. There are, then, two welfare effects of insurance: the welfare gain from shifting the risk and the welfare loss from consuming beyond the optimal point when the individual is ill. True optimality requires that we consider both effects together (Gianfrancesco 1978). Usually investigators focus on the insurance market (Gianfrancesco 1983; Pauly 1990) or the medical care market (Pauly 1972) in isolation from one another.

12.5 EXTRA-WELFARISM

The framework we have used until now includes a number of value judgments and principles. A key principle is that each person is the best judge of his or her own welfare. Welfare, in this framework, depends exclusively on the utility of goods and services as valued by the individuals. If there is any "public" component of goods and services, it is introduced through external demand, which is the value some people place on other people's consumption. Beyond this, there is no justification for publicly provided health care that can be derived from the Paretean welfare framework.

The Paretean framework has come under criticism in recent years on the grounds that it does not include all that people value in life (Culyer 1990; Rice 1992). There are other sources of personal well-being besides goods and services. Many of these other sources of well-being are embodied in the characteristics of people rather than the characteristics of the goods and services that people consume. People value mobility, absence from pain, and absence from distress—and they value these for other people as well as for themselves. While it is true that there are commodities (including medical care) that are linked to these more ultimate sources of well-being, there is no automatic link between them. Consequently, a social evaluation based on commodities consumed and nothing else appears much too narrow.

"Health" is often viewed as a composite of characteristics of people, such as mobility, absence of distress, and so forth. A number of economists have asserted that health is important not only because we want it for ourselves. They regard health as one of several entities that "society" recognizes should be made available to everyone (Culyer 1993) regardless of willingness to pay. This position has often appeared in the health care literature (Fein 1972; Outka 1971). If health really is a socially recognized good, then health *services* cannot be evaluated strictly in terms of their market value. In particular, the distribution of health services must be evaluated on a social basis.

The researchers who hold this position largely avoid the question of who the judge of welfare will be, a question directly addressed in the Paretean framework. They merely assert that some decision maker, chosen (or elected) by society, should be responsible for conducting the evaluation. Thus we are no longer clear, in this extra-welfarist viewpoint, who the judge of welfare is. Indeed, extra-welfarism is consistent with the use of any social judge other than the consumers; the approach merely posits that there are some entities whose social value is determined outside of the consumers themselves. The role of economists is to act as advisors for the distributive organization and uncover the implications of incorporating efficiency and other objectives into the economic analysis. It should be pointed out that people's direct evaluations of their health services can be included in the extra-welfarist economic calculus, as can other (nondirect) evaluations of their health care.

The extra-welfarist position is concerned with how health is distributed among all members of society. Whoever the judge of well-being becomes (the government, a community league, etc.), value judgments must still be made in order to decide how to distribute health services and health. One way to operationalize the extra-welfarist approach (i.e., turn it into an evaluative tool) is to provisionally accept the principle that health care should be distributed according to "need." If need is defined as the ability to benefit from health services (Culyer 1995), then the "decision maker" is faced with the question of how to allocate health services so as to enhance or preserve different individuals' health status. Even if this approach evades the issue (or at least leaves the issue open) of who is to decide on the distribution, it helps make explicit the wide array of distributions that are possible (using the principle of need and other principles as well).

Figure 12–3 is a graph that shows the health of two individuals, A and B, measured along the two axes (Wagstaff 1991). Let us make the following (non-value-laden) assumptions: individual A has a self-assessed health status of h_1 and individual B has a self-assessed health status of h_2. The health status of both can be improved, but there is a limit. Curve H shows the maximum amount of health that can be produced with the resources available for health care (assumed to be fixed for society as a whole). More health can be produced for A, but only at the expense of resources and health for B. With available resources, A's health can be increased up to h_x (with no change in B's health) and B's health can be increased up to h_y (with no change in A's health). The exact shape of the H curve will depend on how effective the additional resources are in improving each individual's health. If very little extra can be done to improve B's health, then the curve will be steeply sloped. Our curve shows that more can be done for both.

Mentioned above was the principle that health resources should be distributed according to need. There are a number of different ways to express "need."

- *Equal health status.* One value judgment is to allocate resources so that everyone ends up with an equal level of health. If this principle is used, then more resources must be provided to A to ensure that in the end both A and B are equally healthy. Equal health implies that each person is on a 45° line from the origin.
- *Maximizing total health regardless of its distribution.* In order to implement this criterion, we must know the trade-off in health status between the two persons. If the health transformation curve, H, favors person A, then resources will be more productive in improving A's health status rather than B's. An optimal point will

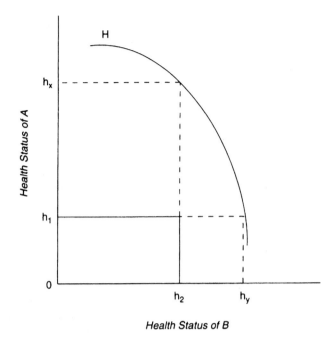

Figure 12–3 Potential health status of two individuals. The health status of A and the health status of B are currently at h_1 and h_2. Through the expending of more resources, their health status can move up to h_x and h_y respectively. However, since the available resources are finite, the limit of improvement for both individuals combined is shown by curve H.

occur on the H curve above the 45° line. The characteristic of the optimal point will be where the additional health per dollar of expenditure will be the same for the two people.

- *Equalizing additional health per dollar.* This criterion is most like the Paretean optimum. According to this criterion, we accept the initial starting point (h_1, h_2) and allocate additional resources so that the total health gain is as large as possible. The optimum point will at a position northeast of the initial position on the transformation curve, H.

The usefulness of the extra-welfarist approach is that it allows us to go further in exploring resource allocation than the Paretean or welfarist position, and if society places special importance on characteristics such as health, then alternative distributions of health care resources need extremely careful evaluation.

12.6 CONCEPTS OF EQUITY

Distributional equity is important in analyzing both access to and consumption of medical care (e.g., differences in utilization among groups) and its financing (e.g., differences in payments), and so it is essential to have measures of equity. We focus here on three types of distributional equity: intergenerational equity, vertical equity, and horizontal equity (Long and Smeeding 1984).

Intergenerational equity, in a financial context, concerns the distribution of payments among different generations. For example, if we divide up the population into retirees (who are generally over 65 and eligible for Medicare benefits), those of working age (say, those 18 to 64), and others, our classification scheme could be regarded as dividing the population along generational lines. Since the Medicare hospital insurance program is financed largely through the flow of payroll taxes into the Hospital Insurance Trust Fund, these taxes will be borne largely by individuals in the working-age group. In other words, the working-age generation is largely financing the care of the generation of retirees. The equity implications of this kind of tax are very different those of the tax used to expand the Medicare program's benefits in 1988. This latter was a 15-percent tax on the taxable income of the retirees, and it proved to be so unpopular that the program expansion was repealed by Congress. This type of tax involves a minimal intergenerational transfer of funds.

Current employment-based private health insurance provides another example of intergenerational transfer. All employees pay a similar health insurance premium, which is based on the average utilization pattern for all workers. If workers were rated separately by age group, according to insurance principles younger workers would have a lower premium than older workers because their utilization is less. The financing method of charging everyone in the plan the same rate (community rating) is in effect intergenerationally inequitable.

The second type of equity, vertical equity, concerns the economic burden experienced by different income groups. For example, imagine we have three income groups: those who make under $20,000, those who make from $20,000 to $40,000, and those who make over $40,000. A tax is progressive if members of a higher income group pay a larger portion of their income in tax than those with a lower income, it is neutral if the portion is the same for all groups, and it is regressive if members of a lower income group pay a higher portion of their income in tax than those with a higher income.

An example of vertical inequity would be a flat tax charged to all individuals regardless of their income level. A fixed premium for Medicare enrollees is such a tax. Lower income groups pay the same rate as higher income groups do, and this premium amounts to a higher portion of their income.

Horizontal equity concerns the degree to which equals are taxed equally. An example of a horizontally inequitable tax is a tax on specific commodities such as alcohol, tobacco products, and hospital care. Consumption or sales taxes on the former two products fall on groups who use these products more heavily. Such taxes have been a popular means of financing health insurance programs for indigents. Even though these taxes are horizontally inequitable, it has been argued that, since these individuals are likely to be less healthy and use the health care system more, they should pay higher taxes. That is, if not just taxes but rather the net of health care services minus taxes paid is considered, then horizontal *inequity* is not present. Another type of tax that has been recommended as a way to pay for medical care for indigents is a tax on hospital admissions. Such a tax will also be inequitable, though to a large extent it will be less visible, because it will be passed on to the third parties who reimburse the providers. (Of course, the insurers, in turn, will pass the tax on by charging higher health insurance premiums.)

12.7 GOALS OF HEALTH POLICY

There are a number of different ways that the goals of health policy can be articulated. At one level, one can articulate a set of environmental conditions that will allow for a smoother operating policy. For example, many feel that if consumers are given a range of health plans to select from and the freedom to choose among those plans, then social goals will be forwarded. At a lower, operational level, there are goals that deal with operating performance, such as efficiency, equity, and public financial constraints. Finally, social goals can be articulated in terms of the health outcomes of a group of individuals. In order for the policy goal to be operational, policies will still have to specify how each person's health status is to be included (e.g., whether everyone is counted the same). In addition, the policy makers should take into account the economic aspects of the policy goals. There are insufficient resources to allow everyone to maximize their health status; therefore, goals have to be set that allow one to rank social measures of health status resulting from different policies.

One might combine policy goals from the different categories. For example, a policy maker might deem equity of resource use to be important. However, once individuals have equal resources available to them (e.g., though spending vouchers), the policy maker might value freedom of choice to allow individuals to select those types of care that they feel would best suit them. As another example, a policy maker might value a population's health status highly but also want to ensure technical efficiency is achieved. The policy maker would select policies that would forward both objectives. Below we discuss briefly each of the goals.

12.7.1 Environmental Conditions

A market is an institution in which free choice is exercised by the participants, who are in pursuit of their own well-being. A social goal that falls under this category is allowing persons the freedom to seek care from whatever health plan they want to join. One might also suggest that anyone who wants to provide health services may do so. Generally, choice in health care markets is not extended to anyone who wants to be a provider. This is a reflection of the fact that other policy goals, such as the protection of quality, are being sought.

12.7.2 Efficiency

In order to achieve economic efficiency, (1) demand must be at an appropriate level, neither too restrictive (e.g., because of monopolistic prices) nor too low (such that there be an excessive demand), and (2) providers must produce an adequate supply of services (3) at an appropriate quality level and (4) at a low cost of production.

12.7.2.1 Demand Barriers

Demand barriers are impediments obstructing the reception of care. Within the context of our present model, price is the prime impediment. One can encourage additional care demanded by lowering the direct price through the purchase of insurance, public programs, or charity. To the degree that additional medical care utilization is thought to be desirable, the extent of financial demand barriers can be measured by the availability of insurance or the direct price faced by individuals.

However, money price is not the only factor related to demand barriers. Waiting costs and travel costs can also obstruct access of care. If medical care consumption is to be encouraged, these costs must be addressed, either through subsidies, relocating facilities to lower travel time and expenses, or expanding facilities and increasing operating hours to decrease waiting time. However, it should be remembered that, from an efficiency standpoint, demand can be too great as well as insufficient.

12.7.2.2 Adequacy of Supply

Adequacy of supply refers to the availability of sufficient resources to provide care at the efficient level (given the level of quality). Adequacy of supply depends on the incentive (reimbursement) system developed, the level of reimbursement, and the adequacy of funds.

12.7.2.3 Technical Efficiency

Technical efficiency is a measure of the cost of producing a given level and quality of output. Technical efficiency is usually expressed in terms of money costs, but care must be taken when comparing costs between facilities to be sure that all other factors (e.g., quality, input prices, and case mix) have been accounted for.

12.7.2.4 Quality of Care

On the assumption that quality is not free, it costs more to achieve a higher quality of care. Therefore quality, like any other characteristic of output, can come in too great or too little a quantity. Quality of care is an often cited policy goal in health care. Regulation and licensing of professionals are often enacted in the name of the protection of quality of care.

12.7.3 Equity

Equity is a very broad concept. We consider two aspects, equity of utilization and equity of finance.

12.7.3.1 Equity of Utilization

A service can be provided efficiently, and yet some individuals who could benefit from more of it simply cannot pay for it. Society, or policy makers, can set utilization goals above those that are provided in a market situation. In this case, the direct price or other barriers to care must be removed. Thus one may lose some efficiency in order to attain a higher degree of equity.

12.7.3.2 Equity of Finance

Equity of finance can refer to direct out-of-pocket prices as well as taxation and premiums, factors that may not directly affect utilization. Health care premiums may be deemed too low, in which case some individuals would be viewed as not paying a fair portion of the cost of medical care. Equity of finance would call for an increase in these premiums.

12.7.4 Public Financial Constraints

Strictly speaking, the government budget does not fall within the scope of our model. Of course, a transfer of funds from A to B is consistent with a tax on A by a government body and subsequent expenditures on medical care for B. But the model says nothing about the size of the tax, the expenditure, or the difference (the contribution to the deficit). In recent years, however, the budget deficit and public spending have come under a great deal of scrutiny, and cutbacks in government programs have been widespread. Typically the rationale for cutting a program's expenditures is not lack of worthiness of the program but the program's contribution to the overall budget deficit. To the extent that cutbacks can be achieved merely through increases in technical efficiency, true savings are provided to society and there are gains in social efficiency. However, cutbacks may also result in reduced supply. This is not necessarily bad if output was greater than the socially optimum level to begin with. However, if the initial output was at the socially optimum level or below it, cutbacks will lead to reductions in social efficiency because the value of the output that is lost is greater than the savings resulting from the cutbacks.

12.7.5 Health Status of the Population

In recent years, many investigators have focused on population-based measures of health status as a goal of policy. Many of the other goals can be viewed as leading to better health, and so these investigators focus on direct measures of health as a policy objective. Of course, the costs of achieving various levels of health status must be considered as well. Thus, one is faced with the constrained objective of maximizing population health subject to resource constraints. Additionally, focusing on this goal does not do away with equity considerations. Once we have more than one individual whose health is measured, we face the problem of how to add up the health status of all the individuals. These problems have been discussed in this chapter, and they need to be addressed in any policy consideration.

EXERCISES

1. Distinguish between Paretean and delegatory value systems, in terms of who determines the preferences.
2. In a world of completely selfish individuals, if we could measure each person's marginal value for his or her own medical care, what conditions must be met in order for the health care market to be at an optimal level of output?
3. What do we mean by the socially optimal level of medical care?
4. In a society with two persons, if one is altruistic and values the other's use of medical care, how will this influence the socially optimal quantity of medical care that is produced.

5. According to the Paretean criterion, if medical care is given away free and in unlimited quantities, will this yield a socially optimal outcome?
6. What is a consumption externality for medical care?
7. Will a freely competitive market without philanthropy yield a socially optimal output when there are consumption externalities?
8. What conditions must be met in order for there to be an optimal degree of insurance coverage?
9. If individuals are fully insured for all health care services, will this necessarily result in a socially optimal amount of insurance coverage?
10. List five goals of health policy.
11. What is the extra-welfarist approach to defining an optimal amount of output and how does it compare with the Paretean approach?
12. Given the following MV information, what is the optimal allocation of care according to the Paretean criteria, when the marginal cost of care is constant at $100.

Person A		Person B	
Quantity of care consumed	MV	Quantity of care consumed	MV
1	$200	1	$150
2	180	2	120
3	162	3	92
4	146	4	66
5	134	5	42
6	122	6	20
7	112	7	0
8	104	8	0
9	98	9	0

BIBLIOGRAPHY

Efficiency Criteria

Arrow, K.J. 1963. Uncertainty and the welfare economics of medical care. *American Economic Review* 53:941–973.

Buchanan, J.M. 1965. *The inconsistency of the National Health Service.* London: Institute of Economic Affairs.

Butler, J.R.G. 1992. Welfare economics and cost-utility analysis. In *Health economics worldwide*, ed. P. Zweifel and H.E. Frech III. Amsterdam: Kluwer Academic Publishers.

Culyer, A.J. 1971. The nature of the commodity "health care" and its efficient allocation. *Oxford Economic Papers* 23:189–211.

———. 1977. On the relative efficiency of the National Health Service. *Kyklos* 25:266–287.

Dor, A., and H. Watson. 1998. Welfare consequences of alternative insurance contracts in the mixed for-profit/nonprofit hospital market. *Southern Economic Journal* 64:698–712.

Evans, R.G. 1997. Going for the gold. *Journal of Health Politics, Policy and Law* 22:427–465.

Feldman, R., and B. Dowd. 1993. What does the demand curve for medical care measure? *Journal of Health Economics* 12:193–200.

Pauly, M.V. 1968. The economics of moral hazard. *American Economic Review* 58:531–537.

———. 1972. *Medical care at public expense.* New York: Praeger.

Peele, P.B. 1993. Evaluating welfare losses in the health care market. *Journal of Health Economics* 12:205–208.

Rice, T. 1993a. Demand curves, economists and desert islands. *Journal of Health Economics* 12:201–204.

———. 1993b. A model is only as good as its assumptions. *Journal of Health Economics* 12:209–211.

———. 1997. Can markets give us the health system we want? *Journal of Health Politics, Policy and Law* 22:383–426.

Thorne, E.D. 1998. When private parts are made public goods. *Yale Journal on Regulation* 15:149–175.

———. 1998. The shortage of market-inalienable human organs: Consideration of nonmarket failures. *American Journal of Economics and Sociology* 57:247–260.

Weisbrod, B.A. 1964. Collective consumption services of individual consumption goods. *Quarterly Journal of Economics* 78:471–477.

Optimal Health Insurance

Blomquist, A., and P.-O. Johansson. 1997. Economic efficiency and mixed public/private insurance. *Journal of Public Economics* 66:505–516.

Chernew, M., et al. 1997. Worker demand for health insurance in the non-group market: A note on the calculation of welfare loss. *Journal of Health Economics* 16:375–380.

Chu, W.H. 1997. Health insurance and the welfare of health care consumers. *Journal of Public Economics* 64:125–133.

Cleeton, D. 1989. The medical uninsured: A case of market failure? *Public Finance Quarterly* 17:55–83.

Gianfrancesco, F.D. 1978. Insurance and medical care expenditure: An analysis of the optimal relationship. *Eastern Economics Journal* 4:225–234.

———. 1983. A proposal for improving the efficiency of medical insurance. *Journal of Health Economics* 2:175–184.

Jack, W., and L. Sheiner. 1997. Welfare: Improving health expenditure subsidies. *American Economic Review* 87:206–221.

Pauly, M.V. 1990. The rational nonpurchase of long-term-care insurance. *Journal of Political Economy* 98:153–168.

Selden, T.M. 1997. More on the economic efficiency of mixed public/private insurance. *Journal of Public Economics* 66:517–523.

Extra-Welfarism

Culyer, A.J. 1989. The normative economics of health care finance and provision. *Oxford Review of Economic Policy* 5:34–58.

———. 1990. Commodities, characteristics of commodities, characteristics of people, utilities, and the quality of life. In *Quality of life: Perspectives and problems*, ed. S. Baldwin et al. London: Routledge.

———. 1991. Conflicts between equity concepts and efficiency in health: A diagrammatic approach. *Osaka Economic Papers* 40:141–154.

———. 1993. Health, health expenditures, and equity. In *Equity in the finance and delivery of health care: An international perspective*, ed. E. van Doorslaer et al. Oxford: Oxford University Press.

————. 1995. *Equality of what in health policy? Conflicts between the contenders.* Discussion paper 142. York, England: University of York, Center for Health Economics.

Pauly, M.V. 1994. Reply to Roberta Labelle, Greg Stoddart, and Thomas Rice. *Journal of Health Economics* 13:495–496.

Rice, T. 1992. An alternative framework for evaluating welfare losses in the health care market. *Journal of Health Economics* 11:85–92.

Wagstaff, A. 1991. QALYs and the equity-efficiency trade-off. *Journal of Health Economics* 10:21–41.

Equity and Other Social Goals

Beauchamp, D.E. 1976. Public health as social justice. *Inquiry* 13:3–14.

Daniels, N. 1982. Equity of access to health care. *Milbank Quarterly* 60:51–81.

Fein, R. 1972. On achieving access and equity in health care. In *Economic aspects of health care,* ed. J.B. McKinlay. New York: Watson Publishing International.

Friedman, L.M. 1971. The idea of right as a social and legal concept. *Journal of Social Issues* 27:189–198.

Goldfarb, R., et al. 1984. Can remittances compensate for manpower outflows. *Journal of Development Economics* 15:1–17.

Hemenway, D. 1982. The optimal location of doctors. *New England Journal of Medicine* 306:397–401.

Lewis, C.F., et al. 1976. *A right to health.* New York: Wiley-Interscience.

Long, S.H., and T.M. Smeeding. 1984. Alternative Medicare financing sources. *Milbank Quarterly* 62:325–348.

Mechanic, D. 1976. Rationing health care. *Hastings Center Report* 9(1):34–37.

Mitchell, B.M., and C.E. Phelps. 1976. National health insurance: Some costs and effects of mandated employee coverage. *Journal of Political Economy* 84:553–571.

Outka, G. 1974. Social justice and equal access to health care. *Journal of Religious Ethics* 2:11–32.

Schwartz, W.B., and P.L. Joskow. 1978. Medical efficacy versus economic efficiency: A conflict in values. *New England Journal of Medicine* 299:1462–1464.

Stoddart, G.L., and R.J. Labelle. 1985. *Privatization in the Canadian health care system.* Ottawa, Ontario: Health and Welfare Department, Government of Canada.

Sudgen, R., and A. Williams. 1978. *The principles of practical cost-benefit analysis.* Oxford: Oxford University Press.

Thurow, L.C., 1985. Medicine versus economics. *New England Journal of Medicine* 313:611–614.

van Doorslaer, E., et al. 1997. Income-related inequalities in health: Some international comparisons. *Journal of Health Economics* 16:93–112.

Whipple, D. 1974. Health care as a right. *Inquiry* 11:65–68.

Financing Health Care

1. Identify the alternative sources of health care funding in the United States.
2. Describe the effect on resource owners of the following means of financing health care: insurance premiums, tax subsidies, and mandated benefits.
3. Define economic incidence and compare the burden of two types of taxes: payroll taxes and sales taxes.
4. Compare the incidence of the following means of financing by income level: insurance premiums, payroll taxes, sales taxes, and income taxes.
5. Define the administrative cost of public and private financing mechanisms.

13.1 INTRODUCTION

There are three major methods of financing health care services—out-of-pocket payments by the consumers, insurance premiums, and taxation—and within each category there are a number of different financing techniques. For example, out-of-pocket payments include deductibles, copayments, and full consumer payments. Insurance premiums can be paid directly by the consumer or paid by the employer or the government. And taxes can be levied on income or on specific products or services. Further, the different financing methods can interact: insurance premiums can be excluded from taxation or can be taxed (as is the case in the United States).

Each method will impact differently on groups with different characteristics, such as income level or family size. Determining how the burden of each financing method will fall is not a straightforward matter. The burden of insurance premiums that are paid out of pocket by consumers will fall on the consumers directly, but income taxes can influence this burden, and when insurance is obtained through the workplace (as is usually the case in the United States), the burden of payment is not clear-cut. Further, different kinds of taxes will have the same impact on groups with varying income levels. Economic analysis is a very useful tool for sorting out the effects of these varying finance methods. In the first part of this chapter, we examine how explanatory economics can be used to analyze the burden of the various financing methods. We also show how these various methods can be assessed in terms of specific criteria or policy objectives.

Different financing methods also have significantly different costs. In the case of private insurance, there are the costs of marketing, rating alternative consuming groups, paying providers, and monitoring utilization. In the case of government finance, there are the costs of collecting taxes and administering public programs. A debate has been occurring in the United States in recent years over whether health care coverage for the population should be financed primarily through private markets (with appropriate subsidies) or public financing. In this chapter, we illustrate how economic analysis can be used to compare these options.

13.2 FINANCING MEANS AND BURDENS IN THE UNITED STATES

Currently in the United States a variety of financing mechanisms are used in health care. These mechanisms and the amounts raised through each are shown in Table 13–1. We use 1997 data in our example because a national survey was conducted in that year that provides thorough information on health insurance expenditures by households. Using data from this survey seems preferable to using data for different years that are not consistent.

As can be seen from Table 13–1, a total of $1,082 billion was spent on health care in 1997. Of this amount, $189.1 billion (roughly 17 percent) was financed by

Table 13–1 Sources of funds for National Health Expenditures, 1997 (billions of dollars)

Private funds	
Out-of-pocket expenses[a]	$ 189.1
Private insurance[a]	346.7
Employment-related	
Employer-contributed[b]	254.7
Employee-contributed[b]	49.5
Non-employment related[b]	42.6
Other private funds[a]	36.3
Government funds	
Federal funds	333.4
Payroll taxes for Part A Medicare (includes revenue from The Hospital Insurance Trust Fund)[c]	112.7
Premiums for Part B Medicare and HMO coverage[d]	19.1
Other federal funds[a]	231.2
State and local government funds[a]	139.2
Total, all sources	$1,082.0

a. Health Care Financing Administration. National Health Expenditures, 1960–1998. Internet site http://www.hcfa.gov/stats/hne-oact/

b. Ratios for employment and non employment-based insurance, and for employer and employee proportion of ratios derived from Vistnes, J., 1992. Private health insurance premiums in 1987: policy holders under the age of 65. AHCRP Publication 92-0061. National Medical Expenditure Survey Summary 5. Rockville, MD: Department of Health and Human Services, Public Health Service, Agency for Health Care Policy and Research

c. Health Care Financing Administration. 1999 Annual Report of the Board of Trustees of the Federal Hospital Insurance (HI) Trust Fund. Internet site: http://medicare.hcfa.gov/pubforms/tr/hi1999/toc.htm.

d. Health Care Financing Administration. 1999 Annual Report of the Board of Trustees of the Federal Supplementary Medical Insurance (HI) Trust Fund. Internet site: http://www.hcfa.gov/tr/smi1999/toc.htm.

out-of-pocket payments by consumers. These payments constituted a larger portion of the funds spent on physician care than on hospital care.

A total of $346.7 billion (32 percent) was financed through private insurance. The majority of private insurance premiums (roughly 82 percent of all premiums) are paid for through employment-provided health insurance, and the rest are paid for through individual purchases that are not employment related. Individually purchased insurance includes Medigap insurance, which individuals over 65 purchase to cover the copayments and deductibles in the Medicare program. Roughly one-half of all premiums purchased directly by individuals (i.e., not obtained through employment) are Medigap premiums.

With regard to health insurance provided through the workplace, the majority of the premiums are paid for by employers, with a smaller amount being paid for directly by employees. However, this does not mean that the employers bear the burden of the majority of the health insurance expenses. For one thing, premiums paid for by employers are workplace benefits that are not subject to income tax. There is therefore a sizable public subsidy given to employees who obtain their insurance in this way; their taxes will be lower than if they paid for their premiums directly. In addition, there is considerable evidence that, when all the wage effects are taken into account, the employees do indeed bear a major share of these premium costs, even if the picture at first glance does not show it that way.

The third form of finance that is used is public finance, or taxation. In 1997, about $472 billion of total financing for health care involved taxation. Most of this amount went to pay for the federal Medicare program, which covers individuals over 65, and the joint federal-state Medicaid program, which is primarily for the lower income groups. These programs are largely but not entirely financed by taxation. With regard to taxation, the major federal tax that pays for the hospital portion (Part A) of Medicare is a payroll tax of 1.6 percent of wages, paid both by employers and employees. In 1997, about $112 billion was collected through this tax. In addition, there is a Medicare "premium" for medical care (physician services) and health maintenance organization (Part B) coverage, which raised $19.1 billion. Most of the remainder of the federal portion was raised through general taxation, the largest portion from direct income taxation. Of the $334 billion spent by governments on health care, $139 billion was raised through state government taxation. Most of state taxation is in the form of direct income and indirect sales taxes.

The above picture does provide an indication of where the money is coming from, but it cannot be used directly to assess the "burden" of medical care financing (defined as the reduction in real income due to payments and taxes). The complexity of the situation and the prominent role played by each of the financing methods calls for a much more detailed analysis. Each financing method imposes different burdens on different groups. We will discuss the pattern of these burdens after examining the positive economics of the burdens.

13.3 ECONOMIC ANALYSIS OF ALTERNATIVE PAYMENT SOURCES

This section presents economic analyses of alternative payment methods. The focus of the analyses is the economic impact of the payment methods on the resource owners (primarily employees and owners of companies). We will examine insurance premiums (in particular, the impact of employer-paid premiums, taxation, and mandated benefits) and taxation (the impact of payroll and sales taxes).

A primary question relates to the economic incidence of a tax, that is, who ends up bearing the economic burden. The group which bears the burden of the tax may be different from the group from which it is originally collected. For example, a government tax on cigarettes may be collected from tobacco retailers. However, to the extent that prices of tobacco products are higher because of the tax, the incidence is on the smokers, who bear the burden of the higher price.

13.3.1 Private Health Insurance

13.3.1.1 Insurance Premiums

Insurance can be obtained through the workplace or by individual purchase. Insurance obtained in the workplace can be paid for directly by the employees (through payroll deductions) or by the employers. There is no controversy over the incidence of premiums paid by employees or by individuals; the purchasers bear the cost of their insurance purchases.

The economic incidence of employer-paid premiums is a little more complicated. The cost of insurance benefit packages are viewed by employers as an expense, much like wages are. An employer has a demand curve for labor and will regard the costs of various forms of compensation as monetarily equivalent. If the marginal employee is worth (has a marginal value of) $50 to the employer, then the employer will be willing to pay up to $50 in compensation, whether in the form of wages or fringe benefits (Kreuger and Reinhardt 1994). If benefits are increased, then the employer will reduce wages. Thus the economic burden of all health insurance benefits will fall on the employee either directly (out of pocket) or indirectly (through a lower wage).

13.3.1.2 Taxation and Insurance Premiums

Health insurance benefits paid by the employer are exempt from personal income and social security taxes. This reduces the cost to the employee of employer-paid health insurance and increases the quantity demanded for health insurance. However, we cannot assume that, once a subsidy is put into place, the quantity demanded and supplied will remain the same. To see why, consider the analysis of a tax subsidy provided below.

In Figure 13–1, the initial demand curve for health insurance (with no tax subsidies) is D_1. According to this curve, when the premium rate is $100, 75 individuals will be willing to shift their risks to insurers. Let us now introduce a 50-percent subsidy. This will in effect lower the out-of-pocket price for insurance at every premium rate. Thus, at a premium rate of $100, the out-of-pocket price to the consumer is $50, and at this price 100 individuals will be willing to shift their risks. The market demand curve will then be D_2.

According to the supply curve for insurance (S in Figure 13–1), insurers will be willing to accept 92 risks at a price of $135. Generally, a higher supplier price will be required to induce the insurers to accept more risks.

Let us initially assume that there is no tax subsidy. Then 100 risks will be shifted at a premium rate of $100. This is the equilibrium price and quantity. Using this

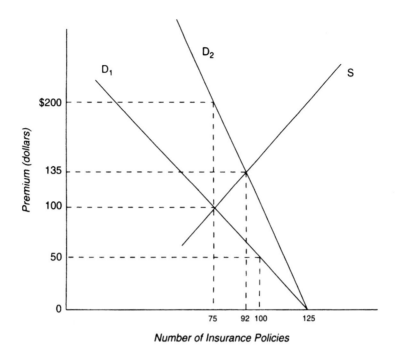

Figure 13–1 The effect of a subsidy on the quantity of health insurance. The demand curve for insurance without any tax subsidy is shown in the above diagram as D_1. This curve shows that, at an unsubsidized premium rate of $100, 75 individuals will demand insurance. Let us introduce a 50 percent subsidy (e.g., at a premium rate of $100, the individual will pay $50). The market demand curve will shift to D_2. The supply curve for insurance is also shown. At a market price of $100, the insurance industry is willing to supply 75 policies (accept 75 risks). Without a subsidy, 75 individuals will shift risks to the insurers. With a 50 percent subsidy, the out-of-pocket premium price would initially drop to $50. There would be a large excess demand at this price, but the industry would not be willing to accept 100 risks at $100. The price would be increased until a new equilibrium is reached—at $135 (and 92 risks shifted).

---

position as a base point, we will now introduce a subsidy on premiums of 50 percent. That is, the individuals are in a 50-percent income tax bracket and are allowed to deduct insurance premiums before calculating income taxes. A preliminary analysis of the effects of the subsidy might be as follows. The premium price would remain the same ($100), but half would be paid ($50) out of pocket by the consumer and half would fall on taxpayers (since the individual would get $50 back from the public purse). This analysis might be applied to 75 insurance policies in order to determine the "shifting" effect. However, a sounder economic analysis would result from supposing that the new quantity on which the subsidy will be based will neither be the old quantity nor the quantity demanded at a premium of $100. In order to determine the likely effects of the subsidy, we must conduct an economic analysis of the type presented in Figure 13–1.

As shown in the figure, the subsidy raises quantity demanded at each price, and so more individuals will seek to shift risks at the premium rate of $100. However, suppliers (insurers) will require higher premiums in order to accept more risks. The premium rate will rise, and less risks will be shifted than were originally indicated by demand conditions alone. In our example, the final premium rate will be $135, and at this price 92 risks will be shifted.

The cost of the premium will be borne half by the consumer and half by the taxpayer. However, the amount of subsidy will be based on the new price of $135. And the quantity of risks shifted will be the new equilibrium quantity. The final equilibrium (and the burden of the subsidy) will depend on the elasticities of demand and supply. In the extreme, if the supply curve were upward sloping, indicating no change in risks shifted, then the analysis would indicate that the premium would rise by the full amount of the subsidy. The taxpayers would pay a subsidy of $100, based on a new premium of $200, with 75 risks still being shifted. It is more likely the supply curve is horizontal, indicating an unlimited supply of risks accepted at a price of $100. Then the consumer would get a full $50 subsidy paid for by the taxpayers; in this case 100 risks would be shifted.

Our analysis does not take into account subsequent effects of the increased insurance coverage on the medical care market. Nevertheless, even this simple analysis indicates that the demand-and-supply analysis should be considered when determining the full effects of a tax subsidy on premiums.

13.3.1.3 Mandated Benefits

Mandated insurance benefits are government-required coverage benefits that individuals privately purchase or employers must provide. Mandated benefits can have a considerable impact on labor markets depending on how they are viewed by consumers, and this impact will in turn affect the incidence of benefits.

We will consider an economic analysis of mandated benefits using a labor market analysis such as that presented in Figure 13–2. In the initial situation, there are no mandated benefits. The demand for labor is shown as D_1, and the supply of labor is shown as $S_{v=0}$. Equilibrium wages are at $8, and equilibrium employment is at 300 workers.

We now introduce mandated insurance benefits that cost $2 per worker. The employer's demand curve for labor in terms of total compensation will remain the same; however, when expressed in terms of the wage rate, the demand curve will shift down by $2, since $2 is added to the wages for each worker to calculate total compensation. The new demand curve for labor, in terms of wages, is D_2.

It would be tempting to say that the employees will bear the entire burden of the mandated benefits and take a $2 reduction in wages, in which case employment would remain the same. Such will be the case only if the workers fully value the benefits (see curve $S_{v=b}$); the new price in this instance would be $6.

If the workers do not value the benefits at all, there will be a reduction in wages (but by less than $2) to $7 (or some such amount, depending on the elasticity of labor supply), and also a reduction in employment. The burden of the mandate will then fall, to some degree, on the workers who lose their jobs. If benefits are only partially valued ($S_{v<b}$), the net result will be somewhere in between.

In an extreme case, such as a vertical supply curve, there will be no employment effect but a full wage effect. In fact, several studies have shown that this result is approximated in reality (Kreuger and Reinhardt 1994), and so the workers bear the full burden of the mandate. In sum, then, mandated benefits may have similar

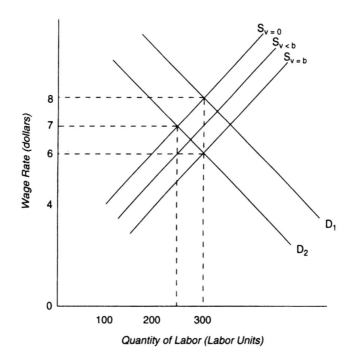

Figure 13–2 The effect of mandated insurance coverage on labor markets. The demand for labor when the employer does not provide any benefits is shown as D_1. For example, at a wage rate of $8, 300 works (the labor units) will be demanded. Let us introduce mandated benefits of $2 per worker. The employer will still value each worker's productivity the same, but at each quantity of labor the total compensation that must be paid by the employer is $2 above the wage rate. Therefore, the demand curve is shifted down by $2 at each quantity of labor (D_2). We posit three alternative supply curves for labor. The first supply surve ($S_{v=0}$) is for the situation where the mandated benefits have no value to the workers. Each employee's supply curve for labor, in terms of the wage rate, remains the same after the benefits are mandated. The second supply curve ($S_{v=b}$) is for the situation where the workers value benefits and wages equally. The supply curve relating wages to the quantity of labor supplied shifts down by the full amount of the mandated benefits ($2 in this case). The third supply curve ($S_{v<b}$) is for the intermediate situation, where the workers place some value on the benefits but less than the $2 that they cost the employer. Initially, without the mandated benefits, the market equilibrium is at a wage of $8 and a quantity of 300 workers employed. When mandated benefits are instituted, the new equilibrium position will depend on the value placed on the benefits by the workers. With full valuation, the new equilibrium will occur where wages fall by $2, but there will be no change in employment. However, if the benefits are not valued at all, then wages will fall (to $7 in this case) and employment will be reduced. If some value (less than $2) is placed on the benefits by the workers, there will be an intermediate result.

---

effects to those that might be posited without a more formal economic analysis, but this is only the case because the supply curve of labor is in reality close to vertical (zero elasticity) in the relevant ranges.

13.3.2 Taxation

Much health care is publicly funded, and much of the funding comes through taxation. However configured, taxes can be regarded as reductions in income or wealth without any attached benefits. While it is true that benefits may come as a result of the use of funds, under taxation these benefits are not directly linked to the taxes. Only full-scale economic analyses using heroic assumptions can link the benefits resulting from the spending of taxes to the costs of the taxes themselves.

Taxation can be direct or indirect. Direct taxes are those that are directly levied on income. They cannot, therefore, be shifted (i.e., the burden cannot be made to fall on someone other than the taxpayer). Indirect taxes on goods and services can be shifted (in essence, avoided) to some degree. Economic analysis is useful in determining the economic impact and burden of taxation. Below we will analyze the burden of two types of taxes commonly used to finance health care: payroll taxes and sales taxes.

13.3.2.1 Payroll Taxes

A payroll tax is a tax that is levied on wages. Medicare uses a payroll (social security) tax of 1.6 percent of total payroll (payable by both the employer and employee) to finance the hospital portion of Medicare. The burden of an employee-paid payroll tax is quite clear: it is paid by the worker. However, because it lowers take-home wages, some workers may decide not to supply labor. Employment will therefore fall. The burden is thus equally shared among workers. The economic effects resulting from the imposition of a payroll tax that is paid by employers is less clear and deserves closer attention.

In Figure 13–3 we introduce the analysis of the effect of a payroll tax on labor and wages. Initially we have a competitive labor market with a given supply of labor (S) and a given demand for labor (D_1). Our output measure is labor hours, and equilibrium in this market occurs with a wage rate of $40 per unit and a quantity of 300 labor hours. Note that we have drawn a very steep supply curve for labor; this indicates that workers will not change their work habits very much when wages increase or decrease. A vertical curve would indicate that they would not change their habits at all. We now introduce an employer-paid payroll tax of 100 percent of wages.

If the employers are in a competitive industry, they cannot raise the price of their output, and so their demand-for-labor curve cannot be increased through higher prices. The employers therefore would have to either absorb the tax themselves or lower wages. At first blush, we might be inclined to say that wages would stay at $40, taxes of $40 would be paid, and employment would remain the same. This is a very unlikely outcome given the forces behind the employment for labor. In Figure 13–3 we present an economic analysis of what will happen.

The effect of this tax is to shift down the demand-for-labor curve, which is based on the marginal revenue of the product that labor produces. At a wage of $20, each employer must pay a tax of $20 (which is 100 percent of the wage). Each worker costs twice as much to the firm. Therefore, whereas the employers formerly demanded 300 labor hours when the wage was $40, they will demand 300 hours of labor at a wage of $20. Note also that because the tax is expressed as a percentage of wages, the new demand-for-labor curve (in terms of wages) is a fixed percentage

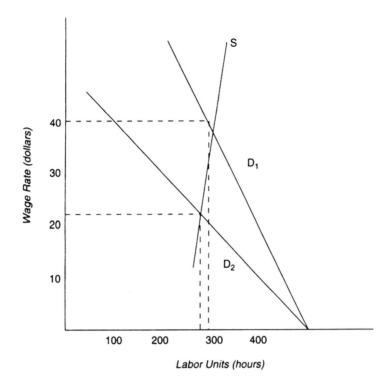

Figure 13–3 The effect of imposing an employer-paid payroll tax. Initially, the demand for labor without a payroll tax is shown in terms of wages. With the given supply curve for labor, equilibrium occurs with a wage of $40 and a quantity of employment of 300 work hours. The effect of a payroll tax of 100 percent of wages is to shift the demand curve in terms of wages down by 50 percent. For example, at a wage rate of $20, the employers pay a tax of $20, for a total payout of $40, and thus the demand with the tax is the same as it would be if the wage was 100 percent higher but there was no tax. The new equilibrium will be determined by the intersection of supply and demand for labor. In this case, the supply curve is almost vertical. There will be very little reduction in employment and an almost 50 percent reduction in wages.

lower than the old one. The higher the wage, the greater the discrepancy between the old and new curves.

With the employers' demand-for-labor curve (in terms of wages) shifting downward, employees will receive lower wages. The equilibrium volume of labor and the corresponding wage rate are just under 300 hours and just over $22. This means that the quantity of labor will hardly have changed but the wage rate will have fallen by almost the full amount of the tax. The workers have not substituted away from working and have borne almost the entire burden of the tax through a reduction in their wage rate. In this case, the supply-of-labor curve is almost vertical, and workers would rather accept lower wages than lose employment. Other situations are possible. For example, if workers were very sensitive to their wage rates and the supply-of-labor curve was close to horizontal, the labor supply would fall when wages fell. In this instance, the workers would avoid the tax entirely by refusing to work at lower wages. At the new wage, the tax would have been shifted to the employers, who also would hire fewer workers.

The effect of the payroll tax, then, will be to reduce employment and wages. How much of the tax will be borne by the workers (through a decrease in wages) will depend on how much they are willing to adjust their wages and their work—information summarized by the supply-of-labor curve.

13.3.2.2 Sales Taxes

A very similar analysis applies to sales taxes. A sales tax is a tax on a product or service. Most states use sales taxes as a major source of revenue. Sales taxes can be general (on all items), modified general (on most items except, e.g., food and children's clothes), and specific (on gasoline, alcohol, tobacco products, health insurance premiums, etc.). In the case of tobacco and alcohol, these taxes may affect consumer behavior with regard to drinking and smoking and thus health status (and health care demand). Certainly this was the rationale for a large tobacco tax that the state of Maine imposed in order to pay for more publicly funded health care benefits in the 1980s.

In order to analyze the effects of sales taxes, we will use the example of a sales tax on prescription drugs. The initial situation, without the sales tax, is shown in Figure 13–4. There is a demand for the drugs, as is shown by the demand curve (D). This is the demand of the consumers of the drugs. And there is also a curve for the supply without the sales tax (S_1). In a competitive market, equilibrium will occur at a price of $4 and a quantity of 200 prescriptions filled.

Let us now impose a sales tax of $2 on each prescription, to be paid by the pharmacists. We might initially imagine that the pharmacists will simply raise the price of each prescription to $6 and collect the tax on each of the 200 prescriptions. But this would occur only if the demand curve for prescriptions was vertical and consumers would demand their prescriptions at any price. This is not a realistic scenario in the case of drugs or most other commodities. There is an elasticity of demand for drugs, as indicated by the downward-sloping demand curve.

The tax will cause the prices charged by the pharmacists to increase (if they pay the tax), and they might at first charge $6 for each prescription (though they would receive $4, as before). But there is a limit to what consumers will pay. In our case, some consumers will refuse to fill their prescriptions, thus avoiding the tax entirely. A new equilibrium will be set at $5, and only 150 prescriptions will be filled. The pharmacists will only receive $3 for each prescription and will supply less (150 at the net-of-tax price of $3).

The market will have shifted part of the tax onto the pharmacists, who now pay one-half of it by receiving a lower price. The consumers end up paying $1 of the prescription tax by reducing the quantity they demand. The burden of the sales tax will thus be shared. We should point out that there are other possible outcomes, depending on the slopes of the supply and demand curves. However, it is not likely that all of the tax will be borne by the consumers.

As pointed out above, sales taxes on a variety of products related to health are very common. Many states impose a tax on health insurance premiums. Such a tax will have an effect on the number of individuals who shift their risks to an insurer, and it can be analyzed using the sales tax model.

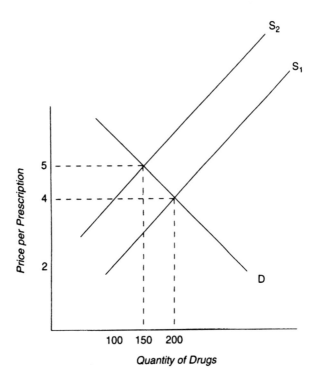

Figure 13–4 Effect of a sales tax. The supply and demand for prescriptions are shown above. Equilibrium without the sales tax is where the price is $4 and the quantity of prescriptions is 200 (where S_1 and D intersect). If a sales tax of $2 per prescription is imposed, to be paid by suppliers, the suppliers' costs will increase by exactly $2, as will the supply curve (S_2). The new equilibrium will take into account the demand elasticity. In the above case, the price will increase by $1 and the quantity sold will be reduced to 150 prescriptions. The consumers will, in effect, have shifted some of the tax onto the suppliers by reducing their demands.

13.4 THE INCIDENCE OF ALTERNATIVE TYPES OF HEALTH CARE FINANCING

In this section we turn our attention to the incidence of alternative types of health care financing. The term *incidence* does not have a precise meaning. We use the term to denote the pattern of distribution of burdens of various financing methods (Due 1957). We will focus on one key characteristic of individuals—their level of income—and four different types of financing: insurance premiums, income taxes, sales taxes, and payroll taxes. Our analysis, though highly simplified, is intended to provide a basic understanding of the major issues.

We assume that there are four income groups each with 100 families (see Table 13–2). Each family in the lowest income group has earnings of $10,000; in the next lowest group, of $20,000; in the next group, of $30,000; and in the highest income group, of $40,000.

Each family incurs health care expenditures of $2,500. There are no differences in health care usage by income level. However, all expenditures are financed, and the out-of-pocket cost is zero. Total medical expenses for all groups equal $1,000,000.

Table 13–2 Income and Expenditures for Four Income Groups

Income Group	Earnings per Family	Number of Families	Total Income	Total Consumption Expenditures	Health Care Expenditures per Family	Total Health Care Expenditures
A	$10,000	100	$1,000,000	$1,000,000	$2,500	$ 250,000
B	20,000	100	2,000,000	1,800,000	2,500	250,000
C	30,000	100	3,000,000	2,400,000	2,500	250,000
D	40,000	100	4,000,000	2,800,000	2,500	250,000
Total		400	10,000,000	8,000,000		1,000,000

Each family's total consumption of commodities, including food but not medical care, is given in Column 5 of Table 13–2. The lowest income group spends all it earns on commodities, the next group spends 90 percent, the third group spends 80 percent, and the highest income group spends 70 percent. What the members of a group do not spend, they save. If they have to pay for medical care, they will reduce other expenditures but will not reduce their savings. If they do pay for medical care itself, it will be through the purchase of insurance.

The financing problem is how to pay for the $1,000,000 in medical care expenses. There are four options: insurance premiums, a sales tax, a payroll tax, and an income tax. Our task is to determine the incidence of each type of financing on the different income groups. The conclusions we will reach are summarized in Figure 13–5.

Premiums. Each family bears the same risk of health expenses, and so it would seem reasonable to charge every family the same premium rate. There are 400 families, and $1 million in health care funds must be raised. Therefore, each family will pay a premium of $2,500.

The burden of the financing method on each family is the premium divided by family income. This would be 25 percent for the lowest income families, 12.5 percent for the families earning $20,000, 8.3 percent for the families earning $30,000, and 6.25 percent for the highest income families. The incidence of premiums is such that the burden decreases steadily as income increases.

Payroll Taxes. In the case of a payroll tax, a fixed percentage of wages is charged, but there is usually a cap above which income is not taxed. We will assume that this cap is $30,000. This means that all wages up to $30,000 are taxed. The members of the highest income group, those earning $40,000, will only pay taxes on the first $30,000 of their wages. Total taxable wages are $9,000,000 for all families. In order to raise the required $1,000,000, a tax rate of 13.1 percent must be levied on all wages below $30,000.

The burden of the tax will be the same for the three groups whose members have incomes at or below $30,000. However, the highest income group only pays $3,330 in payroll taxes per family, for an effective tax rate of 8.325 percent. As shown in Figure 13–5, the burden of the payroll tax is the same for the three lowest groups but falls somewhat for the highest income group.

Sales Taxes. Sales taxes can be imposed on any of a variety of consumption expenditures. We will assume that sales taxes are imposed on all consumption expenditures except medical care expenditures. Total consumption expenditures for all families equal $8,000,000. In order to raise the required $1,000,000 in funds, the overall sales tax rate must be 12.5 percent ($1,000,000/8,000,000). The lowest income group pays $125,000 on its $1,000,000 in expenditures; the next group pays $225,000; the next group, $300,000; and the highest income group pays $350,000.

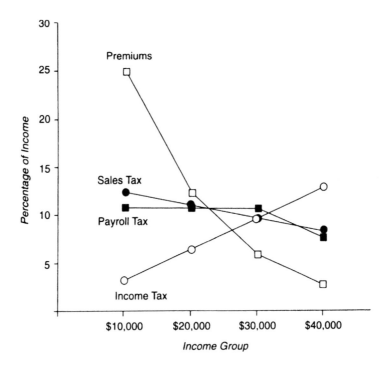

Figure 13–5 Incidence of financing methods. Premiums are the most regressive source of finance, income tax is the most progressive, and sales and payroll taxes fall in between.

The effective tax rate, or burden, for these groups is 12.5 percent, 11.25 percent, 10 percent, and 8.75 percent of income, respectively. The incidence is such that the burden continually falls as income rises. Of course, if certain "necessities" such as food were excluded from the sales tax, this pattern might change.

Income Taxation. The burden of the income tax will depend on the actual tax rates, and these are subject to policy decisions by Congress. We will assume the tax rates are such that the highest income class pays roughly four times the rate of the lowest group. This is very roughly the ratio in the United States today. Specifically, we assume that, given an average overall rate, the lowest group will pay 40 percent of this rate (i.e., 0.4), the second group will pay 80 percent of the rate, the third highest group will pay 120 percent of the rate, and the highest group will pay 160 percent of the rate. Let *x* stand for the overall tax rate. The overall rate can be determined by solving for *x* in this equation:

$$.4(1,000,000)x + .8(2,000,000)x + 1.2(3,000,000)x + 1.6(4,000,000)x = 1,000,000$$

The $1,000,000 is the amount to be collected by the income tax. If we solve for *x*, we will find the average overall rate is 8.33 percent. Based on the ratios determined by "policy," the four groups pay 3.33 percent, 6.64 percent, 9.99 percent, and 13.33 percent of income in income taxes, respectively.

The overall incidence of the funding methods can be compared. Premiums are the most "regressive" and income taxes are the most "progressive." The other two methods fall in between (under our assumptions, they are mildly regressive).

Omitted from our analysis are out-of-pocket expenditures. The use of this type of financing will result in lower overall usage (because of the downward-sloping demand curve for medical care). Thus, if families had to pay out of pocket for health care, total expenditures would likely fall below $1 million. The overall burden would depend on the response of each income group.

Our assessment of financing options will depend on our policy goals. Much of the focus in evaluating types of financing is on considerations of equity. However, efficiency issues need to be addressed as well.

13.5 THE ADMINISTRATIVE COST OF ALTERNATIVE TYPES OF HEALTH CARE FINANCING

There has been a lively debate in recent years about administrative costs associated with the health care financing system in the United States. Much of the debate has been focused on the costs associated with the marketing of health insurance and hospital services, the monitoring of utilization and the regulating of payment by insurers, the billing of third parties by providers, and the collecting of deductibles and copayments from patients by providers. Because of the complexity of the U.S. system of health care finance, more resources are devoted to these functions than in other health care systems, such as those of Canada and the United Kingdom. A study conducted using 1987 data estimated that between $96 billion and $120 billion were spent on administration in the United States, out of a total spent of $488 billion for all health care–related services (Woolhandler and Himmelstein 1991). This study primarily added up the money costs of these functions.

This debate has served to highlight the fact that a health care financing system requires resources and that different systems have different costs. The Canadian system, for example, has lower administrative costs than does the U.S. system. However, the amount of administrative costs is not the only factor that needs to be taken into account when choosing a national health care "system."

Marketing functions serve to inform potential customers about the characteristics of various health plans. Consumers can better select among health plans if they have more information. Regulation and payment functions serve to help ensure that the care that is provided is of a high quality and results in good outcomes. Although these functions are not always completely effective, nevertheless, when we evaluate a financing system, we must look at the benefits of the various financing practices in addition to their costs.

EXERCISES

1. What proportion of total health expenses are made by out-of-pocket, government, and health insurance sources of finance?
2. An employee is worth $100 a week to her employer. The worker demands $20 in health insurance benefits, to be paid by the employer. What would the employer be willing to pay in terms of wages?
3. What is the effect on the market for health insurance of a government tax subsidy on health insurance premiums?

4. What will be the effect of mandated health insurance benefits on the market for labor if the workers do not place any value on these benefits? If they fully value the benefits?
5. What is a payroll tax? How will the imposition of a payroll tax affect the wage rate and the quantity of labor employed?
6. How will the imposition of a sales tax on a commodity affect the price and quantity sold of that commodity? Will the consumer usually bear the entire burden of the tax?
7. How do each of the following methods of financing the health care system impact on persons according to their income group?
   a. income tax
   b. sales tax
   c. payroll tax
   d. insurance premiums

BIBLIOGRAPHY

The Burden of Insurance

Cutler, D.M. 1995. The cost and financing of health care. *American Economic Review* 85 (suppl.): 32–37.

Gruber, J., and A.B. Krueger. 1991. The incidence of mandated employer-provided insurance: Lessons from workers' compensation insurance. In *Tax policy and the economy*, ed. D. Bradford. Cambridge, MA: National Bureau of Economic Research.

Kreuger, A., and U.E. Reinhardt. 1994. Economics of employer versus individual mandates. *Health Affairs* 13:34–54.

Mitchell, B.M., and C.E. Phelps. 1976. National health insurance: Some costs and effects of mandated employee coverage. *Journal of Political Economy* 84:553–571.

Summers, L.H. 1989. Some simple economics of mandated benefits. *American Economic Review* 79:177–183.

Wilensky, G.R., and A.K. Taylor. 1982. Tax expenditures and health insurance: Limiting employer-paid premiums. *Public Health Reports* 97:438–444.

The Burden of Taxation

Aaron, H.J. 1994. Tax issues in health care reform. *National Tax Journal* 47:407–416.

Brandon, W.P. 1982. Health-related tax subsidies. *New England Journal of Medicine* 302: 947–950.

Browning, E.K., and W.R. Johnson. Taxation and the cost of national health insurance. In *National health insurance*, ed. M.V. Pauly. Washington, DC: American Enterprise Institute.

Burman, L.E., and R. Williams. 1994. Tax caps on employment based health insurance. *National Tax Journal* 47:529.

Due, J.F. 1957. *Sales taxation*. London: Routledge and Kegan Paul.

Feldstein, M., et al. 1972. Distributional aspects of national health insurance benefits and finance. *National Tax Journal* 25:497–510.

Gruber, J., and M. Hanratty. 1995. The labor-market effects of introducing national health insurance: Evidence from Canada. *Journal of Business and Economic Statistics* 13:163–173.

Marquis, M.S., and J.L. Buchanan. 1994. How will changes in health insurance tax policy and employer health plan contributions affect access to health care and health care costs? *JAMA* 271:939–944.

Administrative Costs

Himmelstein, D.U., and S. Woolhandler. 1986. Cost without benefit: Administrative waste in U.S. health care. *New England Journal of Medicine* 314:441–445.

Himmelstein, D.U., et al. 1996. Who administers? Who cares? Medical administrative and clinical employment in the United States and Canada. *American Journal of Public Health* 69:172–178.

Woolhandler, S., and D.U. Himmelstein. 1991. The deteriorating administrative efficiency of the U.S. healthcare system. *New England Journal of Medicine* 324:1253–1258.

Chapter 14

Public Health Insurance

1. Identify the key policy goals of public health insurance plans.
2. Describe the Medicare and Medicaid programs in terms of populations covered, services included, financing arrangements, reimbursement strategies, and pro-competition policies.
3. Explain some of the key issues surrounding public health insurance.
4. Outline the goals of the Medicare program in the United States.
5. Identify the key types of policies required for the delivery of a public health insurance program and indicate their effect on the achievement of social goals.

14.1 INTRODUCTION

In this chapter, we use an economic framework to analyze selected aspects of public health insurance coverage in the United States. Health insurance is a key element of the health care system, and public policies related to insurance influence the functioning of the health care market. In this chapter, we show how the economic framework can be used to analyze policy choices, discuss policy goals in relation to the economic framework, and assess policy choices in terms of the social objectives.

In Section 14.2 we present an overview of public health insurance in the United States, focusing on Medicare and Medicaid, the two major national public health insurance plans. In Section 14.3 we discuss the issue of health insurance coverage. In Section 14.4 we present some information on trends in public health insurance. In Section 14.5 we discuss the social goals of Medicare. In Section 14.6 we describe some of the solutions proposed in recent years and explain how each solution contributes to or obstructs the achievement of specific health policy goals. In Section 14.7 we consider alternatives to Medicaid.

14.2 PUBLIC HEALTH INSURANCE

Public health insurance in the United States involves two key programs aimed at target populations. These are the Medicare and Medicaid programs. Some states also have additional public health insurance programs. Often these additional programs will be tied in some way to Medicaid, but in some circumstances they are not. In this chapter we focus on Medicare and Medicaid.

14.2.1 Medicare

14.2.1.1 Who Is Covered

Prior to 1966, there were a variety of health insurance programs oriented toward the retired and aged populations. However, coverage was thin (Aaron 1995) and there were many gaps. To fill these gaps, the Medicare program was instituted with the passage of Title XVIII of the Social Security Act, entitled "Health Insurance for the Aged." Medicare began operation on July 1, 1966. Under Medicare, insurance coverage is extended to individuals 65 and over who are eligible for Social Security benefits, disabled individuals, and persons who have end-stage renal disease. We will focus mainly on the coverage of individuals who are 65 and over. The Medicare program is administered by the Health Care Financing Administration, an agency of the U.S. Department of Health and Human Services.

14.2.1.2 What Is Covered?

Coverage for these individuals is in two parts. Under Part A, also known as hospital insurance (HI), hospitalization and limited (primarily post–acute care) skilled nursing facility (SNF) coverage are provided. Medicare Part A covers 90 days of hospitalization per benefit period (a benefit period is defined by the existence of a preceding specified time during which the enrollee was not a bed patient in a hospital or an SNF); in addition, each enrollee has a lifetime reserve of 60 days. Under Part B, supplementary medical insurance (SMI) is provided; coverage includes ambulatory (noninstitutional) services and supplies, such as physician services, radiology and lab services, drugs, and medical supplies. A listing of what services are and are not covered under Medicare is shown in Exhibit 14–1. We should note that prescription drugs and *long-term* nursing home care are not covered in either parts A or B.

14.2.1.3 Financing Medicare

The basic Medicare plan operates on a fee-for-service basis. Program enrollees pay no premium for Part A; however, there is a deductible tied to the per diem cost of care, which has been rising in recent years. In 2000, it was $776. After the deductible is met, there are no copayments for the next 60 days, and then there is a copayment of $194 per day for days 61 through 90. The public share of HI (exclusive of the deductibles and copayments) is financed primarily through a Social Security tax on worker payrolls. Proceeds from this tax go into a fund called the Hospital Insurance Trust Fund, out of which hospitals and nursing homes are reimbursed. In 2000, this tax amounted to 1.45 percent of the payroll payable by both the employer and employee (2.90 percent in total). The base amount on which this tax is assessed has been increased considerably in recent years. It would be politically unpopular for Congress to change this rate.

Exhibit 14–1 Service Coverage under Medicare Program

Covered under Part A
  Inpatient hospital care
  Skilled nursing facility care
  Postinstitutional home care
  Hospice care
Covered under Part B
  Physician services
  Outpatient hospital care
  Ambulatory surgery
  Clinical diagnostic laboratory services
  Outpatient mental health services
  Home care other than postinstitutional
  Durable medical equipment
  Preventive services (selected screening exams, flu and pneumonia vaccines, diabetes monitoring and education.)
Not covered
  Outpatient pharmaceuticals
  Long-term nursing home care

Source: Reprinted from *Medicare Chart Book*, 2000, Health Care Financing Administration.

The Part B, SMI, program is voluntary; if enrollees choose to participate, they can buy in by paying a premium. The SMI premium was initially set so that the premium covered one-half of the expenditures of the SMI trust fund (out of which providers are reimbursed). Premiums ($45.50 per month in 2000) are tied to Social Security cash benefits The remainder of the SMI fund income comes from general revenues (i.e., public expenditures). In 1966, the first year of Medicare, the SMI premium covered half of all the revenues of the program; by 2000, the share of premiums had fallen to 25 percent, with the remainder of funds coming from general taxation. An enrollee in the SMI program receives benefits subject to an annual deductible (first $100 of reasonable charges in 2000) and a copayment of 20 percent of reasonable charges.

14.2.1.4 Managed Care

Medicare beneficiaries have the option of enrolling in a Medicare managed care plan or a private fee-for-service plan. The enrollee would then pay a monthly premium comprising at least the Part B premium ($45.50 per month in 2000); the managed care plan may charge an additional amount as a premium (usually $50 to $75 per month), so that the total premium might be more than that under Medicare Part B. The managed care plan may also impose copayments on outpatient care (typically $5 to $15 per visit). The plan must cover all deductibles and copayments under Medicare Part A. It must cover all of the services covered by Medicare Parts A and B, but it may also cover other services as well, notably outpatient pharmaceuticals. If the patient is enrolled in a managed care plan, then he or she will be restricted as to his or her choice of providers, including specialists and hospitals. Under point-of-service plans, the enrollee may be given the choice of provider, but he or she would have to pay an additional amount for selecting a nonpreferred provider.

Medicare reimburses the HMO on a per capita basis. A single payment covers all the services listed in Exhibit 14–1. A risk adjustment is made that covers the expected costs incurred by the plan members. Until 1997, payments to the HMO plan were based on the adjusted average per capita cost for fee-for-service enrollees. A different rate was set for each county based on the cost experience of persons in that county. There was a wide variation in capitation rates between counties; in many counties, no coverage was offered at all because the rates were set at a low level. Overall, however, the proportion of Medicare enrollees seeking services from managed care plans has increased considerably since 1993. In 1992, 13 percent of all Medicare enrollees were members of Medicare Risk (HMO) plans; by 1996, this proportion had increased to 33 percent (Health Care Financing Administration 1998). In 1997, the provisions for prepaid Medicare contracts were changed, and new arrangements were set up; these were introduced under a new Part C of Title XVIII of the Social Security Amendments. Under the new rules, the payment rates were made more uniform nationally. These rules are discussed in section 14.2.4.

14.2.2 Medicaid

14.2.2.1 Who Is Covered?

The Medicaid program, originally designed to finance medical care for low-income families who were recipients of financial assistance, was introduced in 1966 under Title XIX of the Social Security Act . Unlike the Medicare program, which is operated under guidelines set by the Social Security Administration, the Medicaid program is a state-federal partnership. Although the form of the program is determined by the federal government, state governments individually decide whether to participate in the program and determine the extent of the program. Who is covered largely depends on criteria established by individual states. In recent years federal guidelines have become more flexible, in part to allow states to impose coverage restrictions.

Individuals covered under the joint federal-state program fall into four groups: (1) cash recipients of the Aid to Families with Dependent Children (AFDC) program (dependent children and adults in AFDC families); (2) cash recipients of Supplemental Security Income (SSI) (aged, blind, and disabled individuals); (3) children and pregnant women in low-income families (i.e., up to 185 percent of the poverty line) who do not receive AFDC; and (4) the "medically needy," many of whom would not qualify on an income basis but who have spent enough on medical care that their incomes net of medical care expenses fall below specific levels. The distribution of total coverage in 1998 was as follows: children, 48%; low-income adults, 23%; individuals over age 65, 19%; blind and disabled individuals, 11%. In this exposition, we will concentrate primarily on the covered population over 65, which falls into categories 2 and 4.

Certain individuals can be eligible for both Medicare (on the basis of age) and Medicaid (on the basis of income and wealth level). For these individuals, Medicaid can "buy into" SMI, paying the SMI premium as well as deductibles and copayments. These enrollees will then be covered by Medicare for SMI and HI benefits and by Medicaid for other benefits, such as skilled nursing care and Medicare copayments and deductibles.

14.2.2.2 *What Is Covered?*

A list of services that must be covered and that optionally may be covered (at the discretion of the state plan) is shown in Exhibit 14–2. Federally required benefits under Medicaid include physician services, inpatient and outpatient hospital services, lab services, and nursing home services in skilled nursing homes. States can put limitations on benefits, such as on the number of inpatient days covered, authorization requirements for specific medical procedures, and so on. In addition, states can provide optional services such as intermediate care facility (ICF) stays, dental care, physiotherapy and, most notably, outpatient prescription drugs.

The financing of Medicaid is based on a formula that incorporates state and national income levels. The minimum federal contribution is 50 percent. The state receiving the highest federal share (Mississippi) receives about 79 percent of its approved program costs from federal funds. Medicaid funds come out of general taxation revenues. Medicaid was originally designed as an open-ended program; that is, the federal share would follow the state share, with no explicit limitations. In recent years, a number of alterations have been proposed that would, in effect, cap the federal contribution. The state's contribution comes out of the state's general revenue funds.

14.2.3 Medigap Insurance for Medicare

The premiums, deductibles, and copayments under Medicare are quite substantial (see below). Indeed most persons under Medicare have some supplementary source of coverage as well as coverage under the basic Medicare plan. In Figure 14–1 we show the proportion of individuals who are covered by Medicare and have supplemental coverage (American Association of Retired Persons 1999). Seven percent have coverage only with the Medicare plan. Another 16 percent who are enrolled in HMO Medicare plans receive additional benefits from their plans. About

---

Exhibit 14–2 Services Covered under Medicaid

Mandatory coverage
  Inpatient hospital services
  Outpatient hospital services
  Rural health clinic services
  Diagnostic services (laboratory and radiology)
  Nurse practitioner services
  Nursing home care
  Home care
  Early screening
  Family planning
  Physician services
  Nurse midwife services
Selected optional services
  Outpatient prescription drugs
  Nonphysician professional services
  Screening and preventive services
  Dental services

Source: Reprinted from *Medicare Chart Book*, 2000, Health Care Financing Administration.

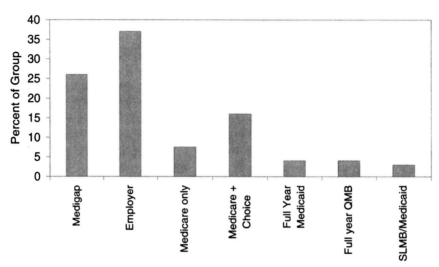

Figure 14–1 Supplemental coverage of Medicaid beneficiaries. Medicare beneficiaries often have supplementary coverage in addition to their Medicare coverage. The most common is through employer benefits for retirees and those working who are Medicare eligible. Over 35 percent of Medicare enrollees have such coverage. Other common forms of coverage are also shown in this diagram. *Source:* From D. Gross and N. Brangan, Out-of-pocket Spending on Healthcare Beneficiaries Age 65 and Older, *AARP Policy Institute Report,* © 1999, AARP. Reprinted with permission.

10 percent receive additional federal coverage, either under Medicaid or from special programs that cover low-income individuals who do not fully qualify for Medicaid additional coverage. About one-third receive some form of benefit through their private retirement plans. Finally, there is an active private market for supplementary insurance to cover the deductibles and copayments of beneficiaries in fee-for-service plans. Over 25 percent of Medicare beneficiaries participate in this market. Enrollees in the SMI program can pay premiums to private insurers for this supplementary "Medigap" coverage. The private insurers then reimburse the providers for the beneficiaries' share of their costs (i.e., the deductibles and copayments). The Medigap insurance market is an extremely active one.

14.2.4 Paying the Providers

14.2.4.1 Fee-for-Service

As stated above, there are two generic types of health care coverage under Medicare: fee-for-service and per capita payment. In the fee-for-service plan the Medicare program sets prices for individual patient contacts. Medicare has developed systems for classifying services for most types of care; these systems now include inpatient hospitalization, outpatient care, home care, and skilled nursing facility care. As shown in Chapter 7, any classification system can divide cases into groups of patients or visits; the patients within each group are assumed to use an equal amount of resources. Each group is assigned *a relative weight,* and a dollar value is assigned to a weighted unit. Medicare adjusts the monetary prices for a variety of factors, including whether the provider is in an urban or rural area, area wage and cost-of-living levels, and provider characteristics (e.g., teaching versus nonteaching units). The result is a complex array of prices.

Inpatient hospital care is funded by the DRG system, first instituted in 1983. There are over 500 different DRGs, each with a basic weight. The weight for a given case will be adjusted if the patient's stay is unusually long (i.e., the patient is an outlier). Overall, however, the sum total of all weighted cases must remain the same so that budget neutrality is achieved. The dollar value per weighted case for fiscal year 2000 was $4,028 for hospitals in large urban areas and $3,963 for hospitals in other areas (*Federal Register* 65, no. 148, August 1, 2000, p. 47126). Adjustments to wage and capital cost levels are made, and indirect medical education costs for teaching hospitals are added.

A recent addition to the Medicare payment system is a prospective payment system for postacute home care. A classification system was developed that is based on the patient's diagnosis and on therapeutic needs (physical, speech-language pathology, and occupational) (Liu et al. 1999). As with inpatient care, a weight is assigned to each group in the class, and a price per weighted unit is set. The Medicare home care payment system replaced a system by which home care providers billed for individual services. It thus represents a bundling of services, in comparison with the payment system prior to 1999, when the prospective payment system was introduced.

Unlike hospital and home care reimbursement, the payment for physicians under Medicare remains on an individual service basis. Physicians are paid by fee category, called *Current Procedural Terminology (CPT)*. Each service is assigned a weight; currently the weighting system is called the *Resource Based Relative Value System (RBRVS)*. The RBRVS contains separate component weights that are supposed to reflect work performed, practice expenses, liability insurance, and regional cost variations. A dollar value is assigned by Medicare that converts the resource-based weights to dollar payments. In 2000, this conversion figure was $36.6137. For example, a routine office visit in Chicago has a relative value of 1.375 units; using the conversion fee listed above, the practitioner would receive $50.33 (American Medical Association 2000).

14.2.4.2 Managed Care

Until 1998, the overall level of payment for a risk (HMO) contract was 95 percent of the fee-for-service level of expenditures in any single county. Beginning in 1998, a blended rate, reflecting local and national costs, was set, subject to a minimum amount per enrollee. In 2000, a risk-adjustment model, called the *Principal Inpatient Diagnostic Cost Group (PIP-DCG)*, was introduced. According to this risk-adjustment model, patients who had been hospitalized in the prior year for specific diagnoses were projected to have higher total costs and thus were entitled to a higher payment (see the Web site www.hcfa.gov/stats/hmorates/45d1999/45d-02.htm). This payment change was made to encourage HMOs to enroll persons with poorer health status and to encourage HMOs to operate in lower cost areas.

14.3 UNCOVERED CARE

Despite the existence of Medicare and Medicaid, many individuals either have no health insurance coverage at all or have large gaps in coverage. According to estimates by the U.S. Bureau of the Census, 16.3 percent of all individuals (about 44.3 million) had no insurance coverage in 1998 (U.S. Bureau of the Census 1999).

A substantial number of this group were young or healthy, but the group included many who were in fair or poor health and also 11 million children (Short et al. 1988; U.S. Bureau of the Census 1999). Further, 24 million of the noncovered individuals were employed, which poses a problem because employment is the usual route through which health insurance is obtained (Monheit and Short 1989).

It should be pointed out that *uninsured* is not the same thing as *unserved*. Many individuals with no insurance still receive medical care: they either pay the full price for this care or receive subsidized or charity care. What is likely, however, is that they receive less care than they would if they had insurance coverage.

In addition to those with no coverage, a substantial number of individuals have gaps in coverage. The Medicare deductibles and copayments can add up to a large amount, and individuals who are covered by Medicare but do not have additional private (Medigap) or Medicaid coverage can, if they become ill, incur substantial out-of-pocket costs, including individuals who need nursing home care. There is very little in the way of long-term care insurance coverage at present, and so individuals in nursing homes (especially intermediate care facilities) will be required to pay for such care themselves unless they "spend down" to the point where both their income less medical expenses and their assets are below the state Medicaid limits.

Lack of coverage has also surfaced as a major policy issue in the area of inpatient hospital care. The burden of treating indigent patients has not fallen evenly on hospitals. Teaching hospitals, public hospitals, and hospitals that partially specialize in certain product lines (e.g., obstetrics) provide larger portions of charity care and have higher rates of bad debt (Mulstein 1984).

14.4 SOME TRENDS IN PUBLIC HEALTH INSURANCE

In recent years, several public insurance trends have captured interest in the public policy arena. In this section we will briefly review these.

14.4.1 Disbursements of the Hospital Insurance Trust Fund

Medicare's HI funding is tied to the growth of the portion of the Social Security tax that is earmarked for the Hospital Insurance Trust Fund. However, there is no automatic link between the growth of trust fund revenues and the growth of fund expenditures, which primarily go to reimburse hospitals (Iglehart 1999; Wolkstein 1984). The revenues are based on a percentage of payrolls and so cannot be increased by more than the increase in payrolls unless the Social Security tax rate is increased or, as happened recently, the base on which the tax is levied is increased (i.e., employment and wages have increased). In the absence of such increases in tax revenues, large deficits in the fund had been experienced, and, until very recently, increasingly large deficits had been predicted.

In Figure 14–2, we show the annual income and expenditures of the trust fund from 1995 through 1998. Income from the fund had been increasing through 1997, but expenditures were increasing by more. The net result was a deficit that grew through 1997 and, until 1997, was predicted to continue into the future. As can be seen from the figure, there was a significant turnaround in outlays in fiscal year 1998, resulting in a surplus of over $7 billion. The fund's income, driven by rising

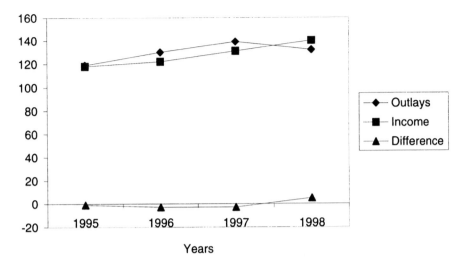

Figure 14–2 Income and outlays of the Medicare Hospital Insurance Trust Fund, 1995–1998. In this figure we show the income and outlays of the Medicare Hospital Insurance Trust Fund. Between 1995 and 1997 outlays exceeded income but due to regulatory changes in 1998, the fund achieved a surplus. *Source:* Reprinted from 2000 Annual Report of the Board of Trustees of the Federal Hospital Insurance and Supplementary Medical Insurance Trust Funds, Health Care Financing Administration.

income levels in the general population, continued to increase. Outlays actually declined in 1998, resulting in the surplus. Future surpluses were also projected. The reason for the budget surplus was the significant reduction in the rates for the payment of hospitals that resulted from the Balanced Budget Act of 1997.

14.4.2 Medicare's SMI Revenues and Expenditures

SMI funds come from two main sources: premiums paid directly by the enrollees (or by Medicaid for those qualifying for Medicaid coverage) and general revenue funds. Originally, the premium rate was set so that premium revenues of the SMI trust fund were one-half of all revenues. From 1973, the growth of premiums was mandated to be no greater than the growth of Social Security cash benefits. As a result, since then the premium share of total fund revenues has fallen to about 30 percent.

Reimbursements from the fund grew by about 23 percent annually from 1966 to 1994 (Health Care Financing Administration 1995). Since the number of enrollees grew by only about 2.2 percent during this period, most of this growth has been in expenditures per enrollee. As in the case of the Hospital Insurance Trust Fund, this growth in expenditures has been a major cause of concern. However, unlike Hospital Insurance Trust Fund outlays, Medical Insurance Trust Fund expenditures can be increased by government appropriations. In Figure 14–3 we show the income and outlays of the fund from 1995 through 1998. Although there was a deficit in 1995 in the fund, incomes were increased in subsequent years. As a result, there was a surplus in each of the following years.

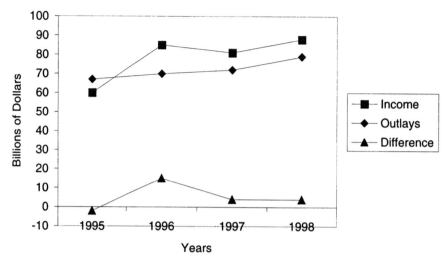

Figure 14–3 Income and outlays of the Medicare Medical Insurance Trust Fund, 1995–1998. This figure shows the income outlays of the Medicare Medical Insurance Fund. For the last three years shown, income consistently exceeded outlays. *Source:* Reprinted from 2000 Annual Report of the Board of Trustees of the Federal Hospital Insurance and Supplementary Medical Insurance Trust Funds, Health Care Financing Administration.

14.4.3 Out-of-Pocket Expenditures for Medicare Enrollees

Because of the Medicare premiums, deductibles, and copayments, Medicare enrollees incur considerable out-of-pocket expenses. Higher income Medicare enrollees seek private insurance options to cover the copayments and deductibles, while many enrollees maintain health insurance through their former employers beyond retirement. As shown in Figure 14–1, about two-thirds of all Medicare enrollees maintain these types of coverage. Some of the remainder have full or partial supplemental Medicaid coverage. However, about 7 percent have no additional coverage beyond Medicare.

The annual out-of-pocket spending of these groups is quite variable. A summary picture is presented in Figure 14–4. In this figure we show the out-of-pocket expenses for two expenditure categories: insurance premiums and out-of-pocket payment for health care services. The highest expenditures were incurred by those with Medigap coverage. These individuals incurred about $3,200 in costs, although, because they had a higher degree of coverage, out-of-pocket costs for services were low. Those with Medicare plus full Medicaid coverage incurred the lowest costs. Other groups shown in Figure 14–4 include those with limited Medicaid coverage. These include Qualified Medicare Beneficiaries (QMB) and Specified Low Income Medicare Beneficiaries (SLMB). Perhaps of greatest concern is the group of individuals who have Medicare coverage only. These individuals may not qualify for Medicaid coverage but may also not be able to afford supplementary coverage. On average, they incurred out-of-pocket expenses of $2,500 annually, of which $2,000 went for direct medical expenses. Individuals with Medicare + Choice, the federal Medicare managed care program, incurred expenses of slightly over $1,500, about one-half in direct expenses. One might be tempted to conclude that managed care is the most economical plan. However, these individuals may have self-selected into the managed care program and may be more healthy than those with fee-for-service coverage.

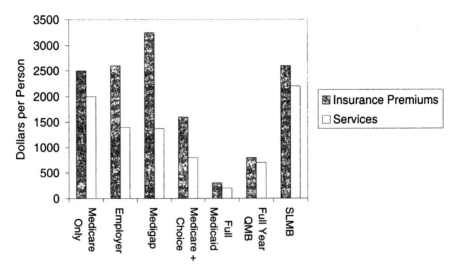

Figure 14–4 Average out-of-pocket spending by Medicare beneficiaries, by type of coverage, 1999. This figure shows both insurance premiums and direct spending for health care services. The highest spending rate was experienced by those with Medigap coverage and the lowest by those with Medicaid. *Source:* From D. Gross and N. Brangan, Out-of-pocket Spending on Healthcare by Medicare Beneficiaries Age 65 and Older, *AARP Policy Institute Report*, © 1999, AARP. Reprinted with permission.

A substantial portion of the out-of-pocket health care expenditures for the over 65 population goes for prescription drugs. Roughly 65 percent of the over 65 population in 1995 had some form of health insurance coverage for prescription drugs. Twenty-nine percent of the Medicare beneficiaries incurred out-of-pocket expenses for prescription drugs of $500 or greater (Gluck 1999). Statistics such as these have raised interest in extending the Medicare program to cover prescription drugs. Coverage problems are magnified for persons with specific conditions. For example, 20 percent of a sample of Medicare beneficiaries who lacked drug insurance and had hypertension did not use any antihypertensive medication. For those with coverage, out-of-pocket expenditures for such medications were still considerable (Blustein 2000).

14.5 GOALS OF MEDICARE

In order to discover what the policy issues are with Medicare, we need to assess the above facts in light of the social goals of Medicare. It was only recently that these goals were stated explicitly (Cutler 2000; U.S. Government Accounting Office 1999). Among these stated goals were affordability, equity, adequacy, feasibility, and acceptance. The definitions of these concepts given below are those of the U.S. Government Accounting Office (GAO), and they differ from the standard economic definitions. *Affordability* refers to the total costs incurred by the program. When stating this goal, the GAO is referring to the public component of the program and its burden on public spending. *Equity* refers to the burden of payments on specific groups. Individuals can be viewed as paying too much if they don't have any sufficient coverage or if their premiums are too high. Individuals can also be paying too little for premiums and copayments; with low direct costs, they would be using too much care (from a strict efficiency viewpoint). *Adequacy* refers to the availability of care. *Feasibility* refers to the ability of Medicare to actually implement changes in policy. *Acceptance* refers to the acceptability of the program to consumers, intermediaries, and providers.

These goals do bear some resemblance to those we presented in Chapter 12. In that chapter, we presented the following as very general economic goals of health policy: economic efficiency (which has demand, technical efficiency, and adequacy-of-supply aspects), equity in utilization and equity in payment, quality of care, and public expenditure control. The economic goal of public expenditure control translates into the GAO goal of affordability. The economic goal of equity of payment translates into the GAO goal of equity. The economic goals of equity in utilization and adequacy of supply translates into the GAO goal of adequacy. The economic goals of quality of care and technical efficiency are not directly addressed in the GAO goals, although quality assurance activities are a very important component of Medicare activities (Medicare Payment Advisory Commission 2000). The GAO goals of feasibility and acceptance are not directly addressed in the economic goals.

In order to assess Medicare policies, we must evaluate Medicare performance in light of the policy goals. As seen in the previous section, the major issues include rising expenditures, hospital trust fund deficits, and large out-of-pocket payments for some groups. These phenomena are related to the goals of affordability, equity of payment, and adequacy of supply. Most importantly, the goals may well conflict with each other (otherwise there would not be an economic problem). In the late 1990s, the Health Care Financing Administration (the agency that administers Medicare) and the Congress instituted a series of reforms designed to address the goal achievement balance under Medicare. The policy initiatives were Medicare Part C and the Balanced Budget Act of 1997. In the following section, we provide an overview of the policies that are available to Medicare.

14.6 POLICY ALTERNATIVES FOR MEDICARE

14.6.1 Economic Analysis and Alternative Solutions

We identify six basic types of policies than can be used to help achieve policy goals. The first set of policies deals with the setting of the broad outline of the program. For example, Medicare can change who is entitled to benefits or what benefits individuals receive. The second set of policies deals with health insurance premiums. Medicare can change Part B premiums, and it can change the out-of-pocket price of supplementary private insurance premiums. As well, Medicare can arrange for supplementary coverage in other programs, such as Medicaid. The third set deals with the direct price of care. Medicaid can change the deductibles and copayments paid by enrollees and in the process impact the demand for care (subject, of course, to the purchase of supplementary insurance). The fourth set deals with provider reimbursement. Medicare can change the basis of reimbursement. For example, home health care was formerly funded on the basis of individual services. Most recently, Medicare developed a home health care classification system that bundled individual services within diagnostic and needs-based groups. In addition to changing the definition of what output they will fund, Medicare can change the rate of payment. Fifth, Medicare can introduce competitive practices into its reimbursement mechanism. It can fund care on the basis of vouchers, encouraging individuals to shop around for their care. And sixth, Medicare can regulate the behavior of providers (i.e., make them provide care based on specific norms set by the program).

14.6.2 The Scope of the Program

Currently, Medicare's main line of business is to provide insurance coverage for persons over 65 years of age. In 1997, Congress set up the Medicare Commission to make recommendations about policies that could affect the future of Medicare. One of the policies recommended by the two committee chairs was to increase the age of Medicare beneficiaries to 67. This proposal did not achieve policy status, but it is an obvious way of changing the number of beneficiaries in the system. One proposal intended to extend the Medicaid mandate was to provide prescription drug insurance coverage (Davis et al. 1999; Soumerai and Ross-Degnan, 1999). Prescription drug coverage can be introduced with a wide variety of features, including additional premiums, copayments and deductibles, prescription limits, and so forth. Its inclusion would add a new dimension to the program, and administrative costs would increase considerably.

14.6.3 Insurance Premiums

Individuals and groups have proposed policies that would both increase and decrease health insurance premiums. Concern over the growth in first-dollar coverage has led some observers to propose a premium tax on Medigap policies. The introduction of such a tax would raise the price of Medigap coverage and reduce the amount of coverage purchased. The reduction in such coverage would lead to a reduction in the use of medical services in the short run.

There is only a premium for Part B Medicare. About one-quarter of Part B revenues come from this premium and the rest from general government revenues. The Balanced Budget Act of 1997, which overhauled Medicare's finances, did not substantially increase the premium; however, the premium is based on Social Security payments, and as such payments increase, so will the Part B premium. In 2000, the premium is $45.50 per month; by 2008, it should increase to $64.80 (McClellan 2000). An increase in the premium influences the goal of equity in payment.

14.6.4 Copayments and Deductibles

Copayments and deductibles serve to regulate demand for covered health care services and to reduce government revenues. Copayments are fixed as a percentage of medical charges, and they increase as charges rise. Copayments and deductibles are based on usage and are not always predictable. Individuals seek predictability by purchasing Medigap insurance coverage, which pays for the copayments and deductibles. The deductible in 2000 was $776 for Part A and $100 for Part B. There was also a 20 percent copayment for Part B. These payments have increased annually, but they have not been a major part of Medicare's cost-cutting plans. Higher copayments reduce availability.

14.6.5 Provider Payments

In 1983 Medicare began paying for inpatient hospitalization on a DRG basis. A price is applied to the DRG weighted units to obtain a given price per weighted unit, which is what the hospitals receive. Every year this price is increased by a given update factor in order to account for inflation and technological change. The update factor is supposed to cover changes in capital input prices, technology changes, and any real changes in the case-mix factor. The Balanced Budget Act of 1997 made changes to Medicare that were projected to result in $116 billion in savings between 1998 and 2002. Two-thirds of these savings were to come from limits in the update factors for inpatient care (Moon et al. 1997). For the first year, there was a freeze on payment rates (Levit et al. 2000).

The Medicare Part A payment strategy also included a switch from fee-for-service to prospective payment systems for home health care and outpatient care. Classification systems have been developed for home health care (Goldberg et al. 1999) and outpatient care (Health Care Financing Administration, 2000). Such systems are expected to increase control over spending in these areas by Medicare. They may also reduce availability.

14.6.6 Managed Care and Competition

In the original Medicare scheme for HMO coverage, the fees paid to HMOs were based on total medical care expenditures per beneficiary. Using the adjusted average per capita cost (AAPCC) method of rate setting, fees were set at 95 percent of the total medical costs for persons in the geographic area (usually the county). Included in the rate was the enrollee's Part B premium. The health plan decided on any benefit package in excess of the standard Medicare A and B coverage (e.g., whether to include drug coverage), additional premiums (if any), and copayments for medical visits. The basic rate was risk adjusted for age, sex, eligibility for Medicaid supplemental coverage, and whether the enrollee was institutionalized. Under the AAPCC formula, there were wide geographic variations in premium rates. In 1997, rates ranged from $250 per month to $760. There were also wide variations in managed care enrollments between states. Only 5 percent of the eligible population enrolled in risk contracts in Arizona in 1997; in California, the statistic was 27 percent. In addition, there was some evidence that Medicare risk plans enrolled persons who were lower users of health services (Brown et al. 1993); as a result, their costs were below the risk premiums set by Medicare, and the HMOs' profits were sometimes considerable.

Many observers have placed high hopes on managed care to achieve acceptable levels of health care for the covered population. The failure of Medicare to achieve a uniformly high degree of managed care coverage was attributed to the wide regional variations in the AAPCC rates and the inability of the risk-rating formula to account for high-cost enrollees. In 1998, Congress enacted a new Part C of Title XVIII of the Social Security Act, creating the Medicare + Choice program. The program had two new features. First, it created a blended national-regional rate for the managed care premium. In this rate, Medicare combined a national rate ($398 per month) with the county rates (the old AAPCC rates). There was to be a floor below which no county-specific rate would fall. This resulted in a severing of the link between fee-for-service costs and managed care rates (McClellan 2000). Second,

Congress instituted a new risk-adjustment variable, called the *Principal Inpatient Diagnostic Cost Group (PIP-DCG)*. According to the PIP-DCG, a patient who is hospitalized in the previous year for a specific (serious) condition will fall into a higher risk category, and the HMO will receive a higher rate adjustment for this patient. The intent of these changes is to encourage HMOs to establish programs in areas that are now poorly served and to accept higher risk patients who have been hospitalized for serious conditions. Other features of the Medicare risk system remained. These include the variable benefits package, additional premiums tied to the benefits package, and consumer premiums and copayments.

Several criticisms have been aimed at the new Medicare + Choice program (Aaron 1999). One is that Medicare + Choice may still not appropriately adjust for risk. The nature of the enrollees of the Medicare program and the circumstances of enrollment make it easier for HMOs to select low-cost enrollees. Medicare enrollees select into the program as individuals rather than within groups, and HMOs can target low-cost individuals for membership much easier than they can target employees who join as a group. In addition, Medicare enrollees have a great variability in cost. In any society most of the people with very high medical costs are older individuals, and in the United States all of the older individuals are in the Medicare program. There are thus considerable benefits to be gained by HMOs from seeking out the lower cost individuals. It is thus particularly important for the Medicare program to have an adequate risk-adjustment mechanism.

A second criticism of the program is that Medicare + Choice offers a services and benefits package. Medicare pays for a basic core of services plus whatever additional services the HMO offers. These extra services are included in the HMO additional premium, if there is one. As a result, Medicare is not paying for a defined group of services, and enrollees may become confused as to what is in the Medicare package and what is extra.

In the coming years, there will be many reform proposals seeking to push Medicare towards becoming a competitive system. In one such proposal, Aaron (1999) suggested that the Medicare risk program become one of a defined (minimum) set of benefits and that any additional benefits should be placed outside the basic Medicare package. HMOs might bid within a region on providing such contracts, and they would have to accept all applicant enrollees. An appropriate risk adjustment would have to be added to the basic premium rate (the accepted bid) to take account of persons who are less healthy. Medicare would pay all HMOs operating in the area the rate that resulted from the bidding process. If an HMO charged more than the accepted rate for the defined benefits package, the enrollee would have to pay the difference. And if the enrollee selected any additional benefits, this would have to be provided through a separate contract, so that the basic components of the plan would not become confused.

It is questionable whether such reforms would solve the problems associated with introducing managed care principles into the Medicare program. Medicare enrollees still join HMOs individually and have high and variable costs. The very significant incentive to select healthier cases will remain as long as the risk-adjustment tools do not permit the identification of high-risk individuals. As well, any attempt to regulate competitive practices will result in an extremely complex set of rules. However, the set of rules may not be any more complex than the set of current fee-for-service rules, in which a multitude of prices and adjustments have been introduced within a complicated regulatory framework. Further, the definition and regulation of the basic product characteristics will prove to be a daunting task. Medical care is a service with many aspects, and the between-patient and between-provider differences are very subtle.

A successful capitation program will better allow Medicare to achieve a greater degree of control over public expenditures. Competition should lead to a greater degree of efficiency in the market. The achievement of the other social goals may be more controversial. The ability of Medicare to ensure uniformly high quality services is still open to question. And the availability of care may be hampered by the continual attempt by managed care plans to enroll low cost patients. Nevertheless, any system must be judged by comparing it to other feasible systems. Currently, fee-for-service is the alternative to Medicare. Fee-for-service may perform better in terms of availability and quality of care, but it is lacking in regard to the goals of efficiency and expenditure control. In the end, the policy maker is faced with a trade-off, and the choice of system will depend on the degree of importance given to each of the social goals.

14.7 POLICY ALTERNATIVES FOR MEDICAID

Medicaid programs are run by the states and financed by them and the federal government. Individual states have a great deal of discretion in the policies they institute to govern the programs, which indeed exhibit substantial variability. Part of this variability is due to the fact that Medicaid serves several very different populations, including the poor aged, poor families with dependent children, and the blind and disabled.

Medicaid's problems are somewhat different from those of Medicare. To begin with, there are a large number of uninsured children in the United States. For example, of the 44 million persons without insurance coverage in 1998, 11 million of these were under 18 years of age. In addition, there are many persons over 65 who have low incomes but no supplementary coverage and who are thus at risk for considerable out-of-pocket expenditures. In 1998, 21 percent of the Medicaid population was over 65 years old and had joint Medicare-Medicaid coverage (Health Care Financing Administration 2000). Until 1990, the growth in total expenditures for Medicaid was moderate. However, beginning in 1990, following the expansion of the program to cover children and women whose incomes were above the poverty level but still low, the growth in expenditures was substantial, although in 1996 and 1997 expenditure growth leveled off. At its inception, the Medicaid program accounted for 2.9 percent of all national health expenditures. In 1998, state and federal outlays for Medicaid totaled $175 billion, accounting for 14.8 percent of the nation's health expenditures.

14.7.1 Scope of the Program

Until 1987, only low-income women (under age 65 and not blind or disabled) and their children who were receiving AFDC payments were eligible for Medicaid enrollment. The Medicaid program expanded eligibility in 1987 to include low-income women and children who were not on the AFDC program. At their discretion, states could offer coverage to families whose incomes reached 185 percent of the poverty level. This expansion of coverage led to a rapid increase in

Medicaid enrollment and expenditures beginning in 1990 (Cutler and Gruber 1996a and 1996b).

Medicaid's scope of coverage is very broad. It usually includes outpatient drugs and dental care. Because the breadth of coverage is wider than that for Medicare, Medicaid also enrolls low-income Medicare enrollees who do not have supplementary coverage.

Although the variety of services was not affected, the state of Oregon instituted a benefit limitation policy in 1994. It created a ranking of the costs and benefits of alternative medical procedures and proposed to pay for only those procedures whose cost-benefit ratios ranked above a certain cutoff point. Near the top of the list were treatments for disorders such as bone cancer and multiple sclerosis, which, it was claimed, yield substantial benefits per dollar of cure. Lower on the list were disorders whose treatments have a lower rate of return, including chronic ulcers and sleep disorders. Thus the scope of the services was to be limited by type of treatment. This program was quite controversial and has generated a great deal of discussion.

14.7.2 Copayments

Generally, Medicaid does not charge recipients for their services. However, states can institute a copayment for some services. As of 1992, 21 states had copayments for prescription drugs, usually ranging from $0.50 to $1.00 per prescription. In addition, some states have mandated limits on the quantity of drugs prescribed and the number of refills. After the enrollee reaches these limits, the drugs are no longer covered. There is evidence that these copayments affect the utilization of drugs, and there is limited evidence that health status is adversely affected (Stuart and Zacker 1999).

14.7.3 Provider Payments

Medicaid programs are noted for the low levels of fees paid to providers (Gruber 1997). Low fee levels discourage providers from serving Medicaid enrollees and thus reduce availability. This is a problem often noted when Medicaid is discussed.

14.7.4 Competitive Bidding by Suppliers

Competitive bidding, which has been implemented by the California and Arizona Medicaid programs, has the objective of providing cost-effective care for indigents. If the buyer has a considerable degree of market power, it can extract a lower price from competitive sellers, and if there is any room for cost reductions, either through increasing efficiency or lowering quality, the reductions will be incorporated into the providers' bids. However, the bidding process is a complex one and may not automatically lead to savings.

14.7.5 Managed Care

Many states are looking to managed care programs in order to consolidate their efforts at provision. In 1998, 53 percent of the Medicaid population was enrolled in managed care plans. The proportion of persons who were enrolled varied by group.

Many older individuals receive long-term care coverage through Medicaid (as well as through their Medicare coverage). Long-term care utilization, for those who need it, is less controllable than other types of care (acute care), and long term care is thus less amenable to HMO-type coverage. Older Medicaid long-term care patients would therefore, tend not to be enrolled in a Medicaid managed care plan. Indeed, only 4.9 percent of Medicaid enrollees who are served by HMOs are over age 65. The majority of Medicaid HMO enrollees are children (51 percent) and parents (22 percent).

Under Medicaid, HMOs face the same issues as under Medicare. There is a wide variation in fee-setting practices and in fees among states (Holahan et al. 1999). In addition, as in the fee-for-service sector, managed care rates in general are quite low (Bruen and Holahan 1999). As well, risk-adjustment factors have not been well developed, and so biased selection in membership may be a problem. In short, Medicaid has problems enrolling members and maintaining the provision of care for these individuals. This policy has the effect of reducing the availability of care for these populations.

EXERCISES

1. What populations are covered by Medicare?
2. What are the most important services covered by Medicare Parts A and B?
3. What are the major sources of funding for Medicare Parts A and B?
4. What populations are covered by Medicaid?
5. What services are covered by Medicaid?
6. What is the major source of funding for Medicaid?
7. What is Medigap and what purpose does it serve?
8. Can a Medicare enrollee join a managed care plan and, if so, what premiums does he or she pay?
9. What are the key characteristics of persons without health insurance in the United States?
10. Why can't the Medicare program increase Part A spending on hospital care by applying for funds out of general taxation revenues?
11. What are the goals of Medicare?
12. List five policies for Medicare and identify what goal(s) each addresses.
13. What are the most important problems faced by Medicaid and what policies might be used to help solve them?

BIBLIOGRAPHY

Medicare

Aaron, H.J., and R.D. Reischauer. 1995. The Medicare reform debate: What is the next step? *Health Affairs* 14, no. 4:8–30.

Aaron, H.J. 1999. Medicare choice: Good, bad, it all depends. In *Medicare reform: Issues and answers*, ed. A.J. Rettenmaier and T.R. Saving. Chicago: University of Chicago Press.

American Association of Retired Persons. 1999. *Out-of-pocket spending on health care by Medicare beneficiaries age 65 and older: 1999 projections.* Washington, DC: American Association of Retired Persons.

American Medical Association. 2000. *Medicare RBRVS*. Chicago: American Medical Association.

Baker, L.C. 1997. The effect of HMOs on fee-for-service health care expenditures: Evidence from Medicare. *Journal of Health Economics* 16:453–481.

Berenson, R., and J. Holohan. 1992. Sources of growth in Medicare physician expenditures. *JAMA* 267:687–691.

Blustein, J. 2000. Drug coverage and drug purchases by Medicare beneficiaries with hypertension. *Health Affairs* 19, no. 2:219–230.

Brown, R.S., et al. 1993. Do health maintenance organizations work for Medicare? *Health Care Financing Review* 15, no. 1:7–23.

Congressional Budget Office. 1983. *Changing the structure of Medicare benefits*. Washington, DC: Congressional Budget Office.

Cutler, D.M. 1999. What does Medicare spending buy us? In *Medicare reform: Issues and answers*, ed. A.J. Rettenmaier and T.R. Saving. Chicago: University of Chicago Press.

———. 2000. Walking the tightrope on Medicare reform. *Journal of Economic Perspectives* 14:45–56.

Davis, K., and D. Rowland. 1984. Medicare financing reform: A new Medicare premium. *Milbank Quarterly* 62:300–316.

Davis, M., et al. 1999. Prescription drug coverage, utilization, and spending among Medicare beneficiaries. *Health Affairs* 18, no. 1:231–243.

Ettner, S.L. 1995. The opportunity costs of elder care. *Journal of Human Resources* 31:189–205.

———. 1997. Adverse selection and the purchase of Medigap insurance by the elderly. *Journal of Health Economics* 16:543–562.

Feder, J. 1995–1996. Some thoughts on the future of Medicare. *Inquiry* 32:376–378.

Fuchs, V.R. 2000. Medicare reform: The larger picture. *Journal of Economic Perspectives* 14:57–70.

Gillis, K.D., and D.W. Lee. 1997. Medicare, access, and physicians' willingness to accept new Medicare patients. *Quarterly Review of Economics and Finance* 37:579–603.

Ginsburg, P.B., and M. Moon. 1984. An introduction to the Medicare financing problem. *Milbank Quarterly* 62:167–182.

Gluck, M.A. 1999. *Medicare prescription drug benefit*. Medicare brief no. 1. Washington, DC: National Academy of Social Insurance.

Goldberg, H.B., et al. 1999. *Case mix adjustment for a national home health prospective payment system: Second interim report*. Cambridge, MA: Abt Associates, Inc.

Goody, B., et al. 1994. New directions for Medicare payment systems. *Health Care Financing Review* 16, no. 2:1–11.

Health Care Financing Administration. 1995. *Medicare and Medicaid statistical supplement*. Baltimore: Health Care Financing Administration.

Health Care Financing Administration.1998. *The profile of Medicare: Chart book 1998*. Baltimore: Health Care Financing Administration.

Health Care Financing Administration. 2000. Medicare program prospective payment system for hospital outpatient services; final rule. *Federal Register* 65, no. 68 (7 April 2000): 18433–18820.

Hsiao, W.C., and N.L. Kelly. 1984. Medicare benefits: A reassessment. *Milbank Quarterly* 62:207–229.

Hsiao, W.C., et al. 1993. Assessing the implementation of physician payment reform. *New England Journal of Medicine* 328:928–933.

Iglehart, J.K. 1999. The American health care system—Medicare. *New England Journal of Medicine* 340:327–332.

Kominski, G.F., and S.H. Long. 1997. Medicare's disproportionate share adjustment and the cost of low-income patients. *Journal of Health Economics* 16:177–190.

Lee, A.J., and J.B. Mitchell. 1994. Physician reaction to price changes: An episode-of-care analysis. *Health Care Financing Review* 16, no. 2:65–83.

Levit, K., et al. 2000. Health spending in 1998: Signals of change. *Health Affairs* 19(1):124–132.

Liu, K., et al. 1999. Medicare's post-acute care benefit. Washington, DC: Urban Institute.

Long, S.H., and Smeeding, T.M. 1984. Alternative Medicare financing sources. *Milbank Quarterly* 62:325–348.

Luft, H.S. 1984. On the use of vouchers for Medicare. *Milbank Quarterly* 62:237–250.

McClellan, M. 2000. Medicare reform: Fundamental problems, incremental steps. *Journal of Economic Perspectives* 14:21–44.

Moon, M., et al. 1997. An examination of key Medicare provisions in the Balanced Budget Act of 1997. Washington, DC: Urban Institute.

Petrie, J.T. 1992. Overview of the Medicare program. *Health Care Financing Review Annual Supplement*, pp. 1–22.

Pope, G.C., et al. 1998. Evaluating alternative risk adjustors for Medicare. *Health Care Financing Review* 20:109–129.

Rice, T., and N. McCall. 1985. The extent of ownership and the characteristics of Medicare supplemental policies. *Inquiry* 22:188–200.

Rice, T. and J. Bernstein. 1999. *Supplemental health insurance for Medicare beneficiaries.* Medicare brief. no. 6. Washington, DC: National Academy of Social Insurance.

Rice, T., et al. 1997. The impact of policy standardization on the Medigap market. *Inquiry* 34:106–116.

Saving, T.R. 2000. Making the transition to prepaid Medicare. *Journal of Economic Perspectives* 14:85–98.

Shih, Y.T. 1999. Effect of insurance on prescription drug use by ESRD beneficiaries. *Health Care Financing Review* 20, no. 3:39–54.

Smits, H.L., et al. 1982. Medicare's nursing home benefit: Variations in interpretation. *New England Journal of Medicine* 307:855–862.

Soumerai, S., and D. Ross-Degnan. 1999. Inadequate prescription drug coverage for Medicare enrollees. *New England Journal of Medicine* 340:722–728.

U.S. Bureau of the Census.1999. *Health insurance coverage, 1998.* Washington, DC: U.S. Bureau of the Census.

U.S. Department of Health and Human Services. 1983. *The Medicare and Medicaid data book.* HCFA publication no. 03156. Baltimore: Health Care Financing Administration.

U.S. Department of Health and Human Services. 1993. *Medicare and Medicaid statistical supplement.* Baltimore: U.S. Department of Health and Human Services.

U.S. Government Accounting Office.1995. *Medicare managed care.* Document no. GAO/HEHS-96–21. Washington, DC: Government Accounting Office.

U.S. General Accounting Office. 1999. *Medicare and budget surpluses.* Publication no. GAO/T-AIMD/HEHS-99–113. Washington: Government Accounting Office.

Wolkstein, I. 1984. Medicare's financial status: How did we get here? *Milbank Quarterly* 62:183–206.

Medicaid

Battistella, R.M. 1989. National health insurance: Dilemmas and opportunities. *Hospital and Health Services Administration* 34:139–156.

Blumberg, L.J., et al. 2000. Did the Medicaid expansions for children displace private insurance? An analysis using the SIPP. *Journal of Health Economics* 19:33–60.

Bradford, W.D. 1995. The effects of a relative value reimbursement scheme on the medical market: Lessons from Medicaid. *Review of Industrial Organization* 10:511–532.

Brecher, C., and J. Knickman. 1985. A reconsideration of long-term-care policy. *Journal of Health Politics, Policy, and Law* 10:245–272.

Bruen, B., and J. Holahan. 1999. *Slow growth in Medicaid spending continues in 1997.* Issue paper. Washington, DC: Kaiser Commission on Medicaid and the Uninsured.

Buchanan, R.J. 1983. Medicaid cost containment: Prospective reimbursement for long-term care. *Inquiry* 20:334–342.

Congressional Budget Office. 1981. *Medicaid: Choices for 1982 and beyond.* Washington, DC: Congressional Budget Office.

Cook, P.J., et al. 1999. The effects of short-term variation in abortion funding on pregnancy outcomes. *Journal of Health Economics* 18:241–257.

Currie, J., and J. Gruber. 1996a. Saving babies: The efficacy and cost of recent changes in the Medicaid eligibility of pregnant women. *Journal of Political Economy* 104:1263–1293.

———. 1996b. Health insurance eligibility, utilization of medical care and child health. *Quarterly Journal of Economics* 110:431–464.

Cutler, D.M., Gruber, J. 1996a. The effect of Medicaid expansions on public insurance, private insurance, and redistribution. *American Economic Review* 86:378–383.

———. 1996b. Does public insurance crowd out private insurance? *Quarterly Journal of Economics* 110:391–426.

Davis, K. 1989. National health insurance: A proposal. *American Economic Review* 79:349–352.

Davis, K., and C. Schoen. 1978. *Health and the war on poverty.* Washington, DC: Brookings Institution.

Ettner, S.L. 1997. Medicaid participation among the eligible elderly. *Journal of Policy Analysis and Management* 16, no. 2:237–255.

Fossett, J.W., and J.A. Peterson. 1989. Physician supply and Medicaid participation. *Medical Care* 27:386–396.

Fox, H.G., et al. 1993. State Medicaid health maintenance organization policies and special-needs children. *Health Care Financing Review* 15, no. 1:25–37.

Gold, M., et al. 1996. Medicaid managed care: Lessons from five states. *Health Affairs* 15, no. 3:153–166.

Gruber, J. 1997. Medicaid and uninsured women and children. *Journal of Economic Perspectives* 11:199–208.

Gruber, J., et al. 1997. Physician fee policy and Medicaid program costs. *Journal of Human Resources* 32:611–634.

Gurny, P., et al. 1992. Payment, administration, and financing of the Medicaid program. *Health Care Financing Review Annual Supplement,* pp. 285–301.

Harrington, C., and J.H. Swan. 1984. Medicaid nursing home reimbursement policies, rates and expenditures. *Health Care Financing Review* 6, no. 1:39–49.

Health Care Financing Administration. 2000. *A profile of Medicaid.* (http://www.hcfa.gov/stats/2Tchartbk.pdf)

Holahan, J. 1975. *Financing health care for the poor.* Lexington, MA: Lexington Books.

———. 1999. Medicaid managed care payment methods and capitation rates. Washington, DC: Urban Institute.

Iglehart, J.K. 1999. The American health care system—Medicaid. *New England Journal of Medicine* 340:403–408.

Joyce, T. Impact of augmented prenatal care on birth outcomes of Medicaid recipients in New York City. *Journal of Health Economics* 18:31–67.

Ku, L., and T.A. Coughlin. 1995. Medicaid disproportionate share and other special financing programs. *Health Care Financing Review* 16, no. 3:27–54.

Levincon, A., and F. Ullman. 1998. Medicaid managed care and infant health. *Journal of Health Economics* 17: 351–368.

Medicare Payment Advisory Commission. 2000. *Report to Congress.* Washington, DC: Medicare Payment Advisory Commission.

Meiners, M.R. 1983. The case for long-term care insurance. *Health Affairs* 2, no. 2:55–79.

Miller, M.E., and D.J. Gengler. 1993. Medicaid case management: Kentucky's patient access and care program. *Health Care Financing Review* 15, no. 1:55–69.

Rask, K.N., and K.J. Rask. 2000. Public insurance substituting for private insurance: New evidence regarding public hospitals, uncompensated care funds, and Medicaid. *Journal of Health Economics* 19:1–31.

Rowland, D. 1995. Medicaid at 30: New challenges for the nation's safety net. *JAMA* 274:271–273.

Shore-Sheppard, L., et al. 2000. Medicaid and crowding out of private insurance: A re-examination using firm level data. *Journal of Health Economics* 19:61–91.

Showalter, M.H. 1997. Physicians' cost shifting behavior: Medicaid versus other patients. *Contemporary Economic Policy* 15:74–84.

Stuart, B. 1972. Equity and Medicaid. *Journal of Human Resources* 7:152–178.

Stuart, B., and C. Zacker. 1999. Who bears the burden of Medicaid drug copayment policies? *Health Affairs* 18, no. 2:201–212.

Stuart, B., et al. 1999. Drug use and prescribing problems in four state Medicaid programs. *Health Care Financing Review* 20, no. 2:63–75.

Tallon, J.R., and D. Rowland. 1995. Federal dollars and state flexibility. *Inquiry* 32:235–240.

Tudor, C.G. 1995. Medicaid expenditures and state responses. *Health Care Financing Review* 16, no. 3:1–10.

Wade, M., and S. Berg. 1995. Causes of Medicaid expenditure growth. *Health Care Financing Review* 16, no. 3:11–25.

Wycoff, P.G. 1985. Medicaid: Federalism and the Reagan budget proposals. *Economic Commentary of the Reserve Bank of Cleveland,* August.

Yelowitz, A.S. 1998. Why did the SSI-disabled program grow so much? Disentangling the effect of Medicaid. *Journal of Health Economics* 17:321–349.

Uninsured Care

Birnbaum, H., et al. 1979. Focusing the catastrophic illness debate. *Quarterly Review of Economics and Business* 19:17–33.

Cafferata, G.L. 1984. *Private health insurance coverage of the Medicare population.* National Health Care Expenditures Study data preview 18. Rockville, MD: National Center for Health Services Research.

Cleeton, D. 1989. The medical uninsured: A case for market failure. *Public Finance Quarterly* 17:55–83.

De Lew, N., et al. 1992. A layman's guide to the U.S. health care system. *Health Care Financing Review* 14, no. 2:151–170.

Hadley, J., and J. Feder. 1985. Hospital cost shifting and care for the uninsured. *Health Affairs* 4, no. 3:67–81.

Levit, K.R., et al. 1992. American's health insurance coverage, 1980–91. *Health Care Financing Review* 14, no. 1:31–57.

Monheit, A.C., and P.F. Short. 1989. Mandating health coverage for working Americans. *Health Affairs* 8, no. 4:22–38.

Mulstein, S. 1984. The uninsured and financing of uncompensated care. *Inquiry* 21:214–229.

Short, P.F., et al. 1988. *Uninsured Americans: A 1987 profile.* Rockville, MD: National Center for Health Services Research and Health Care Technology Assessment.

Wilensky, G. 1987. Viable strategies for dealing with the uninsured. *Health Affairs* 6, no. 1:33–46.

———. 1988. Filling the gaps in health insurance. *Health Affairs* 7, no. 3:133–149.

Reform of the
Health Care Market

1. Define the concept of health care market reform and explain the need for reform in the context of health care and health insurance markets.
2. Explain the operation of an insurance market that is efficient but not "equitable" in the sense that insurance coverage is not universal.
3. Define each of the following policies and describe their effects in terms of equity and efficiency: premium subsidies, cooperative pools, community rating, mandates, and limits on selection.
4. Define managed care.
5. Describe the key characteristics of a health maintenance organization and explain why it is the prototypical managed care organization.
6. Explain how consumer and provider incentives work to achieve cost reduction in a managed care environment.
7. Define *selection bias* and explain how it might cause an HMO to misleadingly appear more efficient than fee-for-service health care provision.
8. Compare the effects of HMOs with the effects of fee-for-service on resource use and quality of care.
9. Explain the conceptual role of consumer sovereignty in hospital markets and identify several reasons why early attempts to achieve it were controversial.
10. Distinguish between employer and individual use of information on health plan performance.

15.1 INTRODUCTION

Health reform is a term that has been applied to insurance and health care markets as well as to the total constellation of health services. In the case of insurance markets, the term refers to specific ways to make the markets perform more like a competitive market, such as by setting rules to prevent insurers from engaging in "biased risk selection," a key factor in market failure, and trying to ensure that insurance is available at a "reasonable" price to those who want it.

In the case of the health care market, the main goal of reform has been to increase consumer choice (i.e., to make the health care markets more sensitive to consumer rather than provider demands). One of the key efforts has been to increase the degree of competition so that the markets work more like the textbook model of a competitive market (see Chapter 8).

The goals that market reforms seek to achieve include equity and efficiency. The insurance market reforms have focused largely on equity (i.e., making insurance affordable to those who want it). Possible strategies include subsidies for high-risk consumers. The reforms are only secondarily concerned with increasing provider efficiency or consumer choice. Health care market reforms have focused on efficiency—on making the markets more like the competitive ideal.

This chapter examines reforms in health care markets and insurance markets and considers the integration of the insurance and health care delivery functions into managed care. Section 15.2 reviews insurance market reforms, focusing on alternative mechanisms that have been proposed to make the insurance markets more sensitive to consumer wants. Section 15.3 looks at the role of managed care in changing provider and buyer incentives to promote greater efficiency and limit cost increases. Finally, Section 15.4 describes some of the developments in information and consumer orientation that have affected health care markets.

15.2 INSURANCE MARKET REFORM

15.2.1 The Need for Reform

The performance of insurance markets can be judged from the vantage point of efficiency or equity. In looking at economic efficiency performance criteria, we are essentially asking whether an optimal degree of risk is being shifted by consumers to insurers. This degree is related to the value of risk shifting to the consumers and the cost of risk shifting to insurers. If individuals are willing to pay for greater amounts of coverage (e.g., coverage for more expensive services), and there are insurers who are willing to provide this coverage at the desired price, but there are some impediments to the shifting of the risks so that it does not take place, then the degree of insurance coverage is not optimal. By the same token, if the value to consumers of shifting additional risks is low (below the cost to insurers of accepting these risks) but consumers purchase insurance anyway because of subsidized out-of-pocket prices or lack of good information, then an excess of coverage will result.

We have seen that an efficient degree of coverage may mean no coverage at all for health care expenditures. If individuals value risk shifting less than they do the cost of insurance, then they will simply not insure. However, these individuals may be very high risk and/or low-income individuals or may work for small companies, and we may think it is inequitable for these individuals to go without insurance coverage. On grounds of equity, we might decide that something should be done to remedy the situation. In this section we examine the causes of market failure in insurance markets and the remedies that have been proposed. We present the analysis using a simple economic model to bring out the essential features of insurance market failure and market reform.

15.2.2 The Basic Model

We set out a basic model of a health insurance market in which there are seven individuals, each with a given degree of risk of being ill. The expected loss for each of these individuals is shown in Table 15–1. Individual 1, the least healthy of the lot, has an expected loss of $12; individual 2 has an expected loss of $8; and so on.

We turn to the assumptions about the demand for insurance. Each individual has a certain willingness to pay for health insurance coverage. Individual 1 is willing to pay $12, which would indicate that he or she is risk neutral (i.e., puts no additional value on the size of the loss). Individual 2 is willing to pay $10 for coverage, individual 3 is willing to pay $9, and so on. Note that individual 1 might be a high-risk person with limited means to pay for health insurance.

In addition to the individuals' demands, we specify personal characteristics or circumstances that will affect the insurance market in a systematic way. One such characteristic is age. In our example, we specify two separate age groups—individuals older than 50 and individuals younger than 50. We would expect, in general, that an individual whose age is above 50 will have greater expected health care costs because of poorer health status. Age is a piece of information that might be used by insurers to set premium rates.

We also specify in our example the individuals' work circumstances, as these are a prime determinant of the cost of providing health insurance and thus of the loading charge. It costs less to provide insurance coverage to individuals in a large group than to individuals who are employed by small companies or who are not employed at all. In our example, we assume that it costs $1 to supply insurance coverage to individuals in a large group and $3 to individuals in smaller employment groups or to those who must purchase insurance individually.

With regard to the supply side of the market, we will assume that there is a single supplier. This supplier knows the risk for each person (a situation referred to as *information symmetry*). The supplier sets a price for each person based strictly on his or her expected loss plus the cost of administration (i.e., the supplier engages in experience rating). Thus, for individual 1, the price will be $15 (the expected loss plus the $3 administrative cost). We also assume that the insurer has sufficient capacity to insure all consumers who are willing to shift their risks.

Table 15–1 The Value and Price of Insurance for Individuals

	Individual						
	1	2	3	4	5	6	7
Willingness to pay for insurance coverage (dollars)	$12.00	$10.00	$9.00	$8.00	$7.00	$6.00	$5.00
Expected loss due to illness	$12.00	$ 8.00	$7.00	$6.00	$5.00	$4.00	$3.00
Age	>50	>50	>50	<50	<50	<50	<50
Employment group type (N = no group; L = large group; S = small group)	N	L	L	L	L	L	S
Cost of administering insurance in absence of pool membership	$ 3.00	$ 1.00	$1.00	$1.00	$1.00	$1.00	$3.00
Model 1 prices (experience rating in absence of pool membership)	$15.00	$ 9.00	$8.00	$7.00	$6.00	$5.00	$6.00
Model 2 prices (complete information asymmetry, first round)	$ 8.00	$ 8.00	$8.00	$8.00	$8.00	$8.00	$8.00
Model 3 prices (25 percent subsidy provided to all individuals, experience rating, and information symmetry)	$11.25	$ 6.75	$6.00	$5.25	$4.50	$3.75	$4.50

We now draw the conclusions of our model regarding the availability of insurance. Each individual will purchase insurance as long as the premium rate is less than or equal to what the individual is willing to pay. In our model, individuals 1 and 7 are not willing to pay up to the premium rates that would be charged by the insurer. Individuals 2 through 6 will obtain insurance at the given premium rates. For all individuals, the outcome is the result of rational decisions. Further, this outcome is economically efficient, in that the net benefits from insurance coverage are maximized. If any additional insurance coverage was secured, the result (given our assumptions) would be a net social loss.

However, just because the outcome is economically efficient does not mean that it is "fair" or even "socially acceptable." All individuals in society (1 through 7) may agree that this outcome is unacceptable and that some solution must be found to ensure that all individuals have some degree of coverage. We will focus on a number of these solutions in subsequent sections of this chapter. However, we first focus on one of the critical assumptions of our analysis—the assumption of information symmetry. There is a considerable literature on what happens when this assumption does not hold. Our simple model will be changed to take the assumption of information asymmetry into account.

15.2.3 Information Asymmetry and Adverse Selection

In a state of information asymmetry, one group of individuals (potentially) engaged in a transaction have better information than another group (potentially) engaged in the transaction. Such a situation can lead to market failure, such that a transaction benefiting both parties never actually takes place. To see how market failure might occur, we return to our previous model, except that we now assume information asymmetry exists. In this case, the information is about the expected loss of the potential purchasers of health insurance. The assumption we make is that the consumers have full information about their risks but the insurer knows nothing about the health status and risks of individual consumers; it only knows about the risks of the entire population.

Given this assumption, the insurer cannot distinguish between insureds in terms of their health status, and it will therefore have to charge each insured the same premium. In total, expected costs are $45 and administrative costs are still the same, $11 for all individuals. Therefore, the insurer must collect $56, or $8 per person. Remember, we are assuming that the insurer has no way of distinguishing between individuals with regard to their risk.

At a price of $8 per person, only four individuals will insure, as the price exceeds the willingness to pay for the other potential insureds. If this situation occurs, then the expected loss per person will be determined by the loss experience of the members of the group who remain in the market. The market will not even insure individuals 1 through 4, because with the other members dropping out the price will have to increase to $9.75 to cover the cost of insuring these individuals. Indeed, the entire market can eventually disappear as people successively drop out. We should note that, except for individual 1, each individual would be willing to pay for the cost of his or her insurance. However, the insurer has no way of finding out each person's risk, and so it must charge a group rate.

15.2.4 Underwriting and Group Rating

The phenomenon of adverse selection occurs in extreme cases of information asymmetry. In fact, insurers or underwriters have numerous ways of distinguishing between high- and low-risk insureds. They know or can obtain information on many characteristics associated with the risk of loss, such as age, gender, and employment (Giacomini et al. 1995). Insurers can also resort to physical exams and tests to determine if individuals have certain conditions that might lead to costly health care. In addition, they have access to the past health records of their potential insureds, and these are often good predictors of future usage. Based on such risk-related information, rates can be set that reflect individual expected costs. Insurers do not have to know exactly how much each person will spend on health care; they must only be able to form separate risk pools and estimate average costs in each pool.

In cases where there are large groups, insurers need only predict the experience of the entire group. For very large groups, health care costs are quite predictable, and therefore information asymmetry does not pose a problem. Indeed, many large employers have realized this and have begun to self-insure. Of course, this does not solve the problem of those who are not members of large groups.

Nevertheless, these phenomena raise the issue of how relevant adverse selection is. Certainly, if information on projected utilization was not available to insurers, this would be a main problem in the market. But the main problem does not seem to be an absence of information. Rather it appears to be what happens when insurers *do* have accurate information about the projected utilization of potential insureds—that is, when they can set very high rates that consumers cannot afford (i.e., are not willing to pay). This leads to a situation where some individuals are selectively excluded from the insurance market. This situation, called "preferred risk selection," will be discussed in subsequent sections.

15.2.5 Subsidies

The absence of insurance coverage can come about in markets with information symmetry and information asymmetry. We will focus our attention on the former, that is, where there is complete information on the part of both groups, the insurers and the insureds. In Section 15.2.2, we concluded (under our assumed conditions) that two individuals would not insure—individuals 1 and 7. We noted that this situation, while efficient, might not be considered equitable. If this is the case, we would have to devise some solution that would increase the amount of insurance purchased by the individuals who do not have insurance.

Let us, for the moment, retain our faith in the market as a mechanism for ensuring that individuals have access to health care when they get sick. At the same time we want to achieve the policy goal of total population insurance coverage. However, because the "unfettered" market excludes some individuals, we must devise a technique to allow all individuals to obtain insurance coverage. One such technique, widely used in the United States, is an insurance premium subsidy provided by government to individuals who purchase insurance. An example of such a subsidy is the income tax deduction for employer-paid health insurance premiums. Such a deduction reduces the cost of the premium by the individual's personal income tax rate. Some states provide subsidies directly to smaller employers in order to induce them to purchase health insurance for their employees.

In our example, let us introduce a subsidy of 25 percent of the premium paid by the individual. In this case, each person pays 25 percent less than before. The postsubsidy premium rates for each individual are shown in Table 15–1. Under our initial assumption of experience rating, individual 1 now pays $11.25 (three-quarters of what was paid before), individual 2 pays $6.75, and so on. In this case, all individuals will purchase insurance. The subsidy is successful in achieving full coverage.

However, the postsubsidy situation may not be efficient from a social point of view. In those cases where the cost of insuring exceeds the individual's willingness to pay in the absence of the subsidy, the social cost of insurance will exceed the social value. Only now the cost has been shifted on to the taxpayer, and so the true cost of insurance coverage is hidden. A second problem with subsidies is they may not be successful. Studies of subsidies provided to small firms that focused on small employers in New York State have indicated that even quite large subsidies may not be sufficient to induce the desired increases in the health insurance coverage that firms provide (Thorpe et al. 1992). Because of the design of the subsidy, there may have been a reluctance on the part of the employers to commit to providing health insurance coverage for their employees. The subsidy was only to last for two years, after which time the employers would have to pay the entire amount. Such a design, because of the greater eventual financial burden, might well deter employers from providing health insurance coverage.

15.2.6 Cooperative Pools

The provision of insurance is less expensive when it is done in the context of a large group, such as employers or professional associations. Individual and small-group policies are much more expensive to administer. As a result, the loading charge for individual and small-group policies is greater than it is for large-group policies.

There has been a recent trend toward the formation of cooperatives or insurance purchasing groups that individuals or smaller employers could join. These are called health insurance purchasing cooperatives (HIPCs). By forming a cooperative, smaller groups can be rated together as a unit and therefore receive the same rate that a larger group with the same risk profile would receive. Purchasing cooperatives have become commonplace, and a number of market reform proposals focus on this trend (Hall 1994; Reinhardt 1993a).

In our analysis, let us assume that individuals 1 and 7 can join the main group. If they do so, the cost of providing them with health insurance falls to $1. If we retained the assumption of experience rating by individual risk, then individual 1, at least, would not be insured. Individual 1 would still not be willing to pay $13, the premium he or she would have to pay. However, the cooperative would have increased insurance coverage (by extending coverage to individual 7) through lowering the cost of provision. This would be an efficient solution and would increase equity.

15.2.7 Community Rating and Biased Selection

One feature that has been included in some health insurance reform proposals is a requirement for community rating. To determine the effects of community rating, let us return to our original model (see Section 15.2.2). We will initially assume that everyone pays the same premium to a single insurer. If the insurer has only to meet its full costs, including administration costs, and if all individuals are to be served, then the single community rate would be $8. At this single rate, individuals 5, 6, and 7 will not insure. This may start a spiral that leads to the eventual drying up of the entire market.

There is another consideration in community rating. Let us assume that there are two insurers, A and B, and they are competing for business at the community rate. We will also change another assumption and suppose that the insurers want to maximize their profits. The implications of these changes are as follows. In order to maximize profits, each of the two insurers will seek out insureds with a low risk of loss and low administrative expenses. They will avoid providing insurance to other individuals. There are numerous ways that the insurers could do this. They could screen applicants and, if provision is not mandatory, refuse to sell insurance to high-cost individuals. Alternatively, they could make it difficult for potentially high cost insureds to reach them by locating in areas where younger, healthier individuals live (Light 1992).

The incentive for insurers to select low-risk individuals is indeed a powerful one, and its relevance needs to be emphasized. A key way for insurers to contain their costs is to make certain that their clients are low risk to begin with. Numerous health insurance reform proposals have been put forward, and most of them at least try to address this issue. However, under community rating, this issue is especially difficult to address because it relates directly to the profits that the insurers can earn.

Another issue relating to community rating is that, if each individual's premium is fixed, there will be no incentive for individuals to reduce their risk through health promotion and disease prevention activities. Under experience rating, individuals can be offered incentives (lower premiums) to engage in behaviors that lead to better health (e.g., no smoking). Such incentives do not exist when everyone pays the same premium.

We can evaluate community rating on two grounds: equity and efficiency. From one point of view, community rating can appear to be the most equitable rating method. After all, everyone pays the same rate. However, if everyone is not in the same risk category, then community rating involves the subsidization of the unhealthy by the healthy. If we subscribe to a notion of equity according to which equals should pay equally and unequals should pay unequally, then community rating might not seem an equitable method. On the other hand, if we view all individuals as "equals" (in the sense that, no matter how healthy or unhealthy, they are all human beings), then community rating will indeed appear fair.

On efficiency grounds, there can be little said in favor of community rating. Community rating discourages individuals from engaging in health promotion activities when the social costs would warrant them to do it. Cost savings from such activities are not passed on to the individuals who engage in them. In addition, community rating encourages insurers to seek out the lowest risk individuals, and this can cause individuals who would otherwise buy insurance not to purchase it, which eventually could lead to a drying up of the health insurance market. In response to these problems, two additional innovations have been introduced. One is a mandate requiring individuals or employers to obtain insurance. The second is risk rating—the assignment of individuals to groups according to their risks and the requirement that they pay different premiums based on these risks.

15.2.8 Mandates

A mandate is a legal requirement that some action be taken, such as the purchasing of health insurance coverage by an individual or an employer. The purpose of a mandate to purchase insurance is to block individuals from leaving the health insurance market. It is maintained that some individuals (primarily low-risk individuals) will not insure until they get older or sick and the risk of their using services increases. Only then do they insure and "take advantage" of their coverage. When low-risk individuals do not participate in the market, this causes higher group premiums and could even result in the eventual disappearance of the market. Under a mandate, everyone must purchase insurance. Many health insurance reform proposals involve introducing a mandate.

Starting with our original example, we will assume community rating and a mandate that all individuals purchase insurance. The premium rate will be $8, and all individuals are mandated to pay this rate.

Such a premium rate might impose a considerable burden on low-income individuals, and so few proposals would stop at a mandate. One way to reduce the burden would be to provide a subsidy for individuals who are designated as low income. The combined reforms would ensure that all individuals were insured and could afford insurance, since those who could not otherwise afford it would be subsidized.

The main objection to a mandate is that it imposes a welfare loss on some individuals. For example, individuals 5, 6, and 7 are not willing to pay $8 for health insurance coverage. Under a mandate, they would have to pay that amount anyway, and so they would suffer an added burden in order that higher risk and/or lower income individuals be able to obtain insurance (Hall 1994). In addition, the mandate does not eliminate the powerful incentive insurance companies have to "cherry pick" or engage in other competitive practices that enable them to select low-risk insureds. Other elements of health insurance reform must be introduced if these practices are to be curbed. The most prominent of these is risk adjustment.

15.2.9 Risk Selection Limitation and Risk Adjustment

Some government policies directly limit insurers' ability to select individual risks. Since past or current health may be a good predictor of future health, a decision to accept a person for coverage or renew a policy may involve examination of the applicant's current health or past claim experience. The existence of a chronic health condition or large past expenses could be the basis for denying coverage. Decisions to deny coverage in such cases have generated significant media and political attention because they can be seen as refusing coverage to people who need it most. Federal legislation in 1996 directly addressed this issue by requiring companies to sell insurance policies to groups willing to purchase them and guaranteeing individuals or groups the right to renew policies.

Risk adjustment is a technique that can be used to modify payments made to prepaid plans on the basis of characteristics of the entire group. The rationale behind this technique is that certain subgroups are more costly to treat (because they use more services) and that health plans should be appropriately compensated for accepting these subgroups as members. Among the variables that have been used in risk-adjustment formulas are age, gender, self-reported health status, and prior period health care use (see Section 7.7).

A problem with risk adjustment, in the present context, is that if a health plan discovers a variable related to health care use, it might be able to profit by selecting low-risk individuals. For example, if body weight was associated with health care utilization, then a health plan might try to select members at least partly on the basis of their weight. Assuming it was successful in attracting lower weight members, it would benefit from having lower costs. Currently, there seem to be a number of risk factors that are not included in the risk-adjustment techniques commonly used. This leaves the door open for health plans to invest in techniques that will identify potentially heavy health care users and avoid them. Such actions would reduce the effectiveness of market reforms.

15.3 MANAGED CARE

15.3.1 Introduction

Managed care is a system of health care insurance and delivery by which the payer attempts to exert direct influence over the economic behavior of the suppliers. Growth of managed care has been a central aspect of health care reform in the United States over the past three decades. In the 1970s, federal legislation endorsed and encouraged the growth of HMOs. Rapid growth of HMO membership occurred during the 1980s, along with the development of other types of managed care organization and the adoption by traditional insurers of some of the techniques of cost control that had been introduced by HMOs. By the 1990s, managed care was a major part of the health care delivery system as well as an important segment of financial markets. A "backlash" began to develop as state and federal governments became aware of growing concerns about quality of care and restriction of consumer choice in the managed care context.

Integration of the insurance function with the health care delivery function in one organization changes incentives for use of resources. Under traditional insurance and fee-for-service medical practice, the providers have little reason to be concerned with the cost consequences of their treatment decisions because the payers bear all the risks of the providers' actions. A managed care organization receives prepayment for members' health care, and since its surplus is the difference between the prepaid amount and the amount spent on health care, it has a clear incentive to provide care as inexpensively as possible. HMOs were initially seen as a possible means of enhancing two types of economic efficiency. Improvements in productive efficiency could result from using different combinations of inputs to produce a given output level (e.g., the substitution of nonphysician providers of care for physicians and the substitution of outpatient treatment for hospitalization). Greater allocative efficiency could result from more careful weighing of the marginal health benefits against the marginal costs of particular treatments. Further, competition among HMOs and between HMOs and traditional insurers had the potential of reducing health care costs through price competition. In addition it was anticipated that HMOs would shift the emphasis from short-term acute care for sickness to prevention and long-term health maintenance. This section reviews some of the economic issues associated with the development of managed care

15.3.2 Types of Managed Care Organization

All managed care organizations employ some form of prepayment and some degree of integration of financial risk bearing with health care delivery. All contract to provide fairly comprehensive health services to members in exchange for an annual premium and often small copayments. However, they differ importantly in their relationships with the health care providers and in the arrangements for dispensing care. The "tightest" type of plan, in terms of ability to control provider decision making, is the staff model HMO, in which physicians are employees of the HMO. A group model HMO is similar, except that the health plan and the physician group are separate legal entities. Usually HMO members make up all or a great majority of the physician group's practice, and the plan and the physician group are in fact managed jointly in many respects. Members of a staff model or group model HMO receive care at one of the HMO's medical office locations, which typically have a number of primary care providers and often some specialty care providers under one roof.

An independent practice association (IPA) type of HMO provides a contrast in several respects. In an IPA, the physicians practice in their own offices as solo practitioners or small groups. The health plan contracts with the physicians to provide care for HMO members. Members of the HMO typically would account for only a small proportion of any physician's practice. Indeed, the physician might well be a provider for several different HMOs. Compared with a staff or group model HMO, an IPA usually offers members a larger number of providers and a larger number of office locations among which to choose from.

A preferred provider organization (PPO) is an arrangement whereby the insurer designates a selected list of providers, including physicians and hospitals. If a patient seeks care from a provider on the list, the insurance coverage will be extensive, with a small or zero copayment. A patient may choose, however, to seek treatment from providers not on the list. In that case, there will still be some insurance coverage but the patient will bear a larger share of the cost.

As the industry evolves, there have grown up various mixed models. The term *network model* is often applied to these. For example, an HMO might offer care through its own health centers but also from a list of physicians in the community. Increasingly popular in HMO contracts is a point-of-service (POS) provision. This provision enables the HMO member to seek care from providers other than the HMO providers but at greater cost. The growth in membership in the various types of managed care organization is summarized in Table 15–2.

Table 15–2 Enrollment in HMOs by model type, 1987, 1990, 1997

Date	Total Enrollment (millions)	Staff Model	Group Model	IPA	Network	Mixed Model
December, 1986	25.8	11.6%	26.5%	38.6%	23.3%	0
January, 1990	32.6	12.2%	28.5%	41.0%	17.8%	0.5%
January 1993	38.7	5.8%	25.1%	40.6%	9.2%	19.3%
January, 1997	58.8	1.4%	14.3%	40.1%	4.9%	39.0%

Source: The Interstudy HMO Trend Report 1987–1997 (Bloomington, Minnesota, 1998), pp. 38–39.

15.3.3 Control of Resource Use

While it is clear that the overall incentive for a managed care organization is to minimize costs, the specific ways it is done make a large difference in terms of the public and political acceptance of this type of organization. Proponents of managed care point to the elimination of unnecessary or low marginal benefit care, the selection of more cost-effective treatment approaches, the encouragement of wellness, and increased access to care through elimination of financial barriers. Critics note the lack of choice of provider and fear that the cost incentives can lead to lower quality care through the elimination or restriction of necessary treatments. We do not take a position in this controversy here but rather describe below some of the factors influencing costs and how they might operate in a managed care environment.

Incentives on both physicians and patients are both relevant. The initial decision to seek care is a patient decision. Specific treatment choices require both physician recommendation and patient consent. Decisions with major resource use implications, such as hospitalization or surgery, are complex, and the physician is the major decision maker.

The method of physician compensation plays an important role and is best viewed in an agency context. Under fee-for-service compensation, the physician earns more by using more resources. This type of compensation can lead to supplier-induced demand and treatments of low marginal benefit. While some managed care organizations (typically IPAs or PPOs) do use it, alternative forms of compensation are common. One is to provide a straight salary. Under salary compensation, a physician's income is not affected by treatment choices made. Capitation is another alternative. Under this scheme, a physician receives a certain sum per assigned patient irrespective of what services are provided to the patient. An extreme form of capitation would pay a primary care physician a certain sum per patient and make him or her financially responsible for all care the patient receives during the time period, including specialty or hospital care. This provides a very strong incentive to limit the care provided and puts the physician at great financial risk if a patient should need treatment for catastrophic illness. The risk is somewhat mitigated if the capitation payment goes to a physician group rather than individual providers, and capitation of this type is often used to pay the physician group in a group model HMO. Individual providers in the group could then be compensated by salary, fees for service, or some other method. Different combinations of compensation schemes are also in use. For example, physicians in an HMO might be paid fees in return for services but have a certain portion of the fees held back by the HMO until the end of the financial year, at which time an amount would be returned to the physician based on the HMO's surplus. Or salary payment could be supplemented by a year-end bonus related to the HMO's financial results.

Under a typical traditional insurance plan, copayments and deductibles to some extent deter utilization of services. For some types of services (e.g., preventive services), coverage may not be included at all, and patients would have to pay the full cost. Managed care tends to rely less on financial incentives to limit utilization and more on administrative arrangements. Such arrangements are particularly important for influencing the use of specialized referral services. In contrast to traditional insurance, where a patient can self-refer to a specialist, many managed care plans will have the primary care provider play a "gatekeeper" role. That is, a referral to a specialist must be authorized by the member's primary care provider in order for the expense to be covered by the HMO. The referral may be limited to a small number of visits to the specialist, after which time the patient care responsibility would return to the primary care provider. Concurrent utilization review for hospitalized patients is another example of a managed care strategy that has the potential to influence utilization more than the relatively laissez faire role of the traditional insurer.

15.3.4 Empirical Evidence: Resource Use, Quality of Care, and Satisfaction

There has been considerable empirical research comparing managed care to traditional insurance over the past 25 years. The subject of study has been something of a "moving target," however. New types of managed care organization have emerged that mix features of the "pure" HMO model with elements of a fee-for-service system, and traditional insurers have adopted methods to influence the delivery of care, methods that have undoubtedly had an effect on economic performance. So it must be kept in mind that we are observing a rapidly evolving industry and that research findings can easily become outdated. Nevertheless, with that caveat we provide below a selective review of some of the findings.

The comparison of care under HMOs to that under traditional insurance has faced substantial methodological challenges. Much early research involved statistical comparisons of hospital admission rates, hospital lengths of stay, or the use of particular expensive procedures between members of an HMO and those of a comparison group with traditional insurance. (For a detailed review, see Luft 1978, Luft 1980.) It was clear in a preponderance of these studies that HMO members seemed to use fewer resources than the comparison group. What was less clear was whether the comparisons were valid in the face of possible selection bias. There was reason to believe that people joining HMOs were different from, and healthier than, the population of people with traditional insurance. If that was the case, it would not be possible to conclude that the observed differences in resource utilization represented greater efficiency.

One way to deal with selection bias in research is to eliminate it through random selection (i.e., to use an experimental study design where people are assigned at random to different types of insurance coverage). This was in fact done in the RAND Health Insurance Study undertaken in the years 1976–1981 in Seattle. The researchers assigned some people to an HMO and others to a variety of fee-for-service insurance plans with different coinsurance rates. They then observed use of health care resources. In the comparison that would best show the HMO effect (i.e., between the HMO group and the traditional insurance with no copayment), there was a clear difference in resource use. Annual hospital admissions (per 100 people) were 8.4 in the HMO group, compared with 13.8 in the traditional insurance group. Annual hospital days (per 100 people) totaled 49 in the HMO group and 83 in the traditional insurance group (Manning et at. 1984).

In a comprehensive literature review covering 37 studies published between 1993 and 1997 comparing managed care and non-managed-care groups, Miller and Luft (1997) found a mixed picture of differences in resource use. HMO hospital use was less than non-managed-care groups in some studies, but about an equal number of studies showed the opposite result. The four studies that looked at specific costly procedures all found somewhat lower use of such procedures in HMOs. Three of the five studies that examined total spending showed that HMOs spent significantly less, with the other two studies finding no such difference.

Quality of care is another dimension along which managed care and nonmanaged care may differ. One could hypothesize a priori that a difference in quality might occur in either direction. Economic incentives to limit resource use could lead HMOs to cut corners, which would lead to a deterioration in quality. On the other hand, lack of financial barriers to early treatment and emphasis on wellness could lead to higher quality in the managed care setting. Studies that have investigated the issue empirically have usually focused on one or two specific diseases or patient groups and used clinical measures of outcome (e.g., risk of dying for ICU patients or blood pressure for hypertensive patients). In the Miller and Luft review, 15 studies examined the quality issue, and the results varied widely: many studies found no significant difference, and about as many found higher quality in HMOs as found lower quality. According to Miller and Luft, "The results show something that is simple, obvious and yet sometimes underemphasized: HMOs produce better, the same, and worse quality of care, depending on the particular organization and particular disease" (p. 15).

Enrollee satisfaction as measured by survey responses has also been a subject of research. The preponderance of the evidence on this issue in the studies reviewed by Miller and Luft showed a somewhat lower level of overall satisfaction among HMO members than those in fee-for-service plans. When the survey questions were broken down into satisfaction with financial aspects and nonfinancial aspects, however, people in HMOs were more satisfied with financial aspects while the reverse was true for nonfinancial aspects.

In a large statistical study, Reschovsky and colleagues (1999) provided new evidence regarding differences between HMOs and nonmanaged care. Unlike most of the studies reviewed by Miller and Luft, which used data from a relatively small number of people in a few plans in one location, the data from this later study came from a large national sample ($N = 60,446$) of people who were interviewed by telephone during 1996 and 1997. The study also is noteworthy in that it examined differences for particularly vulnerable population subgroups (e.g., low-income people, children, racial subgroups, and chronically ill people). The major findings of that study were summarized by the authors as follows (Kemper et al. 1999, pp. 419–420):

- Enrollees in HMOs differ from those not in HMOs but not with respect to health status.
- HMOs provide more primary and preventive care.
- HMOs use less specialist care, but the study did not find evidence of less use of other types of costly care.
- HMOs reduce financial barriers to care but increase provider access problems and organizational barriers.
- Patients assess HMO care as worse than care under non-HMO insurance.
- The study found no consistent evidence that HMO effects differ for vulnerable subgroups.

As is evident from the above, it is hard to generalize about the effects of managed care. Some of the early findings on resource savings attributable to managed care have not held up in the later work. It is also apparent that the worst fears of HMO critics about quality effects are not borne out by research findings. Not all of the possible economic effects of managed care can be captured by the type of study that compares individual managed care organizations to traditional insurance plans, however. HMOs in a market may affect the economic behavior of other market participants and change the nature of competition. We turn to that issue in the next section.

15.3.5 Managed Care in the Market

The entry of new participants into a market can change the structure of the market and the nature of buyer-seller interactions in it. The specific nature of the change will depend, of course, on what the market structure and conduct was like before the entry of the new participants. Managed care represents vertical integration of insurance with medical care and thus has possible effects on two types of market, the market for health insurance and the market for medical care. We consider each of these markets in turn.

In the early years of HMO growth (the 1970s and 1980s), the major issue and subject of research was the effect of HMO market entry on traditional insurers. In a simple theoretical model, entry of new sellers to the insurance market would be expected to shift the supply curve outward and result in lower prices. Particularly if preentry market power was held by the established firms, one would expect price competition to drive prices down. If the entrants had lower costs than established firms, this would have further downward effects on price as established firms imitated the lower cost technology and competition forced prices to reflect marginal costs.

This scenario does not accurately reflect the effects of initial HMO entry into insurance markets in several respects, however. In markets with the possibility of nonprice competition, the rivalry among firms may not take the form of price competition, in which case lower costs and prices would not result. Much of the rivalry between HMOs and traditional insurers was not based on price but rather on product differentiation (McLaughlin 1988). HMOs priced their products somewhat below the traditional insurers and did not fully exploit their cost advantage to lower prices further; instead they offered a more comprehensive benefits package and lower cost sharing. As a consequence, there was considerable pressure on established health insurers to adopt organizational and product innovations, such as expanded benefits packages and utilization review techniques to control costs. (For a review of the early literature, see Frank and Welch 1985.)

As HMOs grew into significant market participants, the focus of research shifted to the effects of managed care on medical care markets. An HMO enters medical care markets as a buyer of services, including hospital and physician services. If the buyer side of these markets was initially competitive (i.e., there were many small buyers), the entry of an HMO as a big buyer would introduce monopsony power. Theory here predicts a downward pressure on price as well as a lower quantity of output. Managed care effects on hospital costs might come from two directions. First, managed care organizations might simply decrease the use of hospital care, substituting outpatient for inpatient care or reducing lengths of stay through administrative techniques like utilization review. Second, they might engage in selective contracting (i.e., directing patients to less expensive and more efficient hospitals).

A number of studies using different research methodologies have explored the relationship between managed care and hospital use and found significant effects. One approach is to examine the relationship between HMO penetration in a market and the rate of hospital cost inflation. One such study, based on California data, examined cost per admission for 298 hospitals during the years 1982–1988. It found that growth in costs per admission was 9.4 percent lower in markets with high HMO penetration than in markets with low HMO penetration (Robinson 1991). Another study (Feldman et al. 1990) estimated demand for hospital admissions by six HMOs in four metropolitan areas. The researchers found that the HMO demand was sensitive to hospital price, with the elasticity for staff-network model HMOs being much greater than that for IPAs. A third study took advantage of a "natural experiment" to examine the effect of a change in benefits for Wisconsin state employees. The change made HMO membership a very attractive choice, and as a result the percentage of state employees enrolled in HMOs grew sharply during the years 1983–1993. Hill and Wolfe (1997) examined the changes in hospital resources that took place over that time period in Madison, Wisconsin, where the state is a very large employer, and they found large decreases in resource use. Finally, two studies by Wholey and coworkers (1995, 1997) examined both HMO penetration and number of HMOs in a market and found that hospital use and premiums were lower where the market was more competitive. This effect was more evident for group model HMOs than for IPAs.

Another type of medical care market where changes might result from the increased presence of HMOs is the market for specialized, expensive, high-technology services. Some empirical studies have found evidence that managed care has decreased the demand for such services, while others have failed to find this effect. The Wisconsin study noted above (Hill and Wolfe 1997) examined two services that required expensive capital equipment, magnetic resonance imaging (MRI) and lithotripsy, a method of treating kidney stones. They noted that after the increase in HMO enrollment, area hospitals were much more likely to obtain the necessary equipment jointly, whereas prior to 1983 the pattern was for individual hospitals to acquire them independently. However, Madison was not much different than comparison cities in the proportion of hospitals with selected high-technology facilities. A study of the growth of an innovative surgical procedure, laparoscopic cholecystectomy, found no difference between HMO enrollees and the general fee-for-service population in the use of this technology (Chernew et al. 1997). One possible effect on market structure results from the pressures of selective contracting by managed care organizations. If HMOs search for the low-cost providers and channel business to them, there is a powerful incentive for providers to seek out and realize economies of scale. A study of mammography found just such a result. HMO market share was associated with consolidation among mammography providers and reductions in cost for mammography services (Baker and Brown 1999).

15.4 INFORMATION AND CONSUMER CHOICE

In a well-functioning competitive market, the principle of "consumer sovereignty" prevails (i.e., the products to be produced are determined by consumer preferences, and appropriate incentives are in place for economic efficiency to be achieved). This market result, however, depends on consumers having adequate information about prices and product characteristics to be able to choose wisely among alternatives. If market-oriented reforms in health care, particularly managed care, are to be effective, potential buyers must be able to assess the characteristics of managed care products. During the period when managed care was experiencing rapid growth, the technology used for developing and disseminating statistical information also advanced greatly. The combination of these changes resulted in a number of initiatives designed to make information about health care organizations more available to consumers with the goal of improving their decision making and at the same time improving market outcomes. This section reviews some of those developments and the issues they raise.

The characteristic of health care organization performance that is perhaps most difficult for consumers to understand is quality, so not surprisingly that characteristic has received the most attention. A number of reporting or rating systems have been introduced that attempt to define quality in a measurable way, develop statistical information about the quality of specific health care organizations, and disseminate that information widely to consumers and employers, often in the form of "report cards." Some of these efforts have been by government agencies while others have taken place in the private sector. Ratings or reports have been developed for health care providers such as hospitals or individual physicians as well as for managed care organizations.

One of the earliest attempts to report widely on hospital performance was the dissemination by HCFA, beginning in 1986, of hospital mortality rates for all hospitals in the United States. These annual reports provided for each hospital the actual mortality rate of Medicare patients as well as that predicted statistically based on characteristics of the admitted patients. Frequently the performance of a particular hospital was the subject of local media attention if it appeared to have an unusually low or high mortality rate compared with other hospitals. The reporting program gave rise to a great deal of controversy and was ended in 1992. Several aspects of the controversy are of continuing interest, since they apply to other similar programs.

First, critics questioned whether the statistical methodology used was adequate to adjust for severity of illness. Certainly hospitals with sicker patients would be expected to have more deaths, so a higher mortality rate in such hospitals would not be indicative of a quality difference but rather a case-mix difference. Indeed, it may be that higher quality hospitals attract the sickest and most difficult to treat patients and have higher mortality rates for that reason. Second, there is a question as to whether it makes sense to consider the hospital's patient population as a whole or whether the analysis should be conducted for individual patient groups. For example, a hospital may be very successful at treating cardiac surgery patients but have less than average success treating cancer patients. An overall assessment would miss these important details. Third, administrative data may not capture clinical information accurately. There may be data errors that occur in the transition from a patient chart to a hospital information system. Moreover, administrative data sets developed mostly for financial or operational purposes may not reflect fully the clinical complexity of a patient's illness and treatment. Finally, of course, there is the question of whether the information provided actually influences the choices of consumers and health care providers. One careful statistical study of the HCFA experience found only very slight evidence of a relationship between the ratings of hospitals and changes in the numbers of patients who used them (Mennemeyer et al. 1997).

Performance measurement and reporting on managed care organizations has been largely a private sector activity. Several different organizations are involved in this field, but the major one is the National Committee for Quality Assurance (NCQA),a private not-for-profit organization that has been reporting on and accrediting managed care organizations since 1991. NCQA was formed initially with the participation of a group of large employers who were concerned about the cost and quality of health care and who believed that a standardized system for evaluating HMOs would help them make better purchasing decisions when administering their employee health benefits. Although NCQA accreditation is voluntary for HMOs, as of 2000 about half of all HMOs in the United States (with enrollments totaling about three-quarters of all HMO members) were accredited by NCQA or seeking accreditation.

Accreditation is different from, although closely related to, performance measurement. NCQA is also the organization that manages the evolution of a major data set for assessing health plan performance. The Health Plan Employer Data and Information Set (HEDIS) includes more than 50 statistical measures of a managed care organization's performance, including survey information on member satisfaction as well as measures based on clinical data on the treatment of specific diseases, such as heart disease, cancer, and diabetes. The goal is to provide a common measure that can be used by purchasers to compare health plans. HEDIS data are often used as the basis for health plan "report cards" made available to consumers by employers and publicized in the media.

Although much effort has gone into the developing systems for analyzing health plan performance, creating statistical reports on performance, and disseminating these reports, the actual effect of these activities is as yet unclear. From an economic standpoint, the important question is whether actual market decisions are made using such information. It is important to recall here that the health plan enrollment decision is really a two-stage process: first, the employer decides to offer particular plans to its workers as choices, and, second, each employee chooses a particular plan from among those in the benefits package. It is reasonable to think that an employer's decision to include a plan in the benefits package would be influenced by performance data, at least in the case of a large employer with sophisticated benefits administrators who have the time and expertise to evaluate the data. Whether smaller employers and individual consumers have the ability and incentive to use such information is less evident. Furthermore, it is hard to know whether the variables chosen by "experts" as measures of plan performance are really what individual consumers care about. One study that examined the influence of HEDIS data on the choices of workers of one large firm found a very weak response to the data in terms of actual plan choice. The researchers suggested that personal experience and word-of-mouth may be more important determinants of individual choices (Scanlon and Chernew 1999). However, the use of performance data is too new for there to be enough evidence for a clear conclusion. This area is an important one for future research.

EXERCISES

1. Explain the relationship between information asymmetry and health insurance market failure.

2. Give an example of a health insurance market outcome that is efficient but not acceptable for reasons of equity. Describe a policy to address it.
3. Explain why individual or small-group insurance tends to be more expensive than large-group insurance.
4. Explain the relationship between community rating and economic efficiency.
5. Give two reasons why a person may lack health insurance, one where an economic efficiency issue is involved and one where no such issue arises.
6. Distinguish between a staff or group model HMO, an IPA, and a PPO with regard to the provider choices and out-of-pocket costs for members.
7. Contrast the incentives for resource use faced by a physician under a salary, under fee-for-service compensation, and under capitation.
8. Explain the problem presented by selection bias for research on the effects of HMOs.
9. Describe the types of effects that the entry of managed care organizations into a market can have on other types of insurance providers.
10. Describe the types of effects that the entry of managed care organizations into a market can have on other types of medical care providers.

BIBLIOGRAPHY

Insurance Market Reform

Abraham, K.S. 1985. Efficiency and fairness in insurance risk selection. *Virginia Law Review* 71:403–451.

Blendon, R.J., et al. 1992. Making the critical choices. *JAMA* 267:2509–2520.

Browne, M.J., and H. Doerpinghaus. 1994–1995. Asymmetric information and the demand for Medigap insurance. *Inquiry* 31:445–450.

Butler, S.M. 1991. A tax reform strategy to deal with the uninsured. *JAMA* 265:2541–2544.

Dranove, D., et al. 1993. Price and concentration in hospital markets: The switch from patient driven to payer driven competition. *Journal of Law and Economics* 36:179–204.

Dranove, D., et al. 1998. Determinants of managed care penetration. *Journal of Health Economics* 17:729–745.

Davis, K. 1991. Expanding Medicare and employer plans to achieve universal health insurance. *JAMA* 265:2525–2528.

Enthoven, A.C. 1993. The history and principles of managed competition. *Health Affairs* 12 (suppl.):24–48.

Enthoven, A.C., and R. Kronick. 1989. A consumer choice health plan for the 1990s. Parts 1, 2. *New England Journal of Medicine* 320:29–37, 94–101.

———. 1991. Universal health insurance through incentives reform. *JAMA* 265:2532–2536.

Flynn, P., et al. 1997. State health reform: Effects on labor markets and economic activity. *Journal of Policy Analysis and Management* 16:219–236.

Giacomini, M., et al. 1995. Risk adjusting community rated health plan premiums. *Annual Review of Public Health* 16:401–430.

Grumbach, K., et al. 1991. Liberal benefits, conservative spending. *JAMA* 265:2549–2554.

Hall, M.A. 1994. *Reforming private health insurance.* Washington, DC: American Enterprise Institute.

Holahan, J., et al. 1991. An American approach to health system reform. *JAMA* 265:2537–2540.

Light, D.W. 1992. The practice and ethics of risk rated health insurance. *JAMA* 267:2503–2508.

Luft, H.S. 1978. How do health maintenance organizations achieve their savings? *New England Journal of Medicine* 298:1336–1343.

———. 1980. Assessing the evidence on HMO performance. *Milbank Memorial Fund Quarterly* 58:501–536.

Pauly, M.V. 1990. The rational nonpurchase of long-term-care insurance. *Journal of Political Economy* 98:153–168.

Pauly, M.V., et al. 1991. A plan for "responsible national health insurance." *Health Affairs* 10, no. 1:5–25.

Reinhardt, U.E. 1993a. An "all-American" health reform proposal. *Journal of American Health Policy* 3, no. 3:11–17.

———. 1993b. Reorganizing the financial flows in American health care. *Health Affairs* 12 (suppl.): 173–193.

Rice, T., et al. 1993. Holes in the Jackson Hole approach to health care reform. *JAMA* 270:1357–1362.

Selden, T.M. 1999. Premium subsidies for health insurance: Excess coverage vs. adverse selection. *Journal of Health Economics* 18:709–725.

Summers, L.H. 1989. Some simple economics of mandated benefits. *American Economic Review* 79 (suppl.): 177–183.

Thomas, K. 1994–1995. Are subsidies enough to encourage the uninsured to purchase health insurance? *Inquiry* 31:415–424.

Thorpe, K.E. 1992. Expanding employment-based health insurance: Is small group reform the answer? *Inquiry* 29:128–136.

Thorpe, K.E., et al. 1992. Reducing the number of uninsured by subsidizing employment-based health insurance. *JAMA* 267:945–948.

Zabinski, D., et al. Medical savings accounts: Microsimulation results from a model with adverse selection. *Journal of Health Economics* 18:195–218.

Managed Care

Baker, L.C. and M.L. Brown, 1999. Managed care, consolidation among health care providers, and health care: Evidence from mammography. *RAND Journal of Economics* 30:351–374.

Chernew, M., et al. 1997. Managed care and medical technology: Implications for cost growth. *Health Affairs* 16, no. 2:196–209.

Feldman, R., et al. 1990. Effects of MHMs on the creation of competitive markets for hospital services. *Journal of Health Economics* 9:207–222.

Frank, R.G., and W.P. Welch. 1985. The competitive effects of HMOs: A review of the evidence. *Inquiry* 22:148–161.

Hellerstein, J.K. 1998. Public funds, private funds, and medical innovation: How managed care affects public funds for clinical research. *American Economic Review* 88, no. 2:112–116.

Hill, S.C., and B.L. Wolfe. 1997. Testing the HMO competitive strategy: An analysis of its impact on medical care resources. *Journal of Health Economics* 16:261–286.

Kemper, P., et al. 1999. Do HMOs make a difference? Summary and implications. *Inquiry* 36:419–425.

Lake, T. 1999. Do HMOs make a difference? Consumer assessments of health care. *Inquiry* 36:411–418.

Manning, W.G., et al. 1984. A controlled trial of the effect of a prepaid group practice on use of services. *New England Journal of Medicine* 310:1505–1510.

McLaughlin, C.G. 1988. Market responses to HMOs: Price competition or rivalry? *Inquiry* 25:207–218.

Miller, R.H., and H.S. Luft. 1997. Does managed care lead to better or worse quality of care? *Health Affairs* 16, no. 5:7–25.

Newhouse, J.P. 1996. Health reform in the United States. *Economic Journal* 106:1713–1724.

Reschovsky, J.D. 1999a. Do HMOs make a difference? Access to health care. *Inquiry* 36:390–399.

———. 1999b. Do HMOs make a difference? Data and methods. *Inquiry* 36:378–389.

Reschovsky, J.D., and P. Kemper. 1999. Do HMOs make a difference? Introduction. *Inquiry* 36:374–377.

Robinson, J.C. 1991. HMO market penetration and hospital cost inflation in California. *JAMA* 266:2719–2725.

Tu, H.T., et al. 1999. Do HMOs make a difference? Use of health services. *Inquiry* 36:400–410.

Wholey, D., et al. 1995. The effect of market structure on HMO premiums. *Journal of Health Economics* 14:81–105.

Wholey, D., et al. 1997. HMO market structure and performance, 1985–1995. *Health Affairs* 16, no. 6:75–84.

Consumer Information

Epstein A.M. 1998. Rolling down the runway: The challenges ahead for quality report cards. *JAMA* 279:1691–1696.

Hannon, E.L., et al. 1992. Clinical versus administrative data bases for CABG surgery: Does it matter? *Medical Care* 30:892–907.

Hirth, R.A. 1999. Consumer information and competition between nonprofit and for-profit nursing homes. *Journal of Health Economics* 18:219–240.

Iezzoni, L.I., et al. 1996. Judging hospitals by severity-adjusted mortality rates: The influence of the severity-adjustment method. *American Journal of Public Health* 86:1379–1387.

Knutson, D.J., et al. 1998. Impact of report cards on employees: A natural experiment. *Health Care Financing Review* 20, no. 1:5–27.

Luft, H.S., et al. 1990. Does quality influence choice of hospital? *JAMA* 263:2899–2906.

Mennemeyer, S.T., et al. 1997. Death and reputation: How consumers acted upon HCFA mortality information. *Inquiry* 34:117–128.

Scanlon, D.P., and M. Chernew. 1999. HEDIS measures and managed care enrollment. *Medical Care Research and Review* 56 (suppl. 2):60–84.

Spoeri R.K., and R. Ullman. 1997. Measuring and reporting managed care performance: Lessons learned and new initiatives *Annals of Internal Medicine* 127:726–732.

Chapter 16

Regulation and Antitrust Policy in Health Care

Ronald P. Wilder

1. Define regulation.
2. Describe two different views on why governments regulate markets.
3. Describe the variables that regulators focus on when regulating health care.
4. Identify the regulatory means that are used by regulators of hospitals, physicians, drugs, health care insurance, and managed care.
5. Explain the rationale for antitrust policy.
6. Describe market changes that have taken place in health care and explain how these might affect antitrust enforcement.
7. Describe the key provisions of antitrust legislation in the United States.
8. Explain how antitrust legislation regulates price fixing.
9. Explain how antitrust legislation regulates mergers.
10. Explain how quality issues in health care affect antitrust policy.

16.1 INTRODUCTION

The regulation of markets takes three general forms. *Direct regulation* refers to intervention in markets by regulatory agencies to control price, quantity, or quality by direct action, such as instituting price controls, establishing professional licensure requirements, or assessing and regulating the quality of services. *Indirect regulation* refers to regulatory activities that affect price, quantity or quality by enforcing the competitive behavior of firms in the market or by changing the structure of the market. Antitrust policy is the leading example of indirect regulation. Governments also intervene in markets through *public ownership* and operation of health care facilities and services (Santerre and Neun 1996). The use of the term *regulation* in this chapter will generally refer to direct regulation. The chapter will focus on regulation of private sector health care providers in the United States and thus will not address public ownership, which is more common in other nations.

16.1.1 The Concept of Economic Regulation

Economic systems based on competitive markets and private enterprise are characteristic of most of the nations of the world, including the United States. In private enterprise systems, scarce resources are allocated and income is distributed primarily on the basis of supply and demand in markets and the resulting price, income, and profitability signals. In these systems, largely unrestricted free markets are the principal determinants of economic outcomes. Under conditions of perfect competition and complete information, the economic outcome meets the social welfare standards of Pareto optimality. In other words, changes in the allocation of resources could not improve the welfare of some members of society without reducing the welfare of other members of society.

In some instances, including health care, the market outcomes may be viewed as suboptimal by society at large. Situations in which a market's price, quantity, or product quality does not meet social welfare norms are said by economists to be cases of market failure. One form of market failure occurs when prices in a market are above marginal costs as a result of monopoly power. Another type occurs when the external effects of the production or consumption of a product, such as pollution, are not captured in the product's price, creating a wedge between the price and social costs of the product. A third form, especially important for health care markets, results from imperfect information. In a market with a low level of information, consumers find it difficult to evaluate the quality of goods and services and to make decisions regarding whether or not to purchase the goods and services.

Economic regulation consists of governmental interventions intended to affect market outcomes in some manner. There are two different views of why economic regulation exists. According to the first view, economic regulation is generally motivated by the objective of reducing the extent of market failure. According to the second view, it is the result of producers or consumers working through the political process to further their own interests.

16.1.2 Regulation of Health Care

The regulation of health care in the United States and Canada is extensive. Much of this activity is directed toward information and quality issues. Quality-of-care regulation frequently takes the form of control of entry into the market, such as by requiring that health care professionals be licensed ant that new drugs be approved by a regulatory agency. Entry by hospitals is also commonly regulated through policy instruments such as the certificate of need, which gives permission to a health care firm to develop the infrastructure to provide care to specific populations. The regulation of price in health care is generally carried out indirectly through antitrust policy and through the effects of government reimbursement rules on the prices of health care services.

16.1.3 Regulation as a Means of Correcting Market Failure

Health care markets are characterized by imperfect information on the price and quality of health care services. The problem of inadequate information can take a number of forms. Consumers tend to have incomplete information about the quality of health care services available from alternative providers and about the probability of a successful outcome for procedures that have a risky outcome. Consumers may also have incomplete information about price, since the out-of-pocket price to consumers may be the result of negotiations between providers and third-party payers.

Information can also be impaired as a result of relationships in which a principal delegates responsibility to an agent. One inherent difficulty with such relationships is that the agent possesses information not available to the principal (the person with ultimate authority) and may have different objectives than the principal. An example of an agency relationship is that between a physician and a patient. In health care, the physician is both a health care provider and an agent of the consumer. The physician's incentives in the provider role may not be aligned with the incentives of the consumer. This agency relationship between physician and consumer is complicated further by the relationship between the physician and the third-party payer or managed care organization, which also involves agency. This complex of relationships has led at least one writer to use the phrase "the doctor as double agent" (Blomqvist 1991).

Consumers may be handicapped by the lack of information about quality of health care services and about quality of alternative providers. Thus incomplete information may prevent socially optimal outcomes in health care markets. The agency relationships between a consumer and his or her physician and between the consumer and other providers may also lead to over- or underconsumption of health care services relative to the social optimum that would be realizable with complete information.

The direct regulation of health care providers, therefore, may be a response of governments to the perception that the consumer lacks information about quality and thus that the workings of competitive, private-enterprise health care markets may not produce the best outcomes in terms of social welfare. Another possibility, as mentioned above, is that regulation is fostered as a means for providers to further their private interests.

16.1.4 Regulation as a Political Good

George Stigler, in his seminal work on the economic theory of regulation (1971), supplemented by work by Peltzman (1976) and others, pointed out that regulatory legislation may redistribute wealth. This effect of regulation is important given that the behavior of legislators is likely to be motivated by their wish to remain in office. If there is competition between special interest groups in the democratic system, that competition may take the form of exchanges of political support for legislation favorable to the objectives of the interest groups. If the political process works in this manner, well-organized interest groups with a high per capita stake in the outcomes of legislation will tend to dominate larger interest groups with a smaller per capita stake.

The economic theory of regulation suggests that providers may be able to dominate the legislative and regulatory process. This suggestion is a hypothesis and not a conclusion of the economic theory of regulation. What are the actual health care-related outcomes of real-world legislative and regulatory processes is an empirical question. Very active lobbying activities are pursued by health care provider groups as well as health care consumer groups.

16.2 REGULATION OF HEALTH CARE

Regulation of health care takes the form of regulation of price, quantity (or utilization), and quality. Sometimes the quality objectives are achieved through control of entry, such as the licensure of physicians. In other instances, quality is regulated by the setting of technical standards, as in the regulation of pharmaceuticals. In the following sections, the regulation of hospitals and long-term care facilities, the regulation of physician services, and the regulation of pharmaceuticals are discussed separately. Indirect regulation through antitrust policy is considered subsequently.

16.2.1 Regulation of Hospitals and Long-Term Care Facilities

Community hospitals are the major providers of acute medical and surgical care. Many hospitals are nonprofit institutions, supported by government or by charitable organizations. In the United States, there has been an increase in the importance of for-profit hospitals during the past two decades. In addition, there has been a large number of hospital mergers as well as formal and informal vertical combinations between hospitals, insurance and managed care companies, and physicians groups (Gaynor and Haas-Wilson 1999).

Direct regulation of hospitals includes supply side measures such as certificate-of-need requirements for the entry of new hospitals or the addition of additional services. Demand side regulations include price controls imposed through the reimbursement practices of government programs such as Medicare and Medicaid. Price controls may also affect the supply side by motivating greater efficiency and reducing lengths of stay. Regulation of hospital service quality includes licensure, peer review, and utilization review.

16.2.2 Regulation of Hospital Quality

Hospitals are licensed by a state licensing agency, usually the state health department. The license requires that a minimum level of facilities and personnel be present. In addition to this direct regulation by state governments, hospitals participate in self-regulation by seeking accreditation from the Joint Commission on Accreditation of Healthcare Organizations (Joint Commission). As of the end of 2000, the Joint Commission accredits nearly 19,000 health care organizations and programs in the United States (Joint Commission 2000).

Hospital quality is also regulated by peer review organizations (PROs), which were established under the Tax Equity and Fiscal Responsibility Act (TEFRA) of 1982, an act that made numerous changes to Medicare. The Health Care Financing Administration (HCFA) administers the PRO program, which is designed "to monitor and improve utilization and quality of care for Medicare beneficiaries." There are 53 PROs, each responsible for a state, territory, or the District of Columbia. The PROs are independent contractors whose mission is to "ensure the quality, effectiveness, efficiency, and economy of health care services provided to Medicare beneficiaries" (Health Care Financing Administration 2000).

16.2.3 Supply Side Regulation of Hospitals

The peer review organizations, in addition to regulating quality, may also review utilization of care. Utilization deemed inappropriate would be denied reimbursement by HCFA. Since the advent of the prospective reimbursement system, however, the PROs have been more focused on quality of service than on excessive utilization.

Certificate-of-need regulation is a form of supply side regulation. Its stated purpose is to restrict the building of hospitals and the addition of major facilities in order to prevent duplication of facilities or excessive capital expenditures. Certificate-of-need regulation for hospitals played an extensive role during the 1970s and 1980s, but the federal requirement that states have certificate-of-need regulation ended in 1986. Since then, several states have ended certificate-of-need regulation for hospitals. A retrospective study of the consequences of ending certificate-of-need regulation found that such regulation had only a modest containing effect on hospital costs (Conover and Sloan 1998).

16.2.4 Demand Side Regulation of Hospitals

Hospital prices and charges are subject to extensive regulation. Rate regulation at the state level was widely practiced during the 1970s and 1980s but has since largely disappeared. Medicare's prospective payment system (PPS), established in the early 1980s, controls hospital charges nationwide, but for Medicare patients only. In addition to their direct effect on hospital charges, Medicare reimbursement rules may influence the charges paid by other payers, such as health insurance companies and HMOs.

Studies of the effectiveness of price regulation of hospitals have generally found that hospitals entered a new competitive era in the early 1980s, as Medicare's PPS, which paid providers prospectively based on diagnosis rather than retrospectively, tended to reduce days of stay and hospital occupancy rates and increase price competition among hospitals (Dranove et al. 1993). The increase in price competition was reinforced by the rapid development of managed care and the greater purchasing power of large payer groups.

16.2.5 Regulation of Long-Term Care Facilities

Long-term care in the United States is provided in nonprofit and for-profit nursing homes, which are regulated by state and federal agencies. Licensing is by state health departments. Nursing homes may also pursue self-regulation by seeking accreditation through the Joint Commission.

Nursing homes are regulated on the supply side by state certificate-of-need regulation that restricts construction and capacity increases. Certificate-of-need regulation was most important in the years directly after Medicare and Medicaid began to cover nursing home costs for some patients. It limited the expansion of nursing home providers and hence the financial burden on states, which finance Medicaid jointly with the federal government (Getzen 1997).

Whatever price regulation of nursing homes exists is primarily a result of the reimbursement systems used by Medicare and Medicaid. Medicaid, which covers the medically needy, generally pays a flat rate per day, although some states are moving to adopt a system in which reimbursement is based on the health status of the patient. Medicare covers skilled nursing services for a limited period of time after certain hospitalizations. Medicare, since the changes introduced by the 1997 Balanced Budget Amendments, uses a prospective payment system in which the daily rate depends on health status of the patient (Folland et al. 2001).

16.2.6 Regulation of Physician Services

Physicians play a central role in health care. They have total or partial control of hospital admissions, specialist referrals, and drug prescriptions. They also advise patients on the necessity or potential benefit of medical services. Traditionally, physicians were paid on a fee-for-service basis. Currently, 80–90 percent of physician fees are paid by third-party payers, who possess some control over price and utilization. Physicians are also subject to regulations intended to ensure high quality of care.

16.2.7 Regulation of Physician Quality and Utilization

The primary regulation of physician quality is through state licensure—the granting of licenses to practice medicine to those who meet specific criteria. Since state legislatures appoint state licensing boards with input from the state medical associations, licensing is a form of self-regulation.

Peer review organizations (PROs) monitor the utilization patterns and the professional quality of hospitals and physicians. In 1986, Congress enacted the Health Care Quality Improvement Act. This act provides legal protections to those participating in peer reviews by granting immunity from testifying in malpractice lawsuits. In addition, the act established the National Practitioner Data Base, which is an information clearinghouse that gathers information on malpractice judgments, disciplinary actions, and license suspensions and revocations. Scheutzow (1999) reviewed the practice of peer review organizations and concluded that, because of the failure to report incidents and other problems, the present peer review process is ineffective.

16.2.8 Regulation of Physician Pricing

Medicare and Medicaid reimburse physicians on a modified fee-for-service basis. In the early years of Medicare and Medicaid, fees were screened on the basis of usual, customary, and reasonable (UCR) payments. The UCR system included the range of fees charged by other physicians in the same geographic area. In 1992, Medicare began using a new method of physician payment. This method, which utilizes the Resource Based Relative Value Scale (RBRVS), includes components for physician time and skill, practice expenses, and professional liability insurance (Medicare Payment Advisory Commission 2000). The reimbursement rules amount to price controls on the services provided to patients covered by Medicare, and in fact they have an effect on the prices charged by managed care plans that insure large numbers of private patients.

16.2.9 Regulation of the Pharmaceutical Industry

The production of pharmaceuticals is regulated by the Food and Drug Administration. The distribution and dispensing of pharmaceuticals is regulated at the state level by the licensing of pharmacists and by requirements that apply to pharmacy operations. At the present time, the prices of pharmaceuticals are not directly controlled, but government agencies such as Medicaid and other large purchasers use their purchasing power to obtain lower prices than those paid by noninsured consumers. In some instances, lower prices are negotiated through the design of drug formularies, which are lists of drugs eligible for prescription under a managed care plan. In order to have a drug included on the formulary, the pharmaceutical manufacturer must agree to charge a discounted price (Abbott 1997).

16.2.10 Food and Drug Administration Regulation of Drugs

The U.S. Food and Drug Administration (FDA), founded in 1906, is one of the oldest federal regulatory agencies. Prior to 1962, the FDA regulated drugs for safety, although there existed a strong element of self-regulation. The 1962 Drug Amendments strengthened the FDA's regulation of drugs for safety and extended its focus to include effectiveness. The approval of a new drug requires extensive testing by the manufacturer and submission of drug studies to the FDA so that the agency can evaluate the drug and reach a judgment as to whether its benefits outweigh its risks. Most new drugs are initially approved as prescription medicines, which means their purchase requires a physician's authorization. The FDA also regulates generic drugs (which compete with brand-name products at the end of the life of drug patents) and over-the-counter drugs (those available without a prescription) (U.S. Food and Drug Administration 2000).

The competition from generic drugs was promoted by a 1984 law that greatly reduced the testing required of generics. Prior to 1984, generic producers were often required to perform tests for safety and effectiveness as part of the approval process. After 1984, they were required only to show the generics were bioequivalent to the name brands. This change promoted the entry of generics and led to lower prices within a relatively short period after patent expiration (Grabowski and Vernon 1992).

Patents on new drugs provide a monopoly position for a period of time that may extend beyond the 20-year standard for American patents (the possibility of extension is to allow for the considerable time required by the regulatory process). The patent right provides an incentive for manufacturers to develop and test new drugs. This incentive must be balanced against the length of time it takes to develop drugs and the risk of failure. The total time lag from the beginning of research and development of a new drug to bringing it to market may be 10 years, and the total development cost may run into the hundreds of millions of dollars. (Abbott 1997).

16.2.11 State Regulation of Pharmacists

In addition to their commercial role as sellers of drugs, pharmacists perform a professional role in monitoring prescriptions. State boards of pharmacy regulate registered pharmacists. In most states, the members of the state board are appointed by the governor, and registered pharmacists generally make up the majority of the members. The state boards regulate pharmacist quality through licensure and through requirements for continuing education. The increasing importance of mail-order pharmacies may restrict the ability of state boards to control the quality of dispensing within state boundaries (Conlan 1997).

16.2.12 Regulation of Health Insurance and Managed Care

In the United States, regulation of insurance is practiced at the state level. This federalist tradition means that state insurance commissions regulate private health insurance companies, both for-profit and nonprofit. The state insurance commissions have oversight control regarding entry and prices for commercial health insurance. Changes in health care markets during the past 25 years have increased competition in these markets. The growing tendency of large employers to self-insure and utilize third-party administrators is a significant trend (Frech, 1993). As a result of this trend, a larger portion of the market escapes regulation.

In fact, state regulators more and more have turned their attention to regulating the behavior of managed care organizations. During the last decade, many state legislatures enacted bills intended to influence the practices of these organizations. Among the provisions were some that placed restrictions on physician communication with patients, placed restrictions on lengths of hospital stay, and mandated the creation of external grievance processes for dissatisfied patients.

Federal legislation that would create a patient bill of rights has been under consideration but has not been enacted as of late 2001. This legislation would extend the federal role in the regulation of private health insurance, especially in regard to the right of patients to sue and the ability of managed care organizations to override the professional judgments of physicians (Pear 2000). Federal regulation of health insurance traditionally has been restricted mostly to Medicare and Medicaid, which are public health insurance programs. The Employee Retirement Income Security Act of 1974 (ERISA) preempts state law related to benefit plans, including health insurance plans, offered by employers. One effect of ERISA has been to free employer self-insured health plans from most state regulatory restrictions, thereby contributing both to the growth of employer-provided plans and to complaints about the lack of patient rights (Havighurst 2000).

16.3 ANTITRUST POLICY

16.3.1 Conceptual Framework

The economist's model of perfect competition is generally used as a benchmark in evaluating market outcomes. The perfectly competitive market, with large numbers of buyers and sellers, free entry and exit, and homogeneous products, yields a long-run competitive equilibrium in which all firms in the market are producing at minimum long-run average cost and in which price is equal to marginal cost. This market equilibrium yields both technical efficiency and economic efficiency. (*Technical efficiency* refers to the tendency of firms in a market to produce goods and services at the minimum long-run average cost, a result of the price competition among firms and of the relatively small scale of each firm in comparison to market demand. *Economic efficiency* refers to the equality of price and marginal cost, which suggests that the allocation of resources could not be improved in a perfectly competitive world by moving resources from their present use to a different one. See Chapter 12 for an exposition of these concepts.)

A second benchmark in examining market outcomes is found in the monopoly market model. In this market structure, because there is a single seller with blocked entry, long-run market equilibrium may yield a price greater than marginal cost. If the monopolist is a profit maximizer, productive efficiency is still achieved (in the sense that average cost is at the lowest level possible given the monopolist's choice of output). The monopolist, however, may not produce at the lowest average cost possible independent of the rate of output selected.

Monopoly markets also raise the possibility of shifts in the distribution of income as compared with a perfectly competitive organization of the market. Under restrictive assumptions, a competitive market in long-run equilibrium that is transformed into a monopoly market as a result of cartelization or merger would be changed in the way shown in Figure 16–1. Total market output would decline from Q_c to Q_m as a result of monopolization. The corresponding equilibrium price would increase from P_c to P_m. Monopoly profits would appear in the amount shown by the area ABDE, while the consumer surplus would decrease from the amount reflected by the area FCD under perfect competition to the area FAE under monopoly. The consumer surplus is the difference between the sum of the marginal valuations over all quantities of the service and the prices paid over all quantities. It is a reflection of the welfare gains made by the consumer from purchasing the product. The difference between these two levels of consumer surplus, measured by the area ABC, is traditionally called the *deadweight loss due to monopoly*.

In sum, the adverse affects of monopoly market structures are related directly to the reduction in market output from Q_c to Q_m. The reduced market output causes redistribution between consumers and producers as well as allocative effects in the form of deadweight loss.

Many real-world markets, including most health care markets, are structured as oligopoly markets. Paucity of sellers and generally large numbers of buyers characterize oligopoly markets. Some health care markets are oligopolies on both sides of the market (i.e., both buyers and sellers are few in number). Economic models of

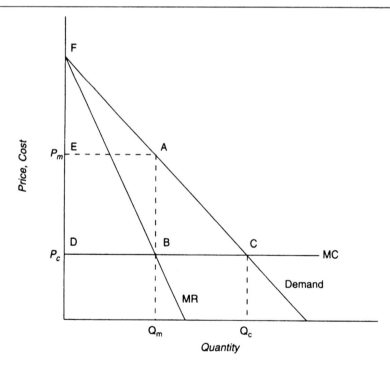

Figure 16–1 Economic analysis of monopolization effects. Under perfect competition, the price is P_c and the quantity is Q_c. Under monopoly, the price is P_m and the quantity is Q_m. Competition yields no monopoly profits and a consumer surplus of *FCD*. Monopoly yields monopoly profits of *EABD* and a consumer surplus of *FAE*.

markets structured as oligopolies tend not to yield general predictions about market outcome. Depending on whether sellers attempt to engage in price collusion and, if not, how they react to one another's price changes, the outcome in oligopoly markets may cover the entire outcome range from monopoly on one extreme to perfect competition on the other.

Antitrust policy economic analysis has traditionally made an attempt to analytically define the boundaries of product markets and geographic markets and to consider whether the structure of markets so defined is close enough to a monopoly structure to suspect that performance in these markets is adversely affected. This approach is reflected, for example, in the merger guidelines that have been developed over the past 25 years by the U.S. Department of Justice and the Federal Trade Commission. More recently, antitrust economists have begun to use simulation as a means of predicting the likely outcome of changes in market structure due to horizontal merger.

It should be noted that, in the previous discussion of competitive and monopoly markets, perfect information on the part of consumers as well as producers is generally assumed. Complete information implies that there is no uncertainty on the part of the consumers regarding product quality. Furthermore, since products are assumed to be homogeneous in a given market, price is the major decision variable for consumers. Clearly, health care markets do not meet this information requirement, partly because of the imperfect ability of consumers to link the acquisition of health care services with improvements in health status and to compare the quality of alternative providers. Additionally, since third-party payers are dominant in most health care markets, the price of a particular health care service may be relatively unimportant to the ultimate consumer of that service. The market structure is further complicated by the role of the physician as the agent of the patient in making decisions about whether a particular service should be purchased.

As a result of these differences between health care markets and standard consumer goods markets, a discussion of antitrust policy in health care markets must take into account their particular economic characteristics. The point of view expressed here favors public policies that oppose monopoly power and promote competitive market structures. In the case of health care markets, however, there are even more caveats concerning this generalization than is true of traditional consumer goods markets. It is often asserted that, in traditional goods and services markets, economies of scale and the possibly greater propensity of firms with monopoly power to engage in research and development may justify market concentration. In health care markets, in addition to those two factors, high seller concentration may also be justified on the basis of access-to-care or quality-of-care considerations.

16.3.2 The Structure of Health Care Markets

16.3.2.1 Hospitals

Hospital services in the United States and Canada have historically been provided by private community hospitals. Community hospitals have traditionally been nonprofit hospitals sponsored by religious organizations, local governments, and charitable organizations. One major structural trend in the 1980s and 1990s in the United States was the rapid growth of for-profit hospital corporations.

Another strong trend in the 1980s and 1990s among U.S. hospitals was the increasing rate of mergers. Many of the mergers were related to the rise of for-profit hospital corporations. Other mergers have occurred among nonprofit hospitals in response to the rise of for-profit hospital corporations or to the increasing market power (on the buyer side) of managed care networks (Schactman and Altman 1995).

The economic analysis of mergers suggests that mergers may be motivated by the pursuit of increased market power, the pursuit of increased efficiency, or both. The effects of changes in Medicare reimbursement policies after the early 1980s provided a ready source of efficiency gains from mergers. The shift to prospective reimbursement for Medicare resulted in shorter inpatient stays and a shift from inpatient to outpatient treatment. The general effect of these shifts was to create overcapacity in many hospitals, increasing the likelihood that efficiency gains could be realized from mergers, especially mergers within the same geographic market. Such horizontal mergers also increase market power in given geographic markets, raising the issue of whether hospital mergers are in the public interest (Gaynor and Haas-Wilson 1999).

16.3.2.2 Physician Services

Physician services have traditionally been produced by physicians practicing alone or in small-group practices. Before 1980, when cost containment was less prominent in the health care sector, physicians played the dominant role in the management of hospitals as well as in the management of physician group practices. The cost-containment trend in hospitals has led to the increased power of hospital administrators in hospital management. The development of managed care networks also tended to reduce the discretionary power of physicians in determining the price and quality of service. One response of physicians to these trends is to form larger practices and other physician networks. Regional and even national physician practice corporations have begun to be established. As in the case of hospitals, the combination of physicians into large networks raises issues of efficiency versus market power.

16.3.2.3 Health Insurers and Managed Care Plans

Employers have traditionally provided health insurance in the United States as a tax-exempt fringe benefit. Before about 1980, most Americans were covered by traditional health insurance, which supported fee-for-service transactions with providers. Health insurers competed with one another to obtain insurance contracts with employers, who provided health insurance as a fringe benefit. Until the 1980s, health care cost containment had a relatively low priority in the U.S. system.

The early 1980s saw the rise of two important health care cost-containment mechanisms. First, Medicare's prospective payment system allowed the program to use its purchasing power to control the pricing and utilization of hospital services and physician services. Second, some states, beginning with California in 1982, began to allow payers to contract selectively with providers. Selective contracting enabled payers to negotiate reduced rates from providers in exchange for volume. Greater coordination of care, utilization review, and other changes caused health maintenance organizations (HMOs) to grow rapidly. As of 2000, HMOs enrolled about 105 million Americans, or about 39% of the population (Standard and Poor's 2000).

The structural change in the payers' markets has important implications for health care competition. In effect, increased market power on the buyer side has evolved in response to market power on the provider side or to rapid price inflation in health care markets resulting from the absence of economizing by consumers due to the existence of third-party payers. Mergers and consolidation among payers also raise potential issues of market power versus efficiency.

16.3.2.4 Pharmaceuticals

The pharmaceutical industry is an oligopoly that includes a relatively small number of large multinational firms with broad product lines along with a large number of small companies with limited product lines. A major competitive dimension is research and development competition—the search for new drugs with broad potential usage. The main incentive for new product development is the patent system, which grants the holder of a patent monopoly rights to manufacture and sell the product for about 20 years. Pharmacy retailers and pharmacy benefits management companies carry out the distribution of pharmaceuticals, with registered pharmacists licensed by state departments of health.

16.3.3 Antitrust Policy: History and Institutions

The most prominent piece of antitrust legislation in the United States is the Sherman Act of 1890. The Sherman Act was a legislative response to rapid changes occurring in American industry. In the last two decades of the nineteenth century, innovations in transportation and communication led to the transformation of local and regional markets into national markets. Business consolidation was a major trend, and near-monopoly conditions arose in some markets. The Sherman Act, building on common law traditions against conspiracy and monopolization, had two major sections:

1) . . . every contract, combination in the form of trust or otherwise, or conspiracy, in restraint of trade or commerce among the several states, or with foreign nations, is declared to be illegal . . .

2) . . . every person who shall monopolize, or attempt to monopolize, or combine or conspire with any other person or persons, to monopolize any part of the trade or commerce among the several states, or with foreign nations, shall be deemed guilty of a felony, . . .

The Clayton Act of 1914, with subsequent amendments, is the other major antitrust legislation in the United States. Two of the more important provisions of the Clayton Act are found in Sections 2 and 7, quoted in part as follows:

2a) . . . it shall be unlawful for any person engaged in commerce in the course of such commerce, either directly or indirectly, to discriminate in price between different purchasers of commodities of like grade and quality

... where the effect of such discrimination may be substantially to lessen competition or tend to create a monopoly.

7) ... no person engaged in commerce or in activity affecting commerce shall acquire, directly or indirectly, the whole or any part of the stock or other share capital and no person ... shall acquire the whole or any part of the assets of another person engaged also in commerce ... where in any line of commerce in any section of the country, the effect of such acquisition may be substantially to lessen competition, or to tend to create a monopoly ...

The Federal Trade Commission Act, also passed in 1914, established the Federal Trade Commission (FTC). The FTC shares in the enforcement of the Clayton Act and enforces Section 5A1 of the FTC Act which holds that "unfair methods of competition in or affecting commerce, and unfair or deceptive acts or practices in or affecting commerce, are declared unlawful ... "

There are two federal agencies that share the enforcement of antitrust law: the Antitrust Division of the U.S. Department of Justice and the Federal Trade Commission. The Department of Justice has primary responsibility for public enforcement of the Sherman Act; the Federal Trade Commission has primary responsibility for enforcement of the Federal Trade Commission Act and of Section 2 of the Clayton Act. The two agencies combine in enforcing the merger provisions of the Clayton Act. In addition, there are areas of overlap in which the agencies share jurisdiction. In addition to public enforcement of the antitrust laws, private enforcement is also important. The importance of private enforcement is related directly to Section 4 of the Clayton Act, which provides that those injured as a result of "anything forbidden in the antitrust laws" may bring private suit and recover triple damages, including attorney's fees. The triple damages provision provides a strong incentive for injured parties to bring private suits, including class action suits.

Because of the time and expense of fully developing cases and bringing them to trial, the majority of antitrust cases are settled by consent decrees. In a consent decree settlement, a court-supervised agreement is worked out between the parties. In the case of criminal suits, a settlement sometimes involves the use of a no-contest plea in order that the defendant may avoid pleading guilty. In private civil cases, financial settlements, generally involving amounts less than those initially requested by the plaintiffs, are common.

16.3.4 Price Fixing and Conspiracy in Restraint of Trade in Health Care Markets

Section 1 of the Sherman Act concerns conspiracy in restraint of trade. The legal tradition in the enforcement of this section is that evidence of direct communication among competitors is sufficient to find a violation. This principle is referred to as the "per se rule." The U.S Supreme Court has strongly stated that whether or not the prices established by conspiracy are reasonable is *not* an issue.

Despite the strong per se tradition in enforcing price fixing, legal precedent was relatively slow in extending the range of antitrust law to the professions. A landmark case in this regard is *Goldfarb v. Virginia State Bar* (1975), in which the Supreme Court stated that the professions are not exempt from the Sherman Act's prohibition of price fixing. The *Goldfarb* case involved fee schedules set for legal fees by a bar association.

That the per se rule also applies to price fixing among physicians was forcefully stated in the U.S. Supreme Court's decision in the case of *Arizona v. Maricopa County Medical Society* (1982). In this case, two physician groups utilized relative value schedules to establish maximum prices for medical services. The Court ruled that this approach to setting maximum physician fees was subject to the per se rule against price fixing.

The Maricopa case clearly establishes that the health care professions fall under the per se rule concerning price fixing and conspiracy in restraint of trade. This is not to say that physicians and other health professionals may not form professional associations and discuss issues of mutual concern. Trade association activities, including some exchange of pricing information, generally do not constitute a violation. However, the use of a common fee schedule setting either maximum or minimum fees would likely be a violation of the Sherman Act.

16.3.5 Mergers in Health Care Markets

A merger is a partial or total combination of two separate business firms. Partial mergers would include such combinations as joint ventures and intercorporate stock purchases. Complete mergers are more common. A complete merger involves the purchase of assets or stock in one corporation by a separate corporation and typically results in the blending of identities and the creation of a single succeeding firm.

Mergers are generally described as falling into one of three categories. The first type of merger is the horizontal merger—the combination of two firms that compete in the same product market and geographic market. A merger of two community hospitals in the same metropolitan area would be an example of a horizontal merger. The second type of merger is the vertical merger, which involves firms that have a buyer-seller relationship. The acquisition of a physician group practice by an HMO would be an example of a vertical merger. The third type of merger is the conglomerate merger, which unites firms that are neither horizontally nor vertically related. The acquisition of a community hospital by a banking corporation would be an example of a conglomerate merger.

Mergers and joint ventures have become very common in health care markets. For-profit hospital corporations such as Columbia/HCA have expanded in size and in geographic scope primarily through merger. Mergers have also been common in physician group practices, as solo practitioners combine to form local and regional group practices.

The enforcement of Section 7 of the Clayton Act by the Department of Justice and Federal Trade Commission focuses on the seller concentration in the market before and after prospective mergers. The Hart-Scott-Rodino Act of 1976 requires that mergers above a threshold size ($100 million in sales or assets on the part of one pre-merger firm and $10 million for the other party) must notify the Federal Trade Commission and Department of Justice in advance of the merger. This provision of the law allows the antitrust authorities to intervene before the merger actually occurs rather than wait until asset ownership has changed hands. This provision also allows for modification of the assets to be acquired if seller concentration in certain markets raises objections to parts of the merger.

Hospital markets tend to be local or regional in scope. In addition, because hospitals differ with respect to the array of services offered, the analysis of hospital mergers must consider both product market definition and geographic market definition. The definitions of geographic market and product market for hospitals are based on the interchangeability or cross-price elasticity of the services offered, as viewed by the consumers. Two or more hospitals are in the same geographic market if consumers (or their physician agents) consider the hospitals to be reasonably interchangeable when making decisions regarding where to seek care. Two or more hospitals are in the same product market if consumers consider their offerings of a given service to be reasonably interchangeable (Wilder and Jacobs 1987).

As noted earlier, the Clayton Act prohibits mergers where "the effect of such acquisition may be substantially to lessen competition, or to tend to create a monopoly." In the case of hospital mergers, a potential anticompetitive effect exists if there is overlap in the product and geographic markets of the hospitals prior to the merger. In general, the question of whether two hospitals are in the same geographic and product markets may be more complicated for hospitals than for non-health-care service firms. The geographic market definition is likely to vary depending on the medical procedure in question. Because patients are likely to be willing to travel greater distances for more complicated, more expensive procedures, the geographic market definition for hospitals is not independent of the procedure in question. In general, the geographic market is much wider for complicated procedures than for simple procedures (Wilder and Jacobs 1987).

Antitrust aspects of hospital mergers must be considered in the light of merger history. During the period 1950–1980, the enforcement agencies treated horizontal mergers very strictly, and modest market concentration levels and modest increases in concentration were often sufficient for horizontal mergers to be successfully challenged. After 1980, horizontal merger enforcement became more lenient, as reflected in the Department of Justice and Federal Trade Commission merger guidelines, the most recent version of which was released in 1992.

In evaluating horizontal mergers, the Justice Department guidelines use the Herfindahl-Hirschman Index (HHI) of market concentration. The HHI is defined as the sum of the squares of the individual market shares of all firms in the market, where market shares are expressed in percentages. For example, one hospital in a market would result in an HHI of 10,000 (100 × 100). Two hospitals of equal size would result in an HHI of 2,500. Ten hospitals of equal size would result in an HHI of 1,000. According to the guidelines, the Justice Department and Federal Trade Commission, in evaluating a proposed merger, consider both the market concentration and the increase in concentration that would result from the merger. The guidelines establish three categories of horizontal mergers:

1. Post-Merger HHI Below 1,000. The agency regards markets in this region to be unconcentrated. Mergers resulting in unconcentrated markets are unlikely to have adverse competitive effects and ordinarily require no further analysis.
2. Post-Merger HHI Between 1,000 and 1,800. The agency regards markets in this region to be moderately concentrated. Mergers producing an increase in the HHI of less than 100 points in moderately concentrated markets post-merger are unlikely to have adverse competitive consequences and ordinarily require no further analysis. Mergers producing

an increase in the HHI of more than 100 points in moderately concentrated markets post-merger potentially raise significant competitive concerns.

3. Post-Merger HHI Above 1,800. The agency regards markets in this region to be highly concentrated. Mergers producing an increase in the HHI of less than 50 points, even in highly concentrated markets post-merger, are unlikely to have adverse competitive consequences and ordinarily require no further analysis. Mergers producing an increase in the HHI of more than 50 points in highly concentrated markets post-merger potentially raise significant competitive concerns, depending on the factors set forth in [other sections] of the guidelines. Where the post-merger HHI exceeds 1,800, it will be presumed that mergers producing an increase in the HHI of more than 100 points are likely to create or enhance market power or facilitate its exercise.... (U.S. Department of Justice and Federal Trade Commission 1992).

If hospital mergers were judged entirely on the basis of the 1992 guidelines, it is unlikely that many hospital mergers in a given geographic market would be approved. In research reported elsewhere, it was found that the HHI for hospitals in a medium-sized metropolitan area market was on the order of 2,600 for all diagnoses together. For individual procedures, the HHI ranged from a low of 2,300 for plastic surgery to a high of 4,600 for surgeries of the nervous system (Wilder and Jacobs 1987).

Hospital mergers have occurred at a rapid rate since 1980. Blackstone and Fuhr state that 40 to 60 hospital mergers per year occurred in the 1980s but that the Department of Justice and Federal Trade Commission challenged fewer than 10 hospital mergers during this decade. In some cases, mergers were not challenged because the hospitals were not in the same geographic market. Many of the mergers and acquisitions were part of the hospital consolidation involved in the formation and growth of firms such as Columbia/HCA. Even when hospital mergers were truly horizontal, the Justice Department and Federal Trade Commission applied somewhat different standards to these mergers than to other horizontal mergers. The variation in standards is apparent in the Department of Justice-Federal Trade Commission Antitrust Guidelines for the Business of Health Care, which were released initially in 1993 and updated in August 1996. The purpose of the guidelines is to provide information concerning the types of mergers, joint ventures, and other competition-related actions that might be challenged by the antitrust authorities. In the area of mergers, the guidelines state that the merger of two small hospitals with low occupancy rates, even if they are in the same geographic market, would not be challenged. The guidelines also state that two or more hospitals of any size could engage in joint ventures to buy high-technology equipment if each hospital by itself could not fully utilize the equipment.

For mergers between larger hospitals, the antitrust agencies state that they will use the "rule of reason" in analyzing mergers. The rule of reason approach considers whether mergers may have a substantial anticompetitive effect and, if so, whether the anticompetitive effect is offset by procompetitive efficiencies (prepared remarks of Commissioner Janet D. Steiger, 1995).

When considering the effect of antitrust policy on hospital mergers, the primary fact to keep in mind is that only a small number of mergers have been challenged by the antitrust authorities out of the hundreds of mergers that have taken place in the past 20 years. Another indication of the effects of antitrust policy on hospital mergers may be seen in the outcome of the antitrust review of the Columbia Healthcare Corporation/HCA Healthcare merger. The merger was allowed after the divestiture of 3 hospitals in Salt Lake City and 4 hospitals in Louisiana, Florida, and Texas. The resulting Columbia/HCA Corporation included 191 hospitals with 39,328 acute care beds. Columbia/HCA subsequently merged with HealthTrust, Inc., forming a national hospital corporation with 320 hospitals and more than 100 outpatient surgery centers. The Federal Trade Commission approved this merger after Columbia/HCA agreed to sell 7 hospitals and end a joint venture with another hospital. In more recent times, Columbia/HCA has come under attack for Medicare billing irregularities, has negotiated a settlement to pay the federal government $754 million plus interest to resolve the overbilling allegations, has spun off and sold some of its hospitals, and has changed its name to HCA—The Healthcare Co. (Kirchheimer 2000).

One reason for the relatively lenient antitrust policy toward hospital mergers is the possibility of efficiency gains. Gaynor and Haas-Wilson (1999) point out that some mergers are rational responses to excess capacity and empty hospital beds resulting from the shift to increased use of outpatient treatment. Mergers may also be driven by changes in reimbursement practices that shift more risk to the provider.

State governments have also become players in the merger policy arena. As of 1998, 20 states had enacted regulatory programs for state approval of hospital actions, including mergers. Under the state action immunity doctrine, state supervision in some circumstances replaces federal antitrust action. This development could, for example, allow some hospital mergers that would otherwise attract federal antitrust action. The effects of state-approved mergers on hospital markets are largely unknown (Hellinger 1998).

The pharmaceutical industry has experienced a number of mergers during the past 15 years. Examples include the Monsanto-Pharmacia Upjohn, Pfizer-Warner Lambert, and Hoechst AG and Rhone-Poulenc Rorer mergers, all of which took place in 1998 and 1999 (Pharmaceutical Researchers and Manufacturers of America 2000). The industry has relatively high seller concentration in some drug submarkets, but the level of concentration in the broadly defined pharmaceutical preparations industry is relatively low. An example of a recent Federal Trade Commission merger complaint is that issued by the agency regarding the Hoechst AG and Rhone-Poulenc merger. This complaint argued that Hoechst's acquisition of Rhone-Poulenc would reduce competition in the market for agents used to treat blood-clotting diseases. A consent decree in 2000 allowed the merger subject to the transfer of Rhone-Poulenc's product in this submarket to a separate firm (U.S. Federal Trade Commission 2000) This case illustrates that the relevant product market in pharmaceutical antitrust cases may be defined quite narrowly.

16.3.6 Antitrust Policy: Monopolization

Section 2 of the Sherman Act makes it illegal to "monopolize, or attempt to monopolize." The use of the verb *monopolize* rather than the noun *monopoly* suggests one of difficulties in enforcing monopoly laws. Conceptually, a monopoly is a single firm with exclusive possession of a market for a good or service. As a practical matter, however, pure monopoly status is highly unusual. Markets with high seller concentration resulting in partial or near-monopoly market structures are the more common objects of monopoly inquiries. As a result, the enforcement of monopoly laws tends to focus on market definition, market share, and specific acts that suggest monopolistic intent.

A good summary of the enforcement tradition in monopoly cases may be found in the U.S. Supreme Court decision in the *Grinnell* case, where Justice Douglas stated that the offense of monopoly "has two elements: 1) possession of monopoly power in the relevant market and; 2) willful acquisition or maintenance of that power . . ." (*U.S. v. Grinnell Corporation*, 384US 563 (1966)).

Relatively little of the antitrust enforcement activity in health care has involved monopolization issues directly. Instead, most enforcement activity has taken place under the conspiracy statute (Section 1 of the Sherman Act) or the antimerger statute (Section 7 of the Clayton Act). As national hospital corporations and health care provider networks grow more important in the United States, however, the likelihood that monopolization issues will become more important will increase.

The major reason that monopolization issues have been less important than other antitrust issues is that the level of seller concentration in most hospital or physician services markets, while relatively high in some instances, does not approach the level that indicates monopoly on the basis of case law. In the most direct statement on the connection between market share and monopoly status, Judge Hand, in the *Aluminum Company of America* case, stated that a market share over 90 percent "is enough to constitute a monopoly; it is doubtful whether 60 or 64 percent would be enough; and certainly 33 percent is not" (*U.S. vs. Aluminum Company of America*, 148F. 2nd 416 (1945)).

Since the *Aluminum Company of America* case in the 1940s, the only very large national corporation whose monopoly status was broken up by antitrust action was AT&T, in a case settled through a consent decree in 1982. A monopolization case against IBM by the Justice Department was dropped at about the same time (in the early 1980s). Because neither of these cases reached the Supreme Court, there is no clear recent judicial statement interpreting monopoly law for today's world.

There are at least three principal market areas within health care in which monopoly issues may come to the fore. First, as national hospital corporations grow and as nonprofit community hospitals merge and engage in joint ventures, the market structure in some local hospital markets may evolve in such a way that a group of jointly owned hospitals will reach a market share of 60 percent. Such market evolution could then make monopolization enforcement under Section 2 of the Sherman Act relevant in some hospital markets.

Physician networks may also become subject to monopolization enforcement. Physicians have been rapidly forming networks that operate as unified firms. Such networks may increasingly accumulate market shares in relevant geographic markets in the 60-percent range or greater. As such market shares arise through continued consolidation, antimonopoly law may become directed toward the larger networks.

HMOs and other managed care organizations may also become the target of monopolization statutes. These organizations tend to increase concentration on the buyer side in markets for hospital and physician services. As the market penetration of HMOs increases, the potential for high market shares on the buyer side of health care markets also increases. Some observers believe that the rapid growth of physician networks and the increasing number of hospital mergers and joint ventures are partly responses to the increased purchasing power of HMOs and other managed care organizations.

The 1996 Department of Justice and Federal Trade Commission statement on health care and antitrust laws addresses the interaction of physician networks and multiprovider networks. In general, the statement indicates that HMOs and other multiprovider networks might violate antitrust laws if the exclusion of some physicians from a dominant network in a local market makes it impossible for them to practice medicine. A similar argument could be directed at a dominant multiprovider network that excludes hospitals in a local market. Efficiency gains may be an offsetting virtue of provider coordination and combination. Antitrust cases considering monopolization issues would also consider efficiency effects.

16.3.7 Quality Competition and Antitrust Policy

Nonprice competition is particularly important in most sectors of the health care market. Quality competition among insurers or managed care organizations is related to attributes such as access to specialists, freedom of choice among providers, and treatment capacity. Quality competition among providers is based on attributes such as credentials, location, and treatment outcomes (Sage and Hammer 1999). Because of incomplete information in health care markets, consumers may be poorly informed about the quality of service. This information problem could mean that antitrust policies that encourages price competition may lead to the provision of lower quality service than is socially optimal (Gaynor and Haas-Wilson 1999).

There is a developing trend toward greater provision of information about health care quality. The Health Care Financing Administration, for example, reports on the characteristics and performance of nursing homes. The Agency for Healthcare Research and Quality sponsors and conducts research with a focus on providing evidence-based information on health care outcomes and quality (Agency for Healthcare Research and Quality 2000). The National Committee for Quality Assurance issues an annual report on the quality of managed care plans (National Committee for Quality Assurance 2000). The committee is funded by government and corporate sponsors. The greater availability of information offers the promise of improved quality competition and a reduction in the likelihood that markets will provide service quality that is suboptimal.

16.3.8 Antitrust Issues Related to Managed Care

One of the most important trends in the health care sector during the past 20 years has been the rise of managed care plans, selective contracting, and integrated health networks. What happened, in a nutshell, is that the market power in the hands of the physicians and hospitals (the suppliers of health care) was met by the growth of market power on the buyer side. The growth of managed care appears to have promoted competitive efficiencies in health care and has likely reduced the rate of increase in health care costs. At the same time, the rise of managed care could eventually result in increased market power on the part of buyers or sellers of health care and ultimately lead to an increase in the prices paid by consumers (Schactman and Altman 1995).

The health care initiatives put forth by the Clinton Administration in 1993—initiatives that seemed likely to result in greater public sector participation in health care—were not politically popular. It is interesting to note, however, that the managed competition approach at the heart of the Clinton plan has been implemented without federal legislation. In other words, the managed care revolution has been a private market response rather than a legislative reaction to increasing health care costs.

The managed care industry has followed a path of consolidation through merger. In 1998, the largest 10 HMO providers accounted for almost two-thirds of the total HMO enrollment in the United States (Standard and Poor's 2000). Because competition takes place in geographic markets at the local or regional level, HMO concentration in specific geographic markets may be higher or lower than at the national level. Feldman and colleagues (1999) found that, while national HMO concentration increased from 1994 to 1997, most local HMO markets were less concentrated in 1997 than in 1994 because of the entry of new firms.

16.3.9 Federal Antitrust Policy Guidelines

A major landmark in health care antitrust policy was the issuing of *The Statements of Enforcement Policy and Analytical Principles Relating to Health Care and Antitrust* by the Department of Justice and Federal Trade Commission in 1993 (revised in 1994 and 1996). These statements reflect the complexity of markets and provider and purchaser institutions in health care. They also indicate that the antitrust authorities are seeking to adapt antitrust policy, which was developed for broad applicability, to the particular economic characteristics of health care markets. The provisions of the statements address the following nine areas:

1. mergers among hospitals
2. hospital joint ventures involving high-technology or other expensive health care equipment
3. hospital joint ventures involving specialized clinical or other expensive health care services
4. providers' collective provision of non-fee-related information to purchasers of health care services
5. providers' collective provision of fee-related information to purchasers of health care services
6. provider participation in exchanges of price and cost information
7. joint purchasing arrangements among health care providers
8. physician network joint ventures
9. analytical principles relating to multiprovider networks

The purpose of the statements is to reduce uncertainty concerning antitrust policy and to establish "antitrust safety zones" (market conditions under which business conduct will not be challenged). For example, the merger of two small hospitals with low occupancy rates would fall into one of the safety zones. A physician network might attract antitrust scrutiny by collusive agreement on price or by excluding some physicians, making it impossible for them to practice in the market.

Physicians criticized the first version of the statements on the grounds that they favored insurance company and hospital networks over those formed by physicians. Statements 8 and 9 regarding physician networks and multiprovider networks were rewritten in the 1996 revision. The new version stated clearly that physician networks "could act jointly, without sharing financial risk, and not be considered as engaged in per se illegal conduct if they were doing something together that had the potential to create significant efficiencies" (Iglehart 1998).

The health care system in the United States has been transformed by structural change, including the rise of managed care, selective contracting, provider networks, and numerous large mergers. These changes have the potential to increase productive efficiency and to slow the rate of health care price inflation. At the same time, the changes may increase market power in some product or geographic markets and may lead to higher consumer prices. In addition, there is increasing concern regarding the quality of health care services, leading to such developments as congressional debates on the legal rights of physicians to form unions and on the patient bill of rights. It is likely that, as greater consolidation among providers and purchasers occurs and as quality-competition tradeoffs are discussed widely, regulation and antitrust issues will become even more important.

EXERCISES

1. Why are physicians sometimes described as "double agents"?
2. If physicians can gain large per capita wealth effects from state regulation and consumers can gain relatively small per capita wealth effects from state regulation, which of the two groups does the economic theory of regulation suggest will control the legislative process that enacts regulatory procedures?
3. If physicians can organize at a low cost to influence state regulation and consumers can organize only at a relatively high cost for this same purpose, which of the two groups does the economic theory of regulation suggest will control the legislative process that enacts regulatory procedures?
4. How can consumers of health care services obtain more information about service quality?
5. Explain how the patent right provides a financial incentive for pharmaceutical manufacturers to develop new drugs.
6. Explain the connection between the Employee Retirement Income Security Act (ERISA) and calls for a patient bill of rights.
7. Suppose that you overhear a foursome of physicians on the golf course discussing the prices they charge for an office visit. Suppose further that you hear them reach an agreement to all charge a fee of $100 for an office visit. What is such an agreement called in antitrust policy and what antitrust law may have been violated?
8. Suppose that emergency room services in the city of Hibiscus are provided by three hospitals. Two of the hospitals each have a market share of 40 percent and the third hospital has a market share of 20 percent. The two largest hospitals plan to merge.
   a. Compute the pre-merger and post-merger HHI for this market.
   b. Based on the 1992 merger guidelines, would this merger likely be challenged by the antitrust authorities?
9. Physician networks have become increasingly popular in the past 25 years. How do the health care antitrust guidelines view physician networks and what benefits of such networks might offset antitrust concerns?

BIBLIOGRAPHY

Regulation

Abbott, T. 1997. The pharmaceutical industry. In *Health economics,* ed. T.E. Getzen. New York: John Wiley & Sons.

Arrow, K. J. 1963. Uncertainty and the welfare economics of medical care. *American Economic Review* 53:941–947.

Blomqvist, A.. 1991. The doctor as double agent: Information asymmetry, health insurance, and medical care. *Journal of Health Economics* 10:411–432.

Conlan, M. 1997. Board games. *Drug Topics* 17 (November): 58–63.

Conover, C., and F. Sloan. 1998. Does removing certificate-of-need regulation lead to a surge in health care spending? *Journal of Health Politics, Policy and Law* 23:455–481.

Dranove, D., and W.D. White. 1987. Agency and the organization of health care delivery. *Inquiry* 24:405–415.

Dranove, D., et al. 1993. Price and concentration in hospital markets: The switch from patient-driven to payer-driven competition. *Journal of Law and Economics* 36:179–204.

Folland, S., et al. 2001. *The economics of health and health care.* 3rd ed. Englewood Cliffs, NJ: Prentice Hall.

Fournier, G.M., and M.M. McInnes. 1997. Medical board regulation of physician licensure: Is excessive malpractice sanctioned. *Journal of Regulatory Economics* 12:113–126.

Frech, H.E., III. 1993. Health insurance: Designing products to reduce costs. In *Industry studies,* ed. L. Deutsch. Englewood Cliffs, NJ: Prentice Hall.

Getzen, T.E. 1997. *Health economics.* New York: John Wiley & Sons.

Grabowski, H., and J. Vernon. 1992. Brand loyalty, entry, and price competition in pharmaceuticals after the 1984 Drug Act. *Journal of Law and Economics* 35:331–350.

Havighurst, C. 2000. American health care and the law—we need to talk! *Health Affairs* 19, no. 4:84–106.

Health Care Financing Administration. 2000. Peer review organizations (PROs). <http://www.hcfa.gov/quality>.

Joint Commission on Accreditation of Healthcare Organizations. 2000. <http://www.jcaho.org>.

Medicare Payment Advisory Commission. 2000. Report to Congress: Medicare payment policy. <http://www.medpac.gov>.

Peltzman, S. 1976. Toward a more general theory of regulation. *Journal of Law and Economics* 19:211–240.

Scheutzow, S.O. 1999. State medical peer review: High cost but no benefit—Is it time for a change? *American Journal of Law and Medicine* 25, no. 1:7–60.

Stigler, G. 1971. The theory of economic regulation. *Bell Journal of Economics* 2:3–21.

U.S. Food and Drug Administration. 2000. *About the Center for Drug Evaluation and Research.* <http://www.fda.gov/cder>.

Health Care Antitrust Policy

Agency for Healthcare Research and Quality. 2000. <http://www.ahrq.gov>.

Blackstone, E., and J.P. Fuhr. 1992. An antitrust analysis of non-profit hospital mergers. *Review of Industrial Organization* 8:473–490.

Dranove, D., and R. Ludwick. 1999. Competition and pricing by nonprofit hospitals. *Journal of Health Economics* 18:87–98.

Dranove, D., and W.D. White. 1998. Emerging issues in the antitrust definition of healthcare markets. *Health Economics* 7:167–170.

Feldman, R., and R.S. Given. 1998. HMO mergers and Medicare: The antitrust issues. *Health Economics* 7:171–174.

Feldman, R., et al. 1999. HMO consolidations: How national mergers affect local markets. *Health Affairs* 18, no. 4: 96–104.

Frech, H.E., and K.L. Danger. 1998. Exclusive contracts between hospitals and physicians. *Health Economics* 7:175–178.

Freudenheim, M. 1994. Health industry is changing itself ahead of reform. *New York Times*, 27 June.

Gaynor, M., and D. Haas-Wilson. 1999. Change, consolidation and competition in health care markets. *Journal of Economic Perspectives* 13:141–164.

Haas-Wilson, D., and M. Gaynor. 1998. Physician networks and their implications for competition in health care markets. *Health Economics* 7:179–182.

Hellinger, F.J. 1998. Antitrust enforcement in the healthcare industry: The expanding scope of state activity. *Health Services Research* 33, no. 5, part 2:1477–1494.

Iglehart, J.K. 1998. The Federal Trade Commission in action: The FTC's Robert F. Leibenluft. Interview. *Health Affairs* 17, no. 5:65–74.

Kirchheimer, B. 2000. Move over Columbia, HCA is back. *Modern Healthcare,* 19 June.

Kuttner, R. 1997. Physician-operated networks and the new antitrust guidelines. *New England Journal of Medicine* 336:386–391.

Lynk, W.J., and L.R. Neumann. 1999. Price and profit. *Journal of Health Economics* 18:99–116.

National Committee for Quality Assurance. 2000. *State of managed care quality 2000.* <http://www.ncqa.org>.

Pear, R. 1996. Doctors may get leeway to rival large companies. *New York Times*, 8 April.

———. 2000. Doctor's antitrust hopes face a roadblock from Lott. *New York Times*, July 1.

Pharmaceutical Research and Manufacturers of America. 2000. *Pharmaceutical industry profile 2000.* <http://www.phrma.org/publications>.

Sage, W.M., and P.J. Hammer. 1999. Competing on quality of care: The need to develop a competition policy for health care markets. *University of Michigan Journal of Law Reform* 32:1069–1118.

Santerre, R.E., and S. Neun. 1996. *Health economics: Theories, insights and industry studies.* Chicago: Dryden Press.

Schactman, D., and S.H. Altman. 1995. *Market consolidation, antitrust, and public policy in the health care industry: Agenda for future research.* Princeton, NJ:Robert Wood Johnson Foundation.

Silvia, L., and R.F. Leibenluft. 1998. Health economics research and antitrust enforcement. *Health Economics* 7:163–166.

Standard and Poor's. 2000. Healthcare: Managed care. *Industry Surveys,* 31 August.

Steiger, J.D. 1995. Prepared remarks of Commissioner Janet D. Steiger, Federal Trade Commission, Health Care Enforcement Issues, before the Health Trustee Institute, Cleveland, Ohio, 9 November.

U. S. Department of Justice and Federal Trade Commission. 1992. *Horizontal merger guidelines,* Washington, DC.

U. S. Department of Justice and Federal Trade Commission. 1996. *Statements of antitrust enforcement policy in health care.* Washington, DC.

U. S. Federal Trade Commission. 2000. *FTC antitrust actions in pharmaceutical services and products.* <http://www.ftc.gov>.

Wilder, R.P., and P. Jacobs. 1987. Antitrust considerations for hospital mergers: Market definition and market concentration. In *Advances in health economics and health services research,* ed. R.M. Scheffler and L.F. Rossiter. Stamford, CT: JAI Press.

Wooley, J.M. 1993. Hospitals: Price-increasing competition. In *Industry studies,* ed. L. Deutsch. Englewood Cliffs, NJ: Prentice Hall.

Economic Evaluation
of Health Services

1. Identify the main research questions in an economic evaluation analysis.
2. Identify the types of analyses that can be used to address each research question.
3. Identify the guidelines that are used to conduct an economic evaluation analysis.
4. Identify the major types of health outcomes that can be used in economic evaluation analysis.
5. Explain how an economic evaluation analysis can be conducted using basic information.
6. Interpret cost-effectiveness ratios and the conclusions that can be drawn from them.
7. Explain how a willingness-to-pay measure can be derived.
8. Explain how to estimate a cost-benefit ratio and how to interpret these findings.

17.1 INTRODUCTION

Economic evaluation analysis involves the quantification of changes in health resource use and outcomes due to the introduction of new interventions. Policy makers are increasingly turning to these analyses in order to acquire information for making decisions about alternatives in health care. Managers of drug formularies, especially publicly funded ones, resort to economic evaluations in order to determine which drugs to pay for. Government policy-makers use health technology assessments, which are based largely on economic evaluations, to shed light on the economic implications of new interventions.

Economic evaluations are used to inform decisions when there is a concern that a market is not yielding the right allocation of resources. The studies attempt to replace poor information or provide missing information on outcomes and their valuations and on the costs of interventions. The direct measure of these concepts can provide important insights as to how resources *ought* to be allocated.

In this chapter we introduce the methods that are used in economic evaluation studies. We first present an overview of the subject, indicating the questions that are posed and the tools that have been developed to answer them. Following this, we present the guidelines for a sound economic evaluation and the key components of three major types of economic evaluation studies: cost-effectiveness, cost-utility, and cost-benefit studies.

17.2 THE PURPOSES OF ECONOMIC EVALUATION

There are several distinct reasons to perform economic evaluation studies. First, we can compare alternative courses of action that are substitute solutions for the same conditions. For example, we might compare two drugs for the treatment of migraine headaches or we might compare the use of drugs versus surgery for treating blocked arteries. Recent studies have shown that the complications of diabetes can be treated effectively with intensive glucose control, which includes frequent monitoring of glucose levels and frequent clinic visits. The alternative intervention is the more conventional treatment, which includes careful diet and exercise but less careful monitoring and less frequent insulin doses (Diabetes Complications and Control Group 1995, 1996). An economic evaluation study would allow us to compare the benefits and costs of the two treatments. Second, we can investigate the question whether a treatment is worthwhile. We might ask, for example, whether we should we treat diabetes at all. Note that there is an important difference between this and the first purpose. In a study of alternatives, we would look at the changes in health that occur as a result of the use of additional resources, but we would not consider whether the changes were worth the cost. In the second kind of study, we would in fact be asking that exact question.

17.3 SELECTING THE RIGHT TYPE OF ANALYSIS

Once we are clear as to our purpose, we can select the appropriate type of study. There are five different types of comparative studies in economic evaluation analysis: cost-effectiveness analysis, cost-utility analysis, cost-minimization analysis, cost-consequence analysis, and cost-benefit analysis (Drummond et al. 1997). In cost-effectiveness analysis we compare the difference in costs to the difference in outcomes (where the outcomes are of a single type, such as years of life following treatment). The formula for cost-effectiveness analysis is

$$(c_2 - c_1) / (q_2 - q_1)$$

where 1 and 2 refer to alternative interventions (e.g., conventional versus intensive treatment for diabetes), c is the cost per person, and q is the outcome. We use cost-effectiveness analysis when we have alternative ways of attaining a single type of outcome, such as life years or quality of life. Associated with cost-effectiveness analysis is cost-consequences analysis. In this type of analysis, we have multiple types of outcome, such as time to death and quality of life, but we do not aggregate the outcomes into a single scale (Bakker et al. 1994). Cost-consequence analysis is similar in purpose to cost-effectiveness analysis, and so we will group them together.

In cost-utility analysis, we compare differences in the "utility" of interventions with differences in cost. The cost-utility formula is

$$(c_2 - c_1)/(u_2 - u_1)$$

where the outcome *(u)* is an index of consumer health status (consumer health status is a composite measure encompassing more than one component of health).

Cost-minimization analysis, in certain circumstances, can be used as a special form of cost-effectiveness or cost-utility analysis. When the outcomes are the same for all of the interventions being studied, then the interventions can be evaluated just by looking at costs. A cost-minimization analysis would then be used. In cost-benefit analysis we replace the health indices with dollar measures of benefits. The assessment is the difference between benefits and costs, all of which are expressed in monetary terms. The formula for the cost-benefit analysis of an intervention is

$$NSB = b - c$$

where NSB is the net social benefit, b stands for the monetary value of the benefits from the intervention, and c is the additional cost of the intervention. There is, of course, an implicit alternative, in that the resources could be used in another way.

There is an appropriate type of analysis for each study objective. If analysts want to compare outcomes and costs for alternative interventions using a single outcome measure (or unweighted multiple outcomes), then they will use cost-effectiveness analysis. If they want to compare costs and outcomes when there is more then one component of outcome, and these are combined into a single index whose weights are a reflection of someone's valuations, then they would use cost-utility analysis. Finally, if they are asking whether the intervention should be adopted (i.e., whether is it worthwhile), then they would use cost-benefit analysis.

17.4 GUIDELINES FOR CONDUCTING A COST-EFFECTIVENESS ANALYSIS

In the past several years, a number of publications have appeared that provide guidance on what steps to take in conducting an economic evaluation analysis in the health care field (Canadian Coordinating Office for Health Technology Assessment 1997; Drummond et al. 1997; Gold et al. 1996; Menon et al. 1996). In this section we present an outline of the elements of cost-effectiveness and cost-utility analyses in the light of what these guidelines recommend. Our exposition will be conducted using an example, that of comparing an intensive treatment of diabetes and the conventional treatment. First, we will briefly present our example, then we will describe the use of the guidelines to conduct economic evaluation analyses.

The example is based on several pivotal clinical trials for diabetes control (Diabetes Complications and Control Trial Research Group 1995, 1996) in which newly diagnosed diabetes patients were randomized to one of two interventions. In the first intervention, called conventional care, the individual tests his or her glucose level daily, takes one or two insulin injections daily, and visits a clinic every three months. In the second intervention, intensive or tight control, the individual tests his or her glucose four times daily, visits a health team often, follows a special diet, exercises regularly, and takes insulin at least four times daily.

Information on deaths and alternative outcomes for the patients in each group are shown in Table 17–1. Alternative outcomes are presented in terms of quality of life, willingness to pay, and quality-adjusted life years (QALYs). The annual cost per person is $5,000 for individuals with tight glucose control and $1,500 for individuals with conventional control. The details of costs are shown in Table 17–2. These include physician visits, inpatient hospitalization, self-care (including the cost of

Table 17–1 Outcome Measures for Alternative Interventions in Diabetes Control

	Year 1	Year 2	Year 3
Tight insulin control			
Survivors	997	994	990
Deaths	3	3	4
Life years	998.5	995.5	992
Quality of life per person	.9	.9	.9
Quality-adjusted life years	898.65	895.5	892.8
Willingness to pay for an additional QALY	$ 40,000	$ 40,000	$ 40,000
Annual cost per person	$ 5,000	$ 5,000	$ 5,000
Annual cost for 1,000 persons	$5,000,000	$5,000,000	$5,000,000
Conventional care			
Survivors	995	990	984
Deaths	5	5	6
Life years	997.5	992.5	987
Quality of life per person	.8	.8	.7
Quality-adjusted life years	798	794	690.9
Willingness to pay for an additional QALY	$ 40,000	$ 40,000	$ 40,000
Annual cost per person	$ 1,500	$ 1,500	$ 1,500
Annual cost for 1,000 persons	$1,500,000	$1,500,000	$1,500,000

insulin), and adverse events not treated on an inpatient basis. Most of the difference in cost between interventions is due to the self-care category.

Using this example, we will outline the various economic evaluation studies that can be conducted.

17.4.1 Perspective

By perspective we mean the viewpoint taken by the investigator. Broadly there are two types of perspective, private and societal. The private viewpoint is that of

Table 17–2 Annual Cost per Person of Alternative Interventions for Diabetes Control

Category	Calculation Details	Cost per Person
Conventional care		
Inpatient hospital care	.10 probability of hospitalization × $2,500 per hospitalization	$ 250
Outpatient visits	1 annual exam × $250 plus 3 visits × $50	400
Self-care	Monitoring supplies, insulin, and supplies for administering insulin	700
Cost of adverse effects	1 visit to an emergency room per year	150
Total		1,500
Intensive therapy		
Inpatient hospital care	.02 probability of hospitalization × $2,500 per hospitalization	$ 50
Outpatient visits	1 annual exam × $250 plus 11 visits × $50	800
Self-care	Monitoring supplies, insulin, and supplies for administering insulin	5,135
Cost of adverse effects	.1 visits to an emergency room per year at $150 per visit	15
Total		5,000

any single provider, patient, or payer or any group of providers, patients, or payers. If the individuals of interest are patients, we want to understand how the intervention impacts these people. If we took the payer's viewpoint, we would be concerned with how much of the payer's own resources are used. The societal perspective is the perspective of all persons. It is an "all resources" perspective, in that it focuses on all resources used by all persons—providers, patients, and caregivers—who are involved in the care. In our diabetes example, we will assume an "all health care resources" perspective, except that we will exclude the non-health-care resource losses (e.g., lost work time) incurred by unpaid caregivers and patients. Most guidelines recommend taking the broadest societal perspective; however, the choice of perspective is a value judgment, and there are uses for studies that take each perspective.

17.4.2 Time Horizons

The time horizon is the period over which costs and outcomes are measured. Most guidelines recommend that the analyses incorporate a long enough timeline to take into account all resources and outcome effects, including downstream events. Sometimes downstream events are hard to identify. For example, if a patient is treated in a neonatal intensive care unit, he or she might experience effects years after the treatment. These events are rarely captured in study databases, and so the investigators must develop a hypothetical model to project such events. In our example, we assume a time horizon of three years.

17.4.3 Outcomes

Outcome measures fall into two major categories, as shown in Exhibit 17–1. These will be termed *clinical* and *holistic*. Clinical outcome measures include complete, partial, or no response in relation to cancer tumors; blood pressure; and cholesterol level. Clinical outcome measures are usually used in clinical trials, since they provide objective evidence of illness.

Clinical outcome measures do not indicate how patients regard their own conditions. A condition with very little objective evidence, such as dyspepsia, may still be of enormous importance to the patient because it produces discomfort.

Clinical outcome measures do not provide information on patients' perceptions of their own conditions. As patient and consumer empowerment has increased, there has been a growing interest in developing outcome measures that

Exhibit 17–1 Measures Used in Economic Studies

Clinical measures
Holistic measures
  Measures based on mortality
    Survival
    Time of survival (life years)
  Health-Related Quality-of-life measures
    Disease-specific indicators
    General health indicators
  Preference-based measures

reflect patients' perceptions. We term these *holistic measures,* in large part because the concept of a holistic measure is so broad, as is the set of the phenomena we want the concept to characterize. As seen in Exhibit 17–1, we have included measures based on mortality in the holistic category. In fact, they would fit into either category. In any case, mortality-related measures are very commonly used because they are easy to obtain and because mortality is of such importance. Mortality measures include the occurrence of death as well as survival time (called *life years*).

The indicator of time until death illustrates the role that the time dimension plays in outcome analysis. Individuals experience different health states through time, and so the benefits and hardships they experience as a result of these health states should include a time dimension. The time-inclusive counterpart of mortality is the number of years of survival. In our example, out of 1,000 persons with diabetes who undertook the tight insulin control intervention, there were 997 survivors at the end of the first year, 994 at the end of the second, and 992 at the end of three years (see Table 17–1). One key outcome would be total deaths within three years, which is 10 for the tight insulin control intervention and 16 for the conventional care intervention. If we add the time dimension and use life years as the outcome measure, then in the first year there are 998.5 life years in the tight insulin control arm (the three individuals who died are assumed to live one-half year each). The total life years for the tight control intervention equal 2,986 over the three-year period, and the total life years for the conventional care arm equal 2,977.

Health-related quality-of-life years may differ from each other because the quality of life that individuals experience can vary considerably. In order to capture the variation in quality of life, a large number of health-related quality-of-life indexes have been developed. Some of the indexes are specific to a particular disease, some are objectively determined indexes oriented toward health status in general, and some are based on consumers' own preferences. A disease-specific index contains items that are relevant to the particular disease, whether it be asthma, cancer, or breast cancer. Objective health status indexes contain items that are relevant to all or many conditions. Both types of indexes will contain a number of questions about aspects of health status. For example, a person might be asked about his or her mobility. The questionnaire might provide five or six levels of mobility (none, ability to sit up in bed, etc.), and the individual marks the level appropriate to his or her condition. The responses determine the index score, although in some quality-of-life indexes there are scores for the separate components. Guidelines on economic evaluations recommend the inclusion of health-related quality-of-life indexes.

Health-related quality-of-life indexes are usually confined to a patient's health status at a given point in time. Extrapolations can be made to cover intervals between responses. However, if patients die during the measurement interval, then the indexes generally do not incorporate this factor into the assessment. Death must be taken into account as a separate indicator. By the same token, mortality measures do not take the quality of life into account. Additionally, none of the measures that have been discussed take into account the consumer's own valuations or preferences for each health state. In order to address these concerns, several different research groups have developed preference-based or utility measures of health outcome (see Table 1–2). These preference-based measures are each based on a set of health dimensions. In the 15-D (15 dimensions of health) measure

(Sintonen 1995) each of the 15 health dimensions has five categories, and there is a description for each category. For example, the five descriptions for the Vitality dimension are as follows:

1. I feel healthy and energetic.
2. I feel slightly weary, tired, or feeble.
3. I feel moderately weary, tired, or feeble.
4. I feel weary, tired, or feeble, almost exhausted.
5. I feel extremely weary, tired, or feeble, totally exhausted.

A score for each category was elicited from a sample of interviewees, each of whom placed his or her own valuation on the category.

A second level of weights, sometimes called *importance weights,* was assigned by a sample group to each of the 15 dimensions (see Table 1–2). All of the importance weights add up to a value of 1.00. As a result, the highest possible score on the 15-D measure is 1.00, which is achieved if a respondent scores at the highest level in each of the categories. Some investigators, both in the 15-D and other preference systems, have assigned a value of 0 to death. This is a very convenient assumption, because it allows investigators to score on a single scale those interventions that have both death and changes in quality of life as outcomes. Within the context of such systems, one can calculate the magnitude of QALYs, which is an extremely convenient outcome measure. In our example, we have assigned, in each of the three years, a QALY value of 0.9 to the persons who practice tight insulin control. Each surviving person would experience a total of 2.7 QALYs over the three years.

There are some deaths in our diabetes example, and the QALY valuation for a deceased persons is zero (deaths are assumed to occur at midpoint in the year). The assignment of a value of zero to death, while convenient, is controversial. When investigators develop weights for alternative health conditions, they usually ask members of a representative group to provide their own values. If patients who have experienced a specific health state are asked for their evaluations, they can provide a value that is based on an understanding of the condition. However, most weights have been developed from surveys of the general population, many of whom have not experienced the health states. In these instances, the valuations are thus projections of what the respondents think they might experience in a given state. The assignment of a value of zero to death is clearly an instance of projection. Individuals who have been surveyed have not experienced the condition, and so its valuation has little basis. Indeed, in all quality-of-life valuation surveys, the investigators did not even ask respondents about what they thought they might experience in death. They made their own extrapolations.

An additional issue in preference-based indicators is whose valuations to include in the measure of outcome. Investigators have alternatively focused on the values of providers (physicians and nurses), the general population, and specific patient groups. In addition, a number of economists have used introspection (inserting valuations of what they think is reasonable) along with sensitivity analyses. There is at present no agreement as to whose values to incorporate into the weights. The patients are the only ones who have actually experienced many of the conditions, but the results of decisions often fall on payers of insurance premiums (employees or employers) or taxpayers.

17.4.4 Efficacy and Effectiveness

When we have two or more interventions, each of which will achieve a given purpose, we must have a method to determine the *differences* in outcomes between these interventions. One method is to use experimental techniques, such as randomized controlled trials. Properly set up, these techniques create carefully specified protocols for selected groups of patients, who are randomized to alternative interventions so that the selection of one intervention or another is beyond the control of the investigators. The investigators can then be sure that the two (or more) groups contain comparable patients. In a randomized controlled trial, the differences in outcomes between interventions yield a measure called *efficacy*. This term refers only to differences between interventions under experimental conditions. Efficacy measures do not always translate into everyday practice. Randomized controlled trials usually follow very tight protocols and monitor patients closely. If the trial is not done in hospital (and most are not), the trial staff must devote considerable resources to monitoring patient adherence to protocols. In many instances, the treatments have unpleasant side effects, and clinical staff try to ensure that the trial protocols are maintained by the patients (e.g., that they take medicines at the prescribed intervals). No such monitoring is possible for practitioners in everyday circumstances. As a result, efficacy measures obtained from clinical trials are not always good indicators of how an intervention will work in actual practice.

The concept of effectiveness is related to differences in outcomes between interventions under nonexperimental conditions. Effectiveness must be determined from data collected from routine operations. Billing data, collected by insurers, provides information that can be used to determine effectiveness. However, administrative or billing data usually does not contain information about quality of life and often does not contain enough clinical information to allow researchers to determine if indeed the patients within each comparison group are truly identical (which they would be in a clinical trial). Thus, unlike in randomized trials, investigators using statistical studies are less sure that the populations that they are comparing are the same. Despite these problems in determining effectiveness, it is this measure of difference, not that of efficacy, that we seek in our cost-effectiveness model. This is because the cost-effectiveness model is used to inform policy or management decisions, both of which are carried out under actual conditions.

In our diabetes example, we assume that the measures of outcomes are similar to those that would be obtained in actual practice conditions. Effectiveness, then, is measured by the difference in outcomes between interventions. There are several different effectiveness measures in our example. One is the number of lives saved during a given time frame. By the end of year 3, there were 992 survivors in the tight insulin control arm, and 984 in the conventional care arm. The difference, 8 lives, is the effectiveness measure. If we sum up all life years in each intervention, then the effectiveness in terms of life years is 9 (2,986 − 2,977). In terms of QALYs, the effectiveness measure is 404.05 years (2,686.95 − 2,282.9). We should note that we have counted a QALY occurring in any year as having the same value as QALYs occurring in other years. Some analysts propose that a discount factor be applied to the benefits that occur in future years. We will discuss this issue below.

17.4.5 Costs

Economic costs are equivalent to the combined value of *resources* used in an intervention. Economic costs should be distinguished from transfer payments, which are unrelated to resources. Transfer payments include taxes, unemployment insurance payments, social security payments, and so on. From the point of view of the payer, such payments would appear as costs; from the viewpoint of recipients, they would appear as revenues. However, they are not payments for resource use and production and so are not indicators of how the economy's resources are being used.

Economic costs are subdivided into direct and lost productivity (also called indirect) costs. Direct costs are equivalent to the combined value of goods and services that are paid for. They can be paid for by insurers, governments, or consumers (out of pocket). To be direct costs, the services must have embodied a resource, and they must have been paid for. Indirect or lost productivity costs are the costs of those services that embodied resources but were not paid for. If a patient travels to a clinic or sits idly in a waiting room, he or she may be losing valuable productive time and income. In effect, the patient's time, which is a resource, is not being paid for; payment has been foregone. The value of time lost will never be objectively observed, but it is real, and an economic value should be imputed to the resource.

Economic evaluation studies call for different perspectives. An insurer is interested mainly in what it pays out, for resources and any other sickness benefits. A patient is interested only in what he or she pays out of pocket and in any time lost from work. The patient will also be interested in sickness-related transfer payments, as these will reduce his or her sickness costs. The broadest perspective, called the societal perspective, is the viewpoint of all social resources. It excludes transfer payments, because these cancel out between payer and recipient. The relationship between the perspective of a study and the cost measures that are included in it is shown in Table 17-3. As can be seen, all resources are included in the societal perspective. In any other perspective, the costs suffered by just certain groups will be the sole focus of attention. Economic evaluation guidelines generally propose that the broadest viewpoint be taken. However, economic evaluation studies are often initiated by special interest groups, such as government drug benefit companies and hospitals. These groups are only secondarily concerned with the societal perspective, however commendable it may be.

The costs that are identified should be the marginal costs of the interventions. These costs are equivalent to the combined value of all additional resources used to deliver the intervention. In our diabetes example, we provide the hypothetical marginal cost of two interventions (see Table 17-2). Each cost estimate was divided into four components: inpatient hospitalization from complications of diabetes, routine outpatient visits, self-care, and adverse events that typically lead to emergency room treatment. Hospital costs are the expected costs of hospitalization, and they are based on the probability of being hospitalized and the cost of a hospitalization. Outpatient costs consist of the physician fees for routine visits. Adverse events costs are the emergency room costs that might result from complications that do not lead to hospitalization or that precede hospitalization. The costs of self-care include the costs of monitoring glucose levels, insulin, and medical supplies. Many of these costs will be out of pocket costs incurred by the patient. We exclude the value of lost productivity in our analysis, which therefore falls somewhat short of taking a full societal viewpoint.

Table 17–3 Costs Included in Economic Evaluation Studies

Perspective of Study	Direct Costs	Indirect Costs	Transfer Payments
Payer	√		√
Provider	√*		√
Patient and caregiver	√†	√	√‡
Societal	√	√	

*Includes only payer portion.
†Includes only out-of-pocket expenses.
‡Includes sickness benefit payments received by patients.

As seen in Table 17–2, intensive insulin therapy costs $5,000 per person per year, whereas conventional therapy costs $1,500. The annual difference between the two interventions ($3,500) is primarily due to the costs of self-care, which total $4,135 for the intensive treatment and $700 for conventional care.

17.4.6 Discounting Future Costs and Benefits

As already discussed in Chapter 4, individuals place a higher value on present utilities than future ones. The discount rate is an expression of the preferences of present over future benefits. All future period costs should therefore be discounted to make them equivalent to costs as of the present time. Let us assume a 5 percent discount rate. The discounted costs of the first year for conventional care (assuming, as is traditional, that the costs occur at the end of the year) are $1,428 ($1,500/1.05). For the second year these costs are $1,361 ($1,500/(1.05)^2), and for the third year they are $1,296. The present value for all three years is the sum of these values, $4,085. The discounted costs for all three years of intensive treatment is $13,615, and the difference in the present value of costs between the two interventions (i.e., $c_2 - c_1$) is $9,532.

There is a controversy over the question whether to also discount nonmonetary benefits. Investigators who wrote on the issue in the 1970s (Weinstein and Stason 1977) stated that benefits and costs should be placed on the same plane and should both be discounted. More recently, some investigators (Parsonage and Neuberger 1992) have claimed that, if we discount the benefits from health promotion activities, many of which are not experienced until years after the intervention, the present value will be reduced significantly. For example, the present value of $1,000 received in 20 years at a discount rate of 5 percent is only $396. Yet a gap of 20 years between health promotion activities and health benefits is not unusual. In light of these findings, a debate has occurred over whether to discount health benefits, since doing so places many health promotion activities on very shaky grounds. The investigators contend that a social time preference discount rate may be less than a private one. In recognition of this, guidelines now recommend conducting a sensitivity analysis that includes a zero (no discount) rate for benefits.

17.4.7 Cost-Effectiveness Ratios

In our diabetes example, a series of cost-effectiveness ratios can be calculated. We calculate three such ratios: cost per life saved, cost per life year saved, and cost per quality-adjusted life year saved. Table 17–4 summarizes the costs and outcomes

Table 17–4 Summary Data for Alternative Cost-Effectiveness Ratios

	Net Discounted Costs for 1,000 persons	Deaths	Life Years	Quality-Adjusted Life Years
Intensive care	$13,615,000	6	2,986	2,686.95
Conventional care	$ 4,083,000	10	2,969	2,282.9
Difference	$ 9,532,000	4	17	404.05

for two groups of 1,000 persons with diabetes. The net discounted costs for 1,000 persons under intensive treatment are $13,615,000 and for persons under conventional care they are $4,083,000. The net difference in costs $(c_2 - c_1)$ is therefore $9,532,000. The difference in deaths equals are four, and so the cost per life saved is $2,383,000 ($9,532,000/4). Similarly, the cost per life year saved is $560,705, and the cost per QALY is $23,564.

The interpretation of these ratios is as follows. With regard to the QALY outcomes, an additional $23,564 in costs will yield an additional quality-adjusted life year. The ratio by itself does not tell us whether it would be worth it to spend the extra resources, and thus it does not provide all the information that we need to choose one type of intervention over the other. It merely says what, in physical terms, we will get for our money.

17.4.7 Sensitivity Analysis

Most evaluations, even those which are based on randomized clinical trials, will be developed using assumed values for some variables. In our analysis, we may have obtained QALY information from different sources than the information for lives saved; for example, the QALY data may have been extrapolated from another study. If we were not sure about our valuation of QALYs for the two populations, we could subject them to a sensitivity analysis to see what would be the effect of making different assumptions. If the results changed appreciably, especially if they resulted in different conclusions, then we would have much less confidence in our analysis (Briggs et al. 1994).

Let us say that the QALY value for the intensive treatment was 0.85 rather than 0.90 for each of the three years. Then the outcome would be 2,537 life years for the three-year period. The value of $q_2 - q_1$ would be 255 QALYs rather than 404, and the cost-effectiveness ratio, if all else remained the same, would be $37,380 per life year saved. This is considerably more than the original ratio; however, whether it would change our recommendation depends on whether the cost-effectiveness ratio exceeded some assumed threshold. We would need to set some standards to determine what was an acceptable cost-effectiveness ratio. In the following section we discuss the setting of standards.

17.4.8 Interpreting the Results

The cost-effectiveness ratio takes on additional meaning if it can be compared to some standard. The development of a standard will require that we make some value judgment about what is an acceptable improvement in cost per QALY. Several investigators (Laupacis et al. 1992) have developed a conceptual tool to help interpret such findings. In Figure 17–1 we present the cost-effectiveness results in graphic form. The two axis represent increases (or decreases) in QALYs and increases (or decreases) in cost. The original coordinates are the levels of cost and the QALY outcome for one of the interventions, say, c_1 and q_1. Let us take c_1 to be \$4,083,000 per 1,000 persons and q_1 to be 2,282 QALYs, which is the value for conventional diabetes care in our example.

Based on the coordinates in Figure 17–1, there are four quadrants, labeled A, B, C, and D. The origin is c_1 and q_1. Relative to these points, c_2 will be the same, greater, or less than c_1; and q_2 will be the same, greater, or less than q_1. At any point in quadrant A, the intensive treatment intervention will cost less and produce more QALYs than the conventional intervention. On both cost and outcome grounds, the intensive intervention is preferred to the conventional one; it is termed *dominant*. On policy grounds, the intensive intervention should be adopted. The same type of reasoning holds for any rate that falls into quadrant C, only in this case the conventional alternative is dominant.

If, relative to c_1 and q_1, the points c_2 and q_2 fall into quadrant D, then intervention 2 (intensive treatment) costs more *and* yields more QALYs. If we want to derive a policy conclusion, a value judgment must be used to set a standard. One group of researchers (Laupacis et al. 1992) proposed the following set of value judgments:

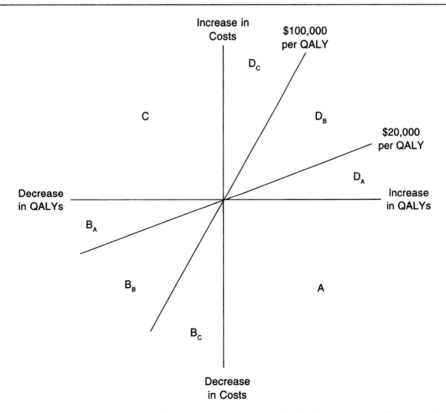

Figure 17–1 Alternative combinations of cost and QALY changes. The position of each point represents a cost-effectiveness ratio. The position of the point will provide a standard that can be interpreted as dominant (quadrants A and C), strong evidence (quadrants D_A and B_A), moderate evidence (quadrants B_B and D_B) and weak evidence (quadrants D_C and B_C).

- If intervention 2 relative to intervention 1 results in a cost-effectiveness ratio that is less than $20,000 per year, then there is *strong* evidence supporting the adoption of intervention 2.
- If intervention 2 relative to intervention 1 results in a cost-effectiveness ratio that is between $20,000 and $100,000 per year, then there is *moderate* evidence supporting the adoption of intervention 2.
- If intervention 2 relative to intervention 1 results in a cost-effectiveness ratio that is greater than $100,000 per year, then there is *weak* evidence supporting the adoption of intervention 2.

These guidelines are presented graphically in Figure 17–1. The line indicating a cost-effectiveness ratio of $20,000 per QALY separates area D_A from the rest of the quadrant D. The line indicating a cost-effectiveness ratio of $100,000 per QALY separates D_C from the remainder of quadrant D. Thus quadrant D is now divided up into three areas related to the values stated. If the cost-effectiveness ratio falls into the area of D_A (cost-effectiveness ratio below $20,000 per QALY), then this provides strong evidence supporting its adoption. If it falls into area D_B (i.e., it is between $20,000 and $100,000), then there is moderate evidence. And if it falls into area D_C (i.e., it exceeds $100,000), then weak evidence for adoption is provided. Similar reasoning holds for ratios that fall into quadrant B.

Analyses such as these make more explicit the value judgments that are related to policy analyses. In this example, the standards were somewhat loosely based on average annual salaries. A low-income person earns about $20,000, and so if the cost per QALY is below that, then the authors conclude that adoption would be warranted. However, these values are by no means universally accepted. Other investigators have chosen the standard of $50,000 to delineate whether an intervention should be recommended (Hirth et al. 2000). A number of investigators have recommended the development and use of community surveys on what the general public is willing to pay for a QALY (Olsen and Donaldson 1998).

17.5 COST-BENEFIT ANALYSIS

Cost-effectiveness analysis and cost-utility analysis provide information about the differences in outcomes in relation to differences in costs. As already stated, they do not provide information on whether the differences in outcomes are worth the differences in cost. To determine whether they are, one must either inject one's own (or somebody else's) valuations of the outcomes or else seek monetary valuations of the outcomes.

17.5.1 Valuation of Outcomes

Among the outcomes for health care are improved health; an ability to work or engage in leisure activities; and desired characteristics of the services themselves, such as convenience. Investigators have placed valuations on all of these.

17.5.2 Human Capital

One method of outcome valuation, called the *human capital approach,* focuses on lost work and lost leisure time. According to this approach, individuals' lost time from work (or leisure) is valued at the opportunity cost of time. This cost can be either the value of lost wages or the amount one must pay someone else to do the replacement work. For example, if a woman has heavy bleeding and loses five days from work, one can place a value on this time by estimating the per diem wage (e.g., $80 per day) and multiplying this wage by the length of time. An alternative way of measuring human capital losses would be through measuring the replacement costs for lost time. If a homemaker was sick for five days and could not engage in housework, then one could estimate the loss by determining the cost of hiring someone else to do the work.

The human capital method, once very popular, has fallen out of favor with economists for several reasons. First, studies in the Netherlands have questioned whether this method commonly overestimates productivity losses (Koopmanschap et al. 1995). According to their friction-cost analyses, companies may replace individuals who are off the job with others; these replacement workers may have been previously unemployed or underemployed. The value of lost production would then be less than stated by the human capital method. Of course, the ease or difficulty of finding replacement workers would depend on overall economic conditions, such as the prevailing unemployment rate.

Second, if a person is sick, he or she loses work time and perhaps income, but there are other benefits lost as well. Individuals may still work but at a lower capacity. Or if they are off work, they may simultaneously lose other benefits usually associated with good health. The lost wage from absence from work, therefore, may not be an understatement of the value of the losses to the individuals after all. For this reason, investigators have sought other means of measuring the value of lost work time.

Third, human capital incorporates a value system that places emphasis on those who are employed. Retirees and unemployed persons are valued at a very low rate, if at all. Yet a large portion of our health resources go to treat those who are not working, including persons who are retired. The human capital approach therefore would not serve as a good method of evaluating lost benefits from interventions that led to improved health but maybe not increased work time. Nevertheless, the human capital approach is still widely used, especially in cost-of-illness studies. Proponents of national economic policies espouse the goal of increasing total productivity and per-worker productivity. Improved health can often lead to the achievement of these goals. This may be why the human capital approach has not completely faded away.

17.5.3 Risk Preference

A second method for evaluating lost benefits is the "risk preference" approach. This approach is based on actual market data rather than inferred values, and so it reflects personal preferences. The widest use of this method has been in the labor market (see Chapter 11). The economic hypothesis states that individuals will demand a risk premium in order to accept more risky occupations. If we can quantify the health risks in various occupations as well as the wages paid in these occupations, then, after we adjust for other variables that might also affect wages (e.g., experience, training, and gender), the wage differential should be related to the risk differential. Put otherwise, the adjusted wage differential measures the extra amount of money that workers demand in return for working in an occupation with a higher risk of injury or death. This measure can be used to evaluate the probability of poor health or death. Somewhat indirectly, one can infer a value per QALY from this information. If there is a 10-percent difference in risk of mortality between two occupations, and the annual pay differential is $5,000, then one can infer a value of $50,000 for the loss of a life ($5,000/.10). In this way, one can estimate some of the benefits from an increased probability of improved health, namely, those associated with longevity. Many other health-related benefits cannot be dealt with through the use of this concept.

17.5.4 Contingent Valuation

A third method of measuring benefits is termed *contingent valuation*. In this method, individuals are asked what they would hypothetically pay if they could achieve the benefits that result from specific interventions. For example, if a person who undergoes kidney dialysis daily could, with no adverse effects, receive dialysis only twice a week, then he or she would benefit enormously. An interviewer could question this person about how much he or she valued (in monetary terms) such an occurrence. The stated value could be construed as the individual's willingness to pay for the improved kidney treatments.

In a contingent valuation study, the responses depend on what the respondents are asked. Much study has gone into this subject. Briefly, here are some guidelines for achieving a valid valuation:

- The effects of the intervention should be clearly stated and understood by the respondent.
- The questionnaire should stress that there are other goods and services competing for the respondent's money.
- The respondent should be told that he or she would have to reduce spending on other things.
- Generally, the respondent should be told that the additional spending would be in the form of higher taxes or product prices.
- The interview should include follow-up questions in order to determine the reasons for the respondent's valuations.

17.5.5 Techniques of Valuation

The valuation techniques described above have been used by investigators in a number of different contexts. One group of investigators surveyed studies in which respondents expressed a willingness to pay in return for specific reductions in risk that would result in expected increases in QALYs. Using the estimates of these studies, the authors calculated a value of life (Hirth et al. 2000). They estimated the age of persons in each study, the expected life years remaining, the QALYs per life year, and thus the number of QALYs. With this information, the investigators could estimate a cost per QALY for each study reviewed. The values arrived at differed widely and seemed to depend on the research approach. According to the human capital approach, the value for cost per QALY was $24,777. Using revealed preference studies, the authors estimated a value of $93,000. And using the contingent valuation approach, they estimated a value of $161,000. Given the large variation between methods, the authors concluded that the goal of determining a cost per QALY was elusive.

In theory, the value of a QALY is most important, as it provides a key to answering a central question in economic evaluation. However, the cost per QALY in practice seems to depend on the context of the analysis and on the method used to obtain information. The values arrived at using the method that is closest to revealed preferences—risk preference—cannot be easily linked to specific health states. As well, there are considerable differences in the results of the various studies. The contingent valuation method suffers from the difficulty of applying it to specific interventions and the difficulty of achieving comparability. This method also elicits hypothetical responses from individuals; faced with actual situations, people may value services differently. It would seem that the contingent valuation method is better suited to answering hypothetical questions about health-related programs than questions about the values placed on specific interventions. Often, respondents would require detailed knowledge about the interventions, and their information needs might tax the interviewing process. A great deal of detail about the results of specific interventions can be obtained from health-related quality-of-life indicators, including preference-based indicators. Willingness-to-pay measures cannot provide such detail. In sum, the best instrument to use depends on the purpose of the investigation.

17.5.6 Cost-Benefit Ratio

Cost-benefit analysis answers the question, Are the costs worth the benefits? If we are looking at a specific intervention, then this question implies that there is an alternative intervention, even if it amounts to "not conducting the intervention." The main point is that there are alternative uses of the resources involved. In a cost-benefit analysis, the alternative should be explicitly considered.

Ignoring discounting, the cost-benefit equation is expressed as

$$NSB = b - c$$

where b refers to the dollar benefits resulting from the intervention and c to the additional costs.

Returning to our diabetes example, assume that, at the current level of treating diabetes (i.e., using the conventional method), the cost per person is as before (i.e., the discounted, three-year value for c is $9,532 per person). This is the additional cost of tight insulin control, assuming that the conventional method would have been used in the absence of tight insulin control. The difference in QALYs per person is 0.404. If the willingness to pay for one additional QALY is $30,000, then the value of b is $12,120 (.404 × $30,000). Thus the net benefits are greater than zero. Since this measure incorporates the worth of a QALY, it provides an answer to the basic question, Is it worth it? In the absence of other considerations, a net present value in excess of zero would yield a recommendation to adopt the intervention.

The contingent valuation we have calculated will almost certainly be derived from studies that elicit answers under hypothetical conditions. The populations who are surveyed may not be representative of all relevant persons. Therefore, like all other measures, the willingness-to-pay measure must be interpreted with care.

EXERCISES

1. A health economist was asked to compare outcomes and costs of two diabetes therapies that affected both the severity of the disease and the survival rate. What evaluation concept should he use?

2. A health economist was asked to compare outcomes and costs for two prophylactic medicines that reduced deaths during surgical operations. The interventions did not influence quality of life. What concept should she use?

3. A health economist was asked whether a new drug that reduced mortality should be used. What concept should she use?

4. Patients who were hospitalized for asthma were placed on a new drug. The drug resulted in an extra day of hospitalization (the length of stay went from 6 to 7 days), which cost $800. There were no other differences in the treatment. The drug cost $300 for the dose. As well, it took an hour of nursing time (wage = $20 per hour) and $10 in supplies to administer it. The mortality rate was 10 deaths per 100 with the drug and 12 deaths per 100 without it. What is the cost-effectiveness ratio for using the drug?

5. In a population of 1,000 persons at the beginning of the year, 40 die during the year. How many life years were there during the year?

6. In one year, 30 persons per 1,000 die of asthma. A new drug reduces that number to 20 1,000. How is outcome defined, and what is the "effectiveness" of the drug?

7. In one year, 60 people per 100 die from complications of diabetes. A new drug will reduce that number to 40 per 100 *if* everyone takes the drug, according to a recently conducted clinical trial. However, 25 percent of those who take the drug will discontinue it, even though this means that their death rate will be the same as the rate for those who don't take the drug. What is the efficacy and effectiveness of the drug?

8. In an asthma center, the nurse took two quality-of-life measurements using the 15-D questionnaire. The scores (on a scale of 1–5) for the first and the second are presented in the table below. The first measurement was taken when the patient entered the clinic, and the second was taken one week later, after the patient received asthma medicine. What is the effectiveness, in quality-adjusted life years, of the asthma medicine?

Health dimension	Score at first visit	Score at second visit
Breathing	2	3
Mental functioning	2	2
Speech	2	3
Vision	2	2
Mobility	2	2
Usual activities	2	2
Vitality	2	4
Hearing	2	2
Eating	2	3
Eliminating	2	3
Sleeping	2	3
Distress	2	2
Discomfort	2	3
Sexual Activity	4	5
Depression	2	2

9. A patient with asthma will live for six months if she does not take her medicine. The quality of life of that patient will be 0.8. If she takes asthma medicine, her quality of life will increase to 0.9 and her length of survival will be seven months. What is the effectiveness of the medicine?

10. Two interventions were each applied to 1,000 persons. Given the resulting data (contained in the table below), determine a cost-effectiveness ratio. The discount rate is 5 percent. Is this a high ratio?

	Year 1	Year 2
Intervention A		
Survivors	980	960
Quality of life	0.9	0.9
Cost per person	$30,000	$6,000
Intervention B		
Survivors	975	970
Quality of life	.85	.85
Cost per person	$20,000	$4,000

BIBLIOGRAPHY

Cost-Benefit and Cost-Effectiveness Analysis: General

Bakker,C., et al. 1994. Cost effectiveness of group physical therapy compared to individualized therapy for ankylosing spondylitis. *Journal of Rheumatology* 21:264–268.

Briggs, A., et al. 1994. Uncertainty in the economic evaluation of health care technologies: The role of sensitivity analysis. *Health Economics* 3:95–104.

Canadian Coordinating Office for Health Technology Assessment. 1997. *Guidelines for economic evaluation of pharmaceuticals: Canada.* Ottawa: Canadian Coordinating Office for Health Technology Assessment.

Cochrane, A. 1972. *Effectiveness and efficiency.* New York: Oxford University Press.

Culyer, A.J. 1985. The scope and limits of health economics. *Okonomie des Gesundheitswesens* (new edition) 159:31–54.

Doubilet, P. 1986. Use and misuse of the term "cost effective" in medicine. *New England Journal of Medicine* 314:253–256.

Drummond, M.F., et al. 1997. *Methods for the economic evaluation of health care programmes.* 2nd ed. Oxford: Oxford University Press.

Drummond, M.F., and Davies, L. 1991. Economic analysis alongside clinical trials. *International Journal of Technology Assessment in Health Care* 7:561–573.

Drummond, M.F., et al. 1987. *Methods for the economic evaluation of health care programs.* Toronto: Oxford University Press.

Gold, M.R., et al. 1996. *Cost-effectiveness in health and medicine.* New York: Oxford University Press.

Haddix, A.C., et al. 1996. *Prevention effectiveness: A guide to decision analysis and economic evaluation.* New York: Oxford University Press.

Hatzriandrou, E.I., et al. 1988. A cost-effectiveness analysis of exercise as health promotion. *American Journal of Public Health* 78:1417–1421.

Hellinger, F.J. 1980. Cost-benefit analysis of health care: Past applications and future prospects. *Inquiry* 17:204–215.

Hirth, R.A., et al. 2000. Willingness to pay for a quality-adjusted life year: In search of a standard. *Medical Decision Making* 20:332–342.

Laupacis, A., et al. 1992. How attractive does a new technology have to be to warrant adoption and utilization? Tentative guidelines for using clinical and economic evaluations. *Canadian Medical Association Journal* 146:473–481.

Luce, B.R., and A. Elixhauser. 1990. *Standards for the socioeconomic evaluation of health care services*. Berlin: Springer Verlag.

Menon, D., et al. 1996. Canada's new guidelines for the economic evaluation of pharmaceuticals. *Medical Care* 34:DS77–DS86.

Parsonage, M., and H. Neuberger. 1992. Discounting and health benefits. *Health Economics* 1:71–79.

Simes, R.J., and P.P. Glasziou. 1992. Meta analysis and quality of evidence in the economic evaluation of drug trials. *Pharmacoeconomics* 1:282–292.

Stoddart, G.L., and M.F. Drummond. How to read clinical journals. VII: To understand an economic evaluation. Parts A and B. *Canadian Medical Association Journal* 130:1428–1433, 1542–1549.

Warner, K.E. 1982. *Cost-benefit and cost-effectiveness analysis in health care*. Ann Arbor, MI: Health Administration Press.

Warner, K.E., and R.C. Hutton. 1980. Cost-benefit and cost-effectiveness analysis in health care. *Medical Care* 18:1069–1084.

Weinstein, M.C., and W.B. Stason. 1977. Foundations of cost-effectiveness analysis for health and medical practices. *New England Journal of Medicine* 296:716–721.

Williams, A. 1974a. The cost benefit approach. *British Medical Bulletin* 20:252–256.

———. 1974b. Measuring the effectiveness of health care systems. *British Journal of Preventive and Social Medicine* 28:196–202.

Diabetes-Related Studies

Diabetes Control and Complications Trial Research Group (DCCT). 1996. Lifetime benefits and costs of intensive therapy as practiced in the Diabetes Control and Complications Trial. *JAMA* 276:1409–1415.

Diabetes Control and Complications Trial Research Group (DCCT). 1995. Resource utilization and costs of care in the Diabetes Control and Complications Trial. *Diabetes Care* 18: 1468–1478.

Gray, A., et al. 2000. Cost effectiveness of an intensive blood glucose control policy in patients with type 2 diabetes: Economic analysis alongside randomized controlled trial (UKPDS 41). *British Medical Journal* 320:1373–1378.

UK Prospective Diabetes Study Group. 1998. Intensive blood-glucose with sulphonylureas or insulin compared with conventional treatment and risk of complications in patients with type 2 diabetes (UKPDS33). *Lancet* 352:857–853.

Health-Related Quality of Life and QALYs

Bakker, C., et al. 1994. Cost effectiveness of group physical therapy compared to individualized therapy for ankylosing spondylitis. *Journal of Rheumatology* 21:264–268.

Erickson, P. 1966. Modeling health-related quality of life: The bridge between psychometric and utility-based measures. *Journal of the National Cancer Institute*, monograph 20, 17–20.

Gudex, C., and P. Kind. n.d. *The QALY Toolkit*. York, England: Center for Health Economics.

Sintonen, H. 1981. An approach to measuring and valuing health states. *Social Science and Medicine* 15C:55–65.

———. 1981. *The 15-D measure of health related quality of life*. West Heidelberg, Australia: National Centre for Health Program Evaluation.

Torrance, G.W., and D. Feeny. 1989. Utilities and quality adjusted life years. *International Journal of Technology Assessment in Health Care* 5:559–575.

Williams, A. 1985. Economics of coronary bypass grafting. *British Medical Journal* 291:326–329.

Value of Health and Life

Blomquist, G. 1981. The value of human life: An empirical perspective. *Economic Inquiry* 19:157–164.

Donaldson, C. 1999. Valuing the benefits of publicly-provided health care: Does "ability to pay" preclude the use of "willingness to pay"? *Social Science and Medicine* 49:551–563.

Fisher, A., et al. 1989. The value of reducing risks of death. *Journal of Policy Analysis and Management* 8:88–100.

Jacobs, P. and K. Fassbender. 1998. The measurement of indirect costs in the health economics evaluation literature. *International Journal of Technology Assessment in Health Care* 14:799–808.

Johanneson, M., et al. 1991. Willingness to pay for antihypertensive therapy: Results of a Swedish pilot study. *Journal of Health Economics* 10:461–474.

Johanneson, M., et al. 1993. Willingness to pay for antihypertensive therapy: Further results. *Journal of Health Economics* 12:95–108.

Koopmanschap, M.A., et al. 1995. The friction cost method for measuring indirect cost of disease. *Journal of Health Economics* 14:171–189.

Landefeld, J.S., and Seskin, E.P. 1982. The economic value of life: Linking theory to practice. *American Journal of Public Health* 72:555–566.

Mooney, G. 1977. *The valuation of human life.* New York: Macmillan.

Muller, A., and T.J. Reutzel. 1984. Willingness to pay for a reduction in fatality risk. *American Journal of Public Health* 74:808–812.

O'Brien, B., and J.L. Viramontes. 1994. Willingness to pay: A valid and reliable measure of health state preference? *Medical Decision Making* 14:289–297.

Olsen, J.A., and C. Donaldson. 1998. Helicopters, hearts, and hips: Using willingness to pay to set priorities for public sector programmes. *Social Science and Medicine* 46:1–12.

Rice, D.P., and T.A. Hodgson. 1982. The value of human life revisited. *American Journal of Public Health* 72:536–538.

Schelling, T.C. 1968. The life you save may be your own. In *Problems in public expenditure analysis*, ed. S.B. Chase. Washington, DC: Brookings Institution.

Shogren, J.F., et al. 1994. Resolving differences in willingness to pay and willingness to accept. *American Economic Review* 84:255–270.

Thaler, R., and S. Rosen. 1975. The value of saving a life. In *Household production and consumption*, ed. M.E. Terleckyj. New York: National Bureau of Economic Research.

Thompson, M.S. 1986. Willingness to pay and accept risks to cure chronic disease. *American Journal of Public Health* 76:392–397.

Viscusi, W.K. 1978. Labor market valuations of life and limb. *Public Policy* 26:359–385.

———. 1993. The value of risks of life and health. *Journal of Economic Literature* 31:1912–1946.

Zeckhauser, R. 1975. Procedures for valuing lives. *Public Policy* 23:419–464.

Specific Cost-Benefit and Cost-Effectiveness Analyses

Berwick, D.M., and A.L. Komaroff. 1982. Cost effectiveness of lead screening. *New England Journal of Medicine* 306:1392–1398.

Bloom, B.S., and J. Jacobs. 1985. Cost effects of restricting cost-effective therapy. *Medical Care* 23:872–880.

Doherty, N., and B.C. Hicks. 1975. The use of cost-effectiveness analysis in geriatric day care. *Gerontologist* 15:412–417.

Elixhauser, A. 1989. The cost effectiveness of preventive care for diabetes mellitus. *Diabetes Spectrum* 2:349–353.

Evans, R.G., and G.C. Robinson. 1980. Surgical day care: Measurements of the economic payoff. *Canadian Medical Association Journal* 123:873–880.

———. 1983. An economic study of cost savings on a care by parent ward. *Medical Care* 21:768–782.

Hammond, J. 1979. Home health care cost effectiveness: An overview of the literature. *Public Health Reports* 94:305–311.

Lave, L.B. 1980. Economic evaluation of public health programs. *Annual Review of Public Health* 1:255–276.

Russell, L.B. 1986. *Is prevention better than cure?* Washington, DC: Brookings Institution.

Scheffler, R.M., and L. Paringer. 1980. A review of the economic evaluation of prevention. *Medical Care* 18:473–484.

Weinstein, M.C. 1983. Cost-effectiveness priorities for cancer prevention. *Science* 221:17–23.

Weisbrod, B.A. 1971. Costs and benefits of medical research. *Journal of Political Economy* 79:527–544.

Weisbrod, B.A., et al. 1980. Alternative to mental hospital treatment. *Archives of General Surgery* 37:400–405.

Economic Evaluation and Technology Assessment

Detsky, A.S. 1985. Using economic analysis to determine the resource consequences of choices made in planning clinical trials. *Journal of Chronic Diseases* 38:753–765.

Drummond, M.F., and G.L. Stoddart. 1984. Economic analysis and clinical trials. *Controlled Clinical Trials* 5:115–128.

Weinstein, M.C. 1981. Economic assessments of medical practices and technologies. *Medical Decision Making* 1:309–330.

Glossary of Health Economics Terms

access. Potential and actual entry of a population into the health care delivery system (U.S. Congress 1988).

acute care. Inpatient diagnostic and short-term treatment of patients.

adjusted average per capita cost (AAPCC). An estimate of the average cost incurred by Medicare per beneficiary in the fee-for-service system, adjusted by county for geographic cost differences related to age, sex, disability status, Medicaid eligibility, and institutional status.

adverse selection. The systematic selection by high-risk consumers of insurance plans with greater degrees of coverage. The insurers who offer these plans end up with insureds who incur greater than normal costs.

agency (agent). A group (individual) that has been delegated authority to make decisions and perform activities on behalf of those doing the delegating. Physicians are often said to act as agents for their patients, indicating that the physicians make decisions about treatments based on their knowledge.

all-payer system. A system of reimbursing providers in which all separate insurers coordinate to set uniform payment policies. Individual providers will then receive the same reimbursement from different insurers for cases with similar characteristics.

alternate level of care (ALC). A non-acute treatment patient occupying an acute care bed would be viewed receiving an alternate level of care—a level other than the appropriate one.

ambulatory care. Care rendered to individuals under their own cognizance any time when they are not resident in an institution.

ambulatory care groups (ACGs). A case-mix classification system incorporating related ambulatory care visits, based on ICD-9-CM diagnostic codes and patient age and sex (Weiner et al. 1991).

ambulatory visit groups (AVGs). A classification system by which ambulatory care visits with associated procedures are classified into similar resource-using groups based on diagnosis, procedure, age, and sex.

appropriateness of care. The extent to which the expected health benefits of a procedure exceed its expected negative consequences by a sufficiently wide margin that the procedure is worth doing. Considerations of cost are excluded (Chassin et al. 1987, 2534).

asymmetric information. An imbalance of information between buyers and sellers of a service, by which one group is better informed than the other.

atypical patients. Patients who exhibit patterns of care different from typical cases, either because they do not complete a full and successful course of treatment in a single institution or because their length of stay exceeds the statistical trim point.

availability. The supply of services, generally in relation to the demand for the services.

average cost (AC). The unit cost for a selected volume of output; total cost divided by total quantity of output. The average cost is equal to the average variable cost plus the average fixed cost.

average fixed cost (AFC). The unit fixed cost for a specific volume of output. The average fixed cost is equal to the total fixed cost divided by the volume of output.

average length of stay. *See* **length of stay**.

average variable cost (AVC). The unit variable cost for a specific volume of output; total variable cost divided by quantity of output.

basis of payment. The unit of output in terms of which the provider is paid. This can be on any of a per day of care, per service provided, per case, or per person (capitation).

bed days. The number of days in a period that beds are available. In a year, bed days are 365 × the number of available beds.

benefit. (1) A dollar value that is placed on health outcomes. (2) The compensation of labor that is additional to wages (e.g., health insurance, life insurance, pension rights, etc.)

biased selection. The deliberate choice, by a provider or insurer, of a group of patients (insureds) with preselected characteristics associated with low utilization of health care.

burden. With reference to a tax, the reduction in real income resulting from the tax (Due 1957, 6).

capacity. Capacity is a measure of the output that can be reached when existing resources are fully and efficiently used.

capital. Human, physical, and financial means of production.

capitation. A payment system in which the entity financially responsible for the patients' health care services receives a fixed periodic sum for each patient that covers the costs of utilization by the patient. The sum can be adjusted for specific patient characteristics, such as age and sex.

case management. A collection of organized activities to identify high-cost patients as early as possible, locate and assess alternative treatment methods, and manage health care benefits for these patients in a cost-effective manner (Scheffler et al. 1991).

case mix. An index or measure of the average level of resource requirements for a group of cases sorted and weighted according to type of case. The weights represent the estimated resource use for each type of case.

case-mix groups (CMGs). A Canadian system for classifying hospital inpatients into groups using similar quantities of resources according to selected patient characteristics such as diagnosis, procedure, age, and comorbidity. CMGs are maintained by the Canadian Institute for Health Information.

charges. A price set for a product by the supplier. Charges may not equal cash received because some payers may receive a discount or fail to pay.

coinsurance. A system of provider payment in which the patient is responsible for a portion of the payment and the insurer or third party is responsible for the rest.

community care. Care provided in a noninstitutional setting, including in the home or in the patient's "neighborhood."

community rating. A method of setting insurance premiums for health care coverage. In this method, all insurers in the group pay the same premium regardless of their risk-related characteristics, such as age or health problems.

comorbidity. A disease or condition that is present at the same time as the principal disease or condition of the patient.

competition. A state of competition exists in a market if no single firm or consumer is large enough to influence the market price. This state usually occurs if there are many buyers and sellers in the market.

competitive price. The price at which demand and supply are in equilibrium in a competitive market.

complements. Two goods or services that are consumed together, such as surgeons' services and operating room services. The economic relevance of complementarity is that a change in the direct price of a complement will cause a shift in the demand curve of the other service.

complications. Adverse patient conditions that arise during the process of medical care.

concentration (market). The extent to which market activity is confined to a limited number of firms.

concurrent review. A process of ongoing review while the patient is undergoing treatment in the hospital, and of certifying the length of stay that is appropriate for the approved admission (Scheffler 1991).

consumer's surplus. The difference between what an individual is willing to pay for a given quantity of a good or service and what is actually paid. This is equal to the area under the demand curve between no consumption and that specified quantity minus the amount paid for all the units (price times quantity).

consumerism. A view that health care should be directly driven by the interests of consumers.

consumption. The use of services to satisfy current wants.

contingent valuation. The valuation that a person would place on a service if he/she had the option of having it available.

continuing care. A system of service delivery that includes all of the services provided by long-term care, home support, and home care. This term reflects within it two complementary concepts, i.e., that care may "continue" over a long period of time and that an integrated program of care "continues" across service components, that is, that there is a continuum of care. Continuing care is still in the process of emerging from its acute care, social services, and public health roots into a separate system of delivery, i.e., a distinct, separate, and major "product line" in the overall health care system (Hollander 1994).

copayments. Out-of-pocket payments for health services made by users as their share of the providers' total reimbursement.

core services. In Canada health services which must be available to every resident of a province (Saskatchewan Health 1993). *See also* **insured services**.

cost. The value placed on the goods and services. *See* **opportunity cost** and **money cost**.

cost benefit. The relationship between the dollar impact of an intervention and its opportunity cost. It can be expressed as a ratio or as a net value (benefits minus costs).

cost curve. The relation between cost and volume of output. It can be specified in terms of total costs, average or unit costs, and marginal costs. *See* **long-run cost curve** and **short-run cost curve**.

cost effectiveness. The relationship between the additional cost and the additional health outcome (expressed in physical terms) of one intervention as compared with another.

cost function. A behavioral relationship between cost (viewed from either a marginal, average, or total perspective) and the variables that influence cost, including volume of output, quality of output, input prices, and variables affecting organizational efficiency. *See* **cost curve, long-run cost curve**, and **short-run cost curve**.

cost sharing. The joint payment or sharing of a price by the consumer and the payer (insurer).

cost shifting. The charging of different prices for differentially insured patients, usually including the subsidization of care for nonpaying patients.

cost utility. The relationship between the additional cost and the additional health outcome (expressed in terms of a utility index) of one intervention as compared with another.

critical care. See **intensive care**.

day procedure groups (DPGs). A classification system for ambulatory patients in which patients are assigned to classes according to principle procedures that use similar resources. The DPG system was developed from New York's PAS system and is used by the Canadian Institute for Health Information.

deductible. A fixed amount that a consumer must spend out of pocket before insurance coverage begins. If the deductible is $200, the individual must pay for the first $200 of medical expenditures out of pocket.

demand. Consumer willingness to purchase alternative quantities of services at various specified prices, represented by the position of the demand curve.

demand curve (schedule). A schedule indicating the quantities of a service that an individual or group is willing to purchase at different prices of that service, all other factors (income, tastes, other prices) held constant.

derived demand. The demand for a factor of production, which is determined by the additional output yielded by that factor.

diagnosis. A determination of the specific physical ailment of an individual.

diagnosis-related groups (DRGs). A system of classifying hospital inpatients into groups using similar quantities of resources according to selected characteristics such as diagnoses, procedure, age, and any complications or comorbidities. DRGs are used for hospital reimbursement in the U.S. Medicare system (Fetter 1991).

direct cost. (1) In social cost accounting, the cost of all resources incurred by providers of health care; usually refers to paid resources. (2) In hospital cost accounting, the cost of resources (doctors, nurses, lab techs) that are directly involved in the provision of care; overhead costs are excluded.

direct price. *See* **out-of-pocket price.**

direct teaching costs. As regards hospital care, the costs in a teaching hospital that can be directly traced to educational rather than patient care functions. These include resident and intern salaries.

discharge planning. The process of assessing a patient's needs for treatment after hospitalization and effecting an appropriate and timely hospital discharge impact of Blue Cross and Blue Shield plan utilization management (Scheffler 1991).

discount (time discount). A constant applied to future costs and benefits in order to value them equivalently to costs and benefits occurring in the present period.

disease prevention. *See* **prevention.**

disequilibrium. A state in which a market is not in equilibrium. As a result of a shift in demand or supply, a market will be in disequilibrium until the price and quantity adjust to the new equilibrium levels. A state of disequilibrium can be permanent if there is some barrier (e.g., government price control) that permanently maintains the price at a level above or below that of equilibrium.

DRG. *See* **diagnosis-related groups.**

economic cost. *See* **opportunity cost.**

economies of scale. Reductions in operating costs associated with larger scale operations.

economies of scope. Reductions in the operating costs of two or more related services (e.g., home care and hospital care) associated with joint production (e.g., production of both services by the same organization).

effectiveness. The relationship between an intervention and its health outcome, usually measured in physical units (e.g., life years saved). Some definitions specify that effectiveness is a measure of the ability of an intervention to bring about an outcome under actual practice conditions.

efficacy. The relationship between an intervention and its health outcome under ideal (usually experimental) clinical conditions.

efficiency. (1) Technical efficiency is a measure of how close a given combination of resources is to producing a maximum amount of output. (2) Allocative or economic efficiency is a measure of how close a given combination of resources is to yielding maximum consumer satisfaction.

elasticity of demand. The quantity of a service demanded in response to the out-of-pocket price of a service or product. Elasticity is calculated by dividing the percent change in the product divided by the percent change in the direct price. The price and quantity in terms of which the change is measured can be the original price and quantity (point elasticity) or an average of the original and the new prices and quantities (arc elasticity).

emergency care. Emergency care involves immediate decision making and action to prevent death or any further disability for patients in a health crisis.

encounter. A single visit to a provider (sometimes used as an output measure).

episode of care. A series of temporally contiguous health care services related to treatment of a given spell of illness or provided in response to a specific request by the patient or other relevant entity (Hornbrook et al. 1985, 171).

episode of illness. A single unbroken interval of time during which the patient suffers from a continuous spell of signs and/or symptoms that are perceived as sickness or ill-health (Hornbrook et al. 1985, 170).

equilibrium. A situation in which all forces are in balance so there is no tendency to change. (1) **consumer equilibrium** occurs where the individual consuming unit has acquired a composition of goods that gives the unit its maximum attainable satisfaction (utility) given the constraints (prices, incomes) it faces. (2) **producer or provider equilibrium** occurs when the firm is producing the level of output that achieves its objectives (e.g., maximum profits, maximum output). (3) **market or competitive equilibrium** occurs when all buyers and sellers simultaneously achieve their maximized positions; demand and supply are therefore in balance at these determined levels of price and quantity.

equity. Fairness (e.g., in the provision of health care). *See* **horizontal equity** and **vertical equity**.

experience rating. A method of setting health premiums for health care coverage. In this method, each insured in the group pays a premium that is based on his or her risk-related characteristics.

extra billing. Billing for an insured health service rendered to an insured person by a medical practitioner in an amount in addition to any amount paid for that service by the provincial or territorial health insurance plan (Canada Health Act 1984).

factors of production. *See* **resources**.

fee-for-service reimbursement. The type of reimbursement in which payment is made for each item or service.

firm. A self-contained organization that engages in the production or provision of a service or product. The production can occur in more than one facility. *See* **plant**.

fixed costs. Costs that remain the same despite changes in the volume of output.

fixed inputs. Inputs that, within a selected range, do not vary with output. Examples include office space and equipment.

flat-of-the-curve medicine. Medical care that has no impact on health status. The allusion is to the curve relating medical care inputs to health status output. Eventually, if medical care is provided in large enough quantities, its additional effectiveness is hypothesized to be zero (i.e., the output will be constant and the curve will be flat).

full cost. The cost that a provider incurs in producing services. The total cost covers *all* inputs, direct and indirect, used in the production of the services.

funding. A payment made to a provider to cover expenses for services rendered. The funding is not necessarily related to the costs incurred for specific patients or services.

global budget. A fixed annual operating grant paid to a provider that is to cover all services provided to all patients who are treated.

gross domestic product (GDP). The money amount of all final goods and services (consumer, investment, and government) produced within defined geographical boundaries. A standard measure of relative health expenditures for a given state, province, or country is total health spending divided by GDP.

group model HMO. A health maintenance organization in which the HMO contracts with an independent group practice to provide care for its members. The contractual arrangements are usually on a per capita basis.

group practice. A medical practice in which several practitioners share some inputs, such as office staff and space.

health. (1) A complete state of physical, mental, and social well being, and not merely the absence of disease or illness (World Health Organization). (2) A state characterized by anatomic integrity; ability to perform personally valued family, work, and community roles; ability to deal with physical, biologic, and social stress; a feeling of well-being; and freedom from the risk of untimely disease (Last 1988, 6).

health care. A range of services and products whose end purpose is the preservation or enhancement of health.

health insurance. The payment for the expected costs of a group resulting from medical utilization based on the expected expenses incurred by the group. The payment can be based on community or experience rating.

health insurance purchasing cooperative (HIPC). An insurance organization that acts as a broker between payers of health insurance (households, businesses, governments) and health care providers. The HIPC sets standards for health care services and seeks competitive bids for these services; the consumers can then select from among the competing providers.

health maintenance organization (HMO). An organization in which a provider or management group takes on the responsibility for providing health services to a specific group of enrollees in exchange for a set annual fee for each enrollee. The HMO can be the provider or it can contract for services with outside providers.

health plan. An organization that acts as an insurer for an enrolled group of members (Prospective Payment Assessment Commission 1993).

health promotion. Education and/or other supportive services that will assist individuals or groups to adopt healthy behaviors and/or reduce health risks, increase self-care skills, improve management of common minor ailments, use health care services effectively, and/or improve understanding of medical procedures and therapeutic regimens (American Hospital Association 1991).

health-related quality of life (HRQOL). A measure of health status that can incorporate physical, emotional, social, and role functioning; pain; and many other factors. It is usually based on the responses of patients to questions in professionally devised instruments.

health status. *See* **health-related quality of life**.

health technology. All procedures, devices, equipment, and drugs used in the maintenance, restoration, and promotion of health.

health technology assessment. A comprehensive form of policy research that looks at the technical, clinical, economic, and social consequences of the introduction and use of health technology.

Herfindahl Index (also called Herfindahl – Hirschman index, or HHI). A measure of market concentration, computed as the sum of the square of firms' market shares.

home care. Care provided in the home, for a wide variety of purposes, including health maintenance, preventive care, and substitution for acute care (Hollander 1994). *See also* **home support**.

home support. Home and community based long-term care services, provided by persons other than professionals, such as nurses or rehabilitation therapists (Hollander 1994).

horizontal equity. Fairness in the treatment of individuals who are at the same level with regard to some scale (e.g., people who are equally wealthy or have the same degree of health).

horizontal integration. The combining under one management of two or more previously independent producers of the same service.

hospice. A combination of services for terminally ill patients and their caregivers that is based on a humanistic philosophy of care.

human capital approach. A method of valuing outcomes that is based on lost productivity.

inappropriate care. *See* **appropriateness of care**.

incidence. The pattern of the distribution of the burden of a tax, among various individuals or groups (Due 1957, 9).

incremental cost. The additional cost resulting from a change in output by one or more than one unit.

indemnity. A type of insurance contract in which the insurer pays for care received up to a fixed amount per episode of illness.

independent practice association (IPA). In this type of HMO, the organization contracts with independent physician practices to provide health care for the enrollees. Payment to providers is usually on a fee-for-service basis.

indigent. An individual who cannot pay for his or her own care.

indirect cost. (1) In social cost accounting, the cost of time lost due to illness (i.e., resources that are not directly paid for). (2) In hospital cost accounting, the cost of resources not directly related to patient care.

indirect teaching costs. The additional costs that a teaching hospital incurs in the process of training interns and residents. These costs cannot be measured directly because they are inseparably joined with treatment costs.

inputs. *See* **resources**.

intensity of care. The amount of resources and services embodied in a unit of care (e.g., a day of hospitalization, a hospital stay, or a physician visit).

intensive care. The clinical speciality that treats patients with threatened or established organ failure through the employment of highly technical equipment by specially trained staff.

intermediate care facility (ICF). A facility providing a lower level of nursing care than a skilled nursing facility. Medicare no longer pays for ICF-level care.

international classification of diseases, ninth revision (ICD-9). A comprehensive disease coding system developed by the World Health Organization.

International Classification of Diseases, Ninth Revision, Clinical Modification (ICD-9-CM). A two-part medical information coding system used in abstracting systems and for classifying patients for DRGs. The first part consists of a comprehensive list of diseases with corresponding codes compatible with the World Health Organization list of disease codes. The second part contains procedure codes that are independent of the disease codes. ICD-9-CM was developed in the United States based on the World Health Organization system, and is the U.S.

coding standard. Some Canadian provinces also use ICD-9-CM diagnosis and procedure codes.

intervention. A task or set of tasks performed by a health professional with the object of influencing health status.

investment. The employment of physical or human capital to create the conditions for further production.

loading charge. The portion of an insurance premium that is over and above the amount expected to cover payment for insured services.

long run. A period over which all inputs can be increased, including capital stock and specialized labor.

long-run cost curve. The relation between the cost of production and volume of output or scale of plant for a period during which all inputs, including capital equipment, have sufficient time to vary.

long-term care. Services that address the health, social, and personal care needs of individuals who, for one reason or another, have never developed or have lost the capacity for self-care. These services may be continuous or intermittent, but it is generally presumed that they will be delivered indefinitely.

managed care. Any system of health service payment or delivery arrangements where the health plan attempts to control or coordinate the use of health services by its enrolled members in order to contain health expenditures, improve quality, or both. Arrangements often involve a defined delivery system of providers who have some form of contractual arrangements with the plan (Physician Payment Review Commission 1994).

managed competition. A manner of funneling payments for health services from a collective insurance fund to competing providers (Enthoven 1993; Reinhardt 1993).

mandate. A legal requirement that certain actions be carried out. For example, the requirement that businesses provide health insurance coverage to their employees.

marginal cost (MC). The change in cost resulting from a change in output by one unit. Since fixed costs do not change with output, marginal cost is related only to variable cost.

marginal productivity. The additional output due to the application of one or more units of an input or resource, holding all other inputs constant. Marginal productivity can be increasing, constant, or diminishing.

marginal revenue (MR). The additional revenue that a firm obtains from selling one more unit of a service.

marginal value product. The money value of additional output that is produced by one extra unit of an input (e.g., labor).

market. A network of buyers and sellers whose interaction determines the price and quantity traded of goods and services.

market structure. Those organizational characteristics of a market that determine the relations of sellers to sellers, buyers to buyers, and sellers to buyers.

Medicaid. A federally aided, state-administered program that provides medical assistance to certain low-income people.

medical care. A component of health care. A process or activity, guided by medical practitioners, in which certain inputs or factors of production (e.g., physician services, medical instruments, and pharmaceuticals) are combined in varying quantities to yield an output (medical care services) or outcome (health status).

Medicare. (1) In the United States, a nationwide, federally administered program that covers hospital and physician care and some related services for eligible persons over age 65, persons receiving Social Security disability insurance payments, and persons with end-stage renal disease. (2) In Canada, the health insurance system that is jointly financed by the federal and provincial governments and administered by the provincial governments.

Medicare + choice. A program of benefits for Medicare beneficiaries which provides choice among different plans, including capitation coverage.

Medigap. A class of insurance policies designed to cover gaps in coverage left by Medicare deductibles, copayments, and uncovered services (such as drugs).

money cost. Expenditures incurred (paid out) at a given volume of output.

monopolistic competition. A state of monopolistic competition exists in a market if there are many sellers but each is able to achieve a certain degree of customer loyalty and thus has some influence over price.

monopoly. A state of monopoly exists in a market if there is a single supplier. The supplier will then have control over prices in the market.

monopsony. A single buyer in a market. The monopsonist generally uses market power to achieve a satisfactory price

moral hazard. The risk to an insurer that its insureds will increase their consumption of insured services because of the reduction in the out-of-pocket price resulting from the insurance coverage.

morbidity. Illness. The morbidity rate is the rate of illness in a population.

mortality. Death. The mortality rate is the rate of death in a population.

most responsible diagnosis. The ICD-9 code identifying the disease or condition considered by the physician to be most responsible for the patient's stay in the institution. In the case where multiple diseases or conditions may be classified as most responsible, it is the one responsible for the greatest length of stay (Canadian Institute for Health Information). This is the Canadian coding convention. For the U.S. convention, *see* **principal diagnosis.**

multiproduct firm. A firm that produces a variety of products with different specifications (e.g., types of medical services).

need. A quantity of services that an expert (doctor, planner, etc.) judges that a patient or group of patients ought to have in order to achieve a desired level of health status (Boulding 1966).

network. A health maintenance organization comprising several different medical groups that are under contract to provide care to enrollees. Usually, the contract is on a fee-for-service basis.

nonprofit (not-for-profit). A nonprofit organization has as its prime purpose the providing of services to a specified population rather than the earning of profits for shareholders.

nursing home. A nursing home is an institution providing supervised, personal care for people who are not ill enough to require hospitalization in an acute care or auxiliary hospital but who require assistance with the activities of daily living.

opportunity cost. The value of the alternative use of resources that was highest valued but not selected. With some exceptions (e.g., when resources are overpaid), this equals the market value of all resources used to produce a given volume of output.

outlier. A patient who has a long length of stay (or a long length of treatment) as compared with other patients with the same diagnosis.

out-of-pocket price. The price that is directly paid for health care services by the consumer and is not subsequently recovered from an insurer or government. The out-of-pocket price is the burden that directly falls on the consumer as a result of his or her use of medical care.

outpatient care. Hospital-provided care that does not involve an overnight stay.

output. An activity or process during which a patient is treated or "cared for" by health care resources with the object of improving the patient's health.

patient days. The number of days that patients are under inpatient hospital or nursing home care during a year.

per capita payment. A fixed annual payment per person made to a provider or health maintenance organization. The totality of payments is intended to cover the cost of care for all enrollees during the year.

per diem payment. A flat-rate payment to a hospital or other institution for each day the patient is an inpatient in the institution.

perspective. The viewpoint (of the person or group) with respect to which economic assessment is taken.

plant. A single facility engaged in production. *See* **firm.**

point-of-service plan (POS). A health maintenance organization plan that allows members to use providers not on the organization's rolls. To gain access to such providers, the members must pay an added premium or out-of-pocket payment.

preadmission certification. The prospective review and evaluation of proposed elective hospital admissions using acceptable medical criteria as the standard for determining the appropriateness of the site or level of care and certifying the length of stay required (Scheffler 1991).

preferred provider organization (PPO). An arrangement in which a group of health providers agrees to provide services to a defined group of patients at an agreed-upon rate for each service (de Lissovoy et al. 1986, 7).

premium. The payment made to an insurance company in return for insurance coverage.

prepaid group practice (PGP). A group practice that charges patients on an annual per capita basis and bears the risk for providing the insured services.

prevention. Any intervention that reduces the likelihood that a disease or disorder will affect an individual or that interrupts or slows the progress of the disorder. Primary prevention reduces the likelihood that a particular disease or disorder will develop in a person. Secondary prevention interrupts or minimizes the progress of a disease or irreversible damage from a disease by early detection and treatment. Tertiary prevention slows the progress of the disease and reduces the resultant disability through treatment of established diseases (Spitzer 1990).

preventive medicine. That aspect of the physician's practice in which he applies to individual patients the knowledge and techniques from medical, social, and behavioral science to promote and maintain health and well-being and prevent disease or its progression (Hilleboe and Lairmore 1965; Last 1988).

price. An amount of money paid or received per unit of a service or commodity.

price discrimination. The charging of different prices for the same product to different customers, made possible by the inability of consumers to resell the product to each other. The charging of different prices is usually due to the existence of different demand conditions for different groups of customers.

price taker. A supplier that has no influence over the price of the services or commodities it sells. However many units it sells, the price is taken as given.

primary care. A type of medical care that emphasizes first contact care and assumes ongoing responsibility for the patient in health maintenance and therapy for illness. Primary care is comprehensive in scope and includes overall coordination of treatment of the patient's health problems.

principal. The person in whose interests an agent is contracted to act.

principal diagnosis. The diagnosis that, after investigation, is found to have been responsible for the patient's admission to the hospital. This is the U.S. coding convention. If a patient is admitted to the hospital for a minor TURP (trans uretheral resection of the prostate) procedure, and it is discovered he has carcinoma of the lung, the prostate diagnosis would be the one coded under this convention. For the Canadian convention, *see* **most responsible diagnosis**.

procedure. An operative or nonoperative intervention.

production. The act of combining resources to yield output.

production function. A quantitative relationship expressing how outputs vary when the quantity of inputs changes. Also called **production relation**.

production relation. *See* **production function**.

productivity. The ratio of physical inputs to physical outputs. The inputs can be one single input (e.g., labor), with others held constant, or all inputs combined.

products of ambulatory care (PACs). An ambulatory care classification system developed in New York State primarily for the funding of nonsurgical, nonemergency ambulatory care visits, based on body parts and purpose of visit (Tenan 1988).

products of ambulatory surgery (PASs). An ambulatory surgery classification system developed in New York State for funding ambulatory surgery procedures, based on similar resource-using procedures (Kelley et al. 1990).

profit. Total revenue minus total cost. Accounting profit is defined as total revenue for a period's sales minus costs matched to those sales. Economic profit is total revenue minus economic costs.

prospective payment. Payment to (usually institutional) providers based on predetermined rates unrelated to current or past costs.

provider. A supplier of health care services.

public health. The combination of science, practical skills, and beliefs that is directed to the maintenance and improvement of the health of all the population. It is one of the efforts organized by society to protect, promote, and restore the people's health through collective or social actions (Last 1988).

quality-adjusted life year (QALY). A numerical assessment of the proportion of an individual's state of full health experienced over a year. QALY values generally range from 0 (assigned to death) to 1 (full health), though certain states of health can be valued at less than 0. QALY values can be directly derived from individuals' utility measurements or can be based on existing values of health states.

quality of care. The degree to which the process of medical care increases the probability of outcomes desired by patients, and reduces the probability of undesired outcomes, given the state of medical knowledge (U.S. Congress 1988).

quality of life (QOL). The degree to which an individual enjoys everything. It has been defined, by a philosopher, as the possession and enjoyment of all the real goods in the right order and proportion. Nonphilosophers, *see* **health-related quality of life (HRQOL)** or **health status** for terms only slightly less stratospheric.

quantity demanded. The quantity of a service that an individual or group is willing to buy at one specific rate.

quantity supplied. The amount of a service a supplier or market is willing to supply at any one price.

rate. The price per unit charged by an institution for its services.

rate setting. The setting of institutional prices by a paying or regulatory agency.

refined diagnosis-related groups (RDRGs). Also called **refined group numbers (RGNs).** A classification system in which resource use patterns and secondary diagnoses are used to refine the assignment of patients to severity classes (RDRGs).

regulation. (1) A regulation is a law or rule imposing government or government-mandated standards and significant economic responsibilities on individuals or organizations outside the government establishment. (2) The process of regulation is carried out by government or mandated agencies through such means as setting or approving prices, rates, fares, profits, interest rates, and wages; awarding licenses, certificates, and permits; devising safety rules; setting quality levels; enacting public disclosure of financial information regulations; and enacting prohibitions against price, racial, religious, or sexual discrimination (U.S. Domestic Council 1977).

reimbursement. The payment made by an insurer to a provider for specific services provided to an insured patient. Reimbursement is usually associated with payments based on a service-by-service, or patient-by-patient basis.

relative value. A value placed on a specific unit of service (e.g., a follow-up office visit, a blood test, or an inpatient cholecystectomy) expressed in relation to some standard (e.g., a minute of lab test time or physician care).

resource-based relative value system (RBRVS). A resource weights service classification system that aims at setting resource weights according to the total relative cost of each service, including "psychological" costs of the provider, time costs, and training costs.

resource intensive weights (RIW). Canadian relative weightings for inpatient groups. RIWs combine Canadian length of stay and U.S. cost per day data to form hybrid cost per case weights. Separate weights are calculated for "typical" and "atypical" cases.

resource utilization groups (RUGs). Clusters of nursing home residents, defined by residents' characteristics, that explain resource use (Fries et al. 1994, 668).

resources. Resources are defined as the means used in producing services. Resources can include physical capital (beds and equipment) and human capital (physicians, nurses, etc.). Also called *inputs* and *factors of production*.

retrospective payment. Payment to a provider for services provided based on actual costs incurred by the provider. Since the payment is based on costs incurred, the amount to be paid must be determined after the service has been provided (i.e., retrospectively).

retrospective review. A review of claims after the episode of care is concluded and the claim is submitted to the insurer (Scheffler et al. 1991).

returns to scale. The relationship between total output and scale of operations, which are measured as proportional increases in all resources. Because all resources are allowed to increase in proportion, this is a long-run relationship.

revenue. Income earned from the provision of services. Gross revenues equal income earned overall, while net revenues equal income earned minus costs or expenses.

risk. Uncertainty as to loss; in the case of health care, the loss can be due to the cost of medical treatment or other losses arising from illness. Risk can be objective (relative variations between the difference between actual and probable losses) and subjective (psychological uncertainty relating to the occurrence of an event) (Greene 1977). *See also* **risk averse**, **risk neutral**, and **risk taker**.

risk averse. A person is said to be risk averse if losses of a given amount create more disutility than the utility that comes from gains of the same amount (and so losses will tend to be avoided).

risk factor. Behavior or condition that, based on evidence or theory, is thought to directly influence the level of a specific health problem.

risk neutral. A person is said to be risk neutral if he or she values losses and gains of the same amount equally.

risk pooling. The sharing of the costs incurred by members of a population. The payment method can vary but will not be based on the risk of individuals.

risk taker. A person is said to be a risk taker if, for that person, the utility of gains is greater than the disutility of losses of equal value. A risk taker is therefore predisposed to gamble.

second surgical opinion. Patients are sometimes required to get a second or even a third consulting opinion for specified nonemergency surgical procedures (Scheffler et al. 1991).

secondary care. Specialist-referred care for conditions of a relatively low level of complication and risk. Secondary care can be provided in an office or hospital and can be diagnostic or therapeutic.

selective contracting. A procedure whereby an insurer can legally exclude providers from its list of participating providers (Melnick and Zwanzinger 1988, 2669).

sensitivity analysis. Determining the extent to which the conclusions or results of a model depend on the model' assumptions.

short run. A period in which all of the inputs cannot be adjusted (increased or reduced). Those inputs that cannot be adjusted are called "fixed" and include capital stock. *Short run* also refers to lengths of time insufficient for new firms to enter a market or industry.

short-run cost curve. The relation between cost and volume of production of a plant during a short adjustment period in which only some inputs are variable (and the rest are fixed).

shortage. An excess of supply over demand at a given price.

signout case. A patient who leaves the hospital against medical advice.

single-payer system. A reimbursement system in which there is a single payer or one dominant payer.

single-product firm. A production unit that produces a single, homogeneous product. Exists only in economic theory.

skilled nursing facility (SNF). A facility that provides short-term, subacute posthospitalization care and rehabilitative care.

social cost. The cost to all members of society of any activity or service. Can be the sum of private and external costs or of direct and indirect costs.

solo practice. A one-doctor medical practice.

staff model HMO. A health maintenance organization whose practitioner staff are employees of the health plan. Usually the practitioners are paid on a salary rather than fee-for-service basis.

standardized mortality rate (SMR). A single mortality rate for a large group of individuals who are in different age and sex categories. The total rate for the entire group is made up of the rates in different age and sex subgroups, which are weighted or averaged according to a given structure of a standard population (e.g., the population of an entire country or the population in a base year).

substitutes. Goods or services that compete with each other, such as Aspirin and Tylenol. The direct price of one of the substitutes will cause a shift in the demand curve for the other.

substitution effect. The shift from one product to another as a result of a price change, after compensating for any increase or reduction in real income that accrues from the price change.

supplier-induced demand. The amount of shift in the demand for services resulting from the suppliers' influence on consumers' tastes (intensity of desire for the services).

supply. A supply curve. The quantity supplied at each price.

supply curve. (1) For a single firm, the quantity the firm is willing to supply of a service at alternative prices of the commodity. (2) For the market, the relationship between the quantity that all firms are willing to supply and alternative prices of the service.

supply function. (1) For a single provider, a quantitative relationship between the quantity the supplier is willing to supply and a series of variables that influence the supplier's behavior, such as price, technology, case mix, quality, and input prices. (2) For a market, the quantitative relationship between the quantity that all suppliers in the market are willing to supply and a series of variables that influence all of the suppliers' behavior, including price, technology, case mix, quality, input prices, and the number of suppliers in the market.

surplus. (1) For a nonprofit firm, total revenue minus total expense (the counterpart of profit for a for-profit firm). (2) For a market, the excess of quantity supplied over quantity demanded at a given price.

tastes. Consumer preferences for goods and services expressed in terms of an index of satisfaction or utility. Taste is a catchall concept for everything other than prices and incomes that affect demand, including health status, age, sex, level of education, and so on.

technology. *See* **health technology**.

technology assessment. *See* **health technology assessment**.

tertiary care. Highly specialized care administered to patients who have complicated conditions or require high-risk pharmaceutical treatments or surgery. Tertiary care is provided in a setting that houses high-technology services, specialists and subspecialists, and intensive care and other highly specialized services.

third-party payment. Payment by a private insurer or government to a medical provider for care given to a patient.

time cost. The value of time required to conduct an activity. This variable has two components: value per unit of time and time actually spent in the activity. Value per unit of time is taken as equivalent to lost earnings or the value placed on forgone leisure activities.

total costs (TC). The sum of fixed and variable costs. All of the costs required to produce a specified level of output.

total fixed costs (TFC). All of the fixed costs required to produce a specified level of output.

total product. The total amount of output produced.

total variable costs (TVC). All of the variable costs required to produce a specified level of output.

transaction costs. The costs of reaching an agreement and coordinating activity among participants in a market. These include the costs of searching for potential buyers or sellers and for product quality and cost; negotiating an agreement; monitoring that the agreement conditions are met; and enforcing the terms of the agreement.

transfer case. A hospital inpatient who is admitted from or discharged to another institution.

transfer payment. A payment made to an individual that is unrelated to resource use.

trim point. A point, calculated using a statistical formula, applied to all lengths of stays (or cost per case) within a single DRG (or CMG) in order to separate outlier cases from the rest.

typical patient. A patient who receives a full, successful course of treatment in a single institution and is discharged when he or she no longer requires acute-care services.

utility. (1) An index comparing various levels of an individual's satisfaction with alternative quantities of specified goods, services, or situations under certainty. The index that allows the quantification of differences between the levels is called *cardinal utility* (Pigou 1960). (2) A ranking of alternative bundles of goods and services under certainty, on the basis of better, equal, or worse, with no indication as to *degrees* of satisfaction (ordinal utility). (3) A ranking of alternative risky situations on the basis of an individual's own preferences regarding probabilities (von Neumann-Morgenstern utility) (Torrance et al. 1995).

utilization. The actual use of services by consumers (the services must be demanded and supplied).

utilization management. A set of techniques used by or on behalf of purchasers of health care benefits to manage health care costs by influencing patient care decision-making through case-by-case assessments of the appropriateness of care prior to provision (Institute of Medicine 1991).

value judgment. A pronouncement that states or implies that something is desirable (or undesirable) and is not derived from any technical or objective data but instead from considerations of ultimate value, i.e., ethical considerations (Nath 1973).

variable costs. Costs that change in response to changes in output. Variable costs can be expressed as total, average, or marginal.

variable inputs. Inputs that can vary in quantity during a specified time period.

vertical equity. Fairness in the treatment of individuals who are at different levels with regard to some scale (e.g., people who fall into different income classes).

vertical integration. The combining under one management of activities at different stages of the production process.

volume. The number of cases (or other service units) provided.

wants. Consumer tastes or desires.

willingness-to-pay approach. A method of valuing an outcome that is based on the consumer's own preferences.

BIBLIOGRAPHY

American Hospital Association. 1991. *Health statistics.* Chicago: American Hospital Association.

Boulding, K. 1966. The concept of need for health services. *Milbank Quarterly* 44:202–223.

Chassin, M.R., et al. 1987. Does inappropriate use explain geographic variations in the use of health care services? *JAMA* 258:2533–2537.

de Lissovoy, G., et al. 1986. Preferred provider organizations. *Inquiry* 23:7–15.

Due, J.F. 1957. *Sales taxation.* London: Routledge and Kegan Paul.

Enthoven, E. 1993. The history and principles of managed competition. *Health Affairs* 12 (suppl): 24–48.

Fetter, R.B., ed. 1991. *DRGs: Their design and development.* Ann Arbor, Mich.: Health Administration Press.

Fries, B., et al. 1994. Refining a case mix measure for nursing homes. *Medical Care* 7:668–685.

Greene, M.R. 1977. *Risk and insurance.* 4th ed. Cincinnati: South-Western Publishing Co.

Hilleboe, H.E., and Lairmore, G.W. 1965. *Preventive medicine.* 2nd ed. Philadelphia: W.B. Saunders.

Hollander, M.J. 1994. The cost effectiveness of continuing care services in Canada. Ottawa: Queen's University of Ottawa Economic Projects.

Hornbrook, M.C., et al. 1985. Health care episodes. *Medical Care Review* 42:163–218.

·Institute of Medicine. 1991. Quoted in Scheffler, R.M., et al. The impact of Blue Cross and Blue Shield plan utilization management programs, 1980–88. *Inquiry* 28:263–275.

Kelley, W.P., et al. 1990. The classification of resource use in ambulatory surgery. *Journal of Ambulatory Care Management* 13(1):55–63.

Last, J.M. 1988. *Public health and human ecology.* New York: Appleton and Lange.

Melnick, G.A., and Zwanzinger, J. 1988. Hospital behavior under competition and cost containment policies. *JAMA* 260:2669–2675.

Physician Payment Review Commission. 1994. *Annual report to Congress, 1994.* Washington, DC: Physician Payment Review Commission.

Pigou, A.C. 1960. *The economics of welfare.* London: Macmillan.

Reinhardt, U.E. 1993. Reorganizing the financial flows in American health care. *Health Affairs* 12 (suppl):172–193.

Saskatchewan Health. 1993. *A guide to core services*. Regina, Saskatchewan: Saskatchewan Health.

Scheffler, R.M., et al. 1991. The impact of Blue Cross and Blue Shield plan utilization management programs, 1980–88. *Inquiry* 28:263–275.

Spitzer, W.O. 1990. The scientific admissibility of evidence on the effectiveness of preventive interventions. In *Preventive disease*, ed. R.B. Goldbloom and R.S. Lawrence. New York: Springer-Verlag.

Tenan, P.M., et al. 1988. PACs: Classifying ambulatory patients and services for clinical and financial management. *Journal of Ambulatory Care Management* 11(3):36–53.

Torrance, G., et al. 1995. Multi-attribute preference functions. *Pharmaco-Economics* 7:503–520.

U.S. Congress, Office of Technology Assessment. 1988. *The quality of medical care*. Pub. no. OTA-H-386. Washington, D.C.: U.S. Government Printing Office.

U.S. Domestic Council. 1977. *The challenge of regulatory reform*. Washington, D.C.: U.S. Government Printing Office.

Weiner, J., et al. 1991. Development and application of a population-oriented measure of ambulatory care case mix. *Medical Care* 28:452–472.

Answers to Odd-Numbered Questions

CHAPTER 1

1. Quality can be judged from a structure, process, or outcome perspective. The training of physicians is a structure-related quality issue, the types of procedures done is a process-related quality issue, and the health status of patients after the treatment is an outcome-related quality issue.
3. Morbidity is the rate of illness (the proportion of people in a given population who are ill), whereas utilization concerns the services provided to treat illness. Hospitalization is often used to measure both, although hospitalization is influenced by factors such as availability of care and practice patterns as well as illness.
5. A health-related quality-of-life index is a composite measure of different components of health. Level values measure the level of each component. Social importance weights measure the relative importance persons place on each component.
7. If the study group has relatively many old or ill persons in it, the mortality rate is liable to be high merely because of the underlying poor health status of the group, in which case it would be wrong to interpret the rate as indicating poor performance on the part of the health care providers.
9. Health status is positively influenced by medical care; however, as more medical care is provided to a given population, eventually additional units of medical care will improve their health at an increasingly lower rate. The "flat of the curve" describes the situation where large amounts of care are already available.

CHAPTER 2

1. A premium is a payment to an insurer in return for the insurer's acceptance of the financial risk associated with health care (if and when it is consumed). A deductible is a payment by the consumer for care that has been provided.
3. Medicare primarily serves the elderly (individuals over 65) and those with end-stage renal disease. Part A covers hospitalization and posthospitalization care (home care and nursing home care). There is no premium, but there are deductibles and copayments.

5. Medicaid covers low-income populations, including the aged (for services not covered by Medicare). There are no deductibles but occasionally there are small copayments. There are no premiums because the low-income persons could not afford them.

7. In a preferred provider organization, consumers can obtain services from providers who are not PPO members, although they must pay a differential price. In a traditional HMO, members must use providers designated by the HMO.

9. An opportunity cost is the value of services that are given up by choosing alternative courses of action. Opportunity cost is a broader concept than paid expenses or money costs.

11. A cost-of-illness study measures the direct and indirect costs of illness for a population. Using the prevalence approach, costs are related to the health care provided in a certain year. If death occurs during that year, future costs are attached to that death. Using the incidence approach, costs (including related future costs) are assigned to the reporting or occurrence of the illness.

CHAPTER 3

1. Demand is the relationship between price and quantity demanded. Quantity demanded is the amount demanded at a certain price.

3. (a) It will shift demand to the right. (b) It will shift demand to the right. (c) It will shift demand to the left. (d) It will shift demand to the right. (e) It will shift demand to the right.

5. It will shift demand to the right.

7. The elasticity is $[(Q2 - Q1)/(Q2 + Q1)]/[(P2 - P1)/(P2 + P1)] = (-10/55)/(.05/.275) = -1$.

9. (a) No effect on demand would occur. (b) There would be a movement along the curve, not a shift. (c) The demand curve would shift to the right. (d) No effect on demand would occur. (e) The demand curve would shift to the left.

11. The current quantity of visits is 3,000,000 x 2.4 per million, or 7,200,000. Q2 is the unkown quantity and using the elasticity formula (with an elasticity value of –0.2), we can solve for Q2 as follows:

$$-0.2 = \frac{[(3,000,000 \times 2.4) - Q2]/[(7,200,000 + Q2)/2]}{.50/.25}$$

.2 (7,200,000 +Q2) = (7,200,000 – Q2)
Q2 = 4,800,000

CHAPTER 4

1. The reduction in health status will eventually cause an increase in demand for health care.

3. Her travel costs equal $125 (4 hours × $20 = $80; 150 miles × 0.3 = $45). Her waiting costs equal $20 (1 hour × $20). The total is $145.

5. Information asymmetry occurs when the agent has better information than the principal. The principal cannot then effectively monitor the agent.

7. Supplier-induced demand occurs when physicians directly cause a shift in the demand curve by influencing their patients' belief in the efficacy of health care. The problem arises from the fact that physicians act as agents for their patients in addition to being suppliers of health care.

9. The present value of exercise = $1,900 + ($1,900/1.1) + $2,000/(1.1)^2 = $5,280. The present value of medicine = $2,000 + $1,900/1.1 + $1,900/(1.1)^2 = $5,297.

CHAPTER 5

1. The total product for May = 100. The total product for June = 120. The marginal product = 20/2 = 10 patients per nursing hour.
3. (a) It will shift the curve upward. (b) It will shift the curve downward. (c) It will shift the curve downward. (d) There will be no effect. (e) It will shift the curve downward. (f) There will be no effect. (g) There will be no effect.
5. The average and marginal costs are as follows:

Total Cost	Marginal Cost	Average Cost	Quantity
$100		$100	1
160	$60	80	2
200	40	66.7	3
260	60	65	4
360	100	72	5

7. The fixed costs total $4,200 (office = $2,000; phones = $200; secretary = $2,000). The variable costs are shown in the following table:

	Variable Costs at 1,200 Visits	Variable Costs at 1,300 Visits
Nurses	30 × $4,000 = $120,000	$130,000
Supplies	$20 × 400 = $8,000	$20 × 430 = $8,600
Totals	$128,000	$138,600

9. The fixed costs total $200.
11. The fixed costs total $17,000 (physician: $50 × 200 hours = $10,000; nurse: $15 × 200 hours = $3,000; secretary: $10 × 200 hours = $2,000; rent: $2,000). The variable costs equal $10,000 (supplies: $10 × 1,000).
13. The costs are shown in the following table:

Visits	Hours	Total Fixed Costs	Total Variable Costs	Total Costs	Marginal Costs
1	2	$150	$41	$191	
2	4	$150	82	232	$41
3	8	$150	163	313	81
4	14	$150	284	434	121
5	22	$150	445	595	161
6	32	$150	646	796	201

15. The costs are shown in the following table:

Quantity	Total Cost	Total Fixed Cost	Total Variable Cost	Marginal Cost
0	$100	$100	$ 0	$—
1	120	100	20	20
2	150	100	50	30
3	200	100	100	50
4	300	100	200	100

CHAPTER 6

1. Two thousand operations.
3. Eighty dollars.
5. (a) Four units. (b) Four units.
7. (a) At $10, the quantity supplied is zero. (b) At $20, the quantity supplied is zero. (c) At $30, the quantity supplied is four.
9. (a) The quantity of visits will equal 100. (b) The supply curve will move in the direction of Supply$_1$. (c) No change will occur. (d) The supply curve will move in the direction of Supply$_1$. (e) The supply curve will move in the direction of Supply$_2$. (f) The supply curve will move in the direction of Supply$_1$.

CHAPTER 7

1. Insurers must incur contract costs. These are the costs of negotiating contracts, monitoring performance, and enforcing the terms of the contracts.
3. A salary basis of payment encourages a reduction in services. Per service payment encourages an increase in services, visits, and patients. Per visit payment encourages a reduction in services per visit and an increase in visits and patients. Per patient payment encourages a reduction in services and visits and an increase in patients.
5. RBRVS is a fee-for-service system based on a detailed analysis of time costs. Implementation of the system led to a reduction in surgical fees relative to fees for nonsurgical services.
7. In prospective reimbursement, payment is based on predetermined rates. Payment can be made on the basis of services, days, and cases.
9. The answers are contained in the following table:

	Degree of Risk Incurred by Insurer	Degree of Risk Incurred by Hospital
Retrospective reimbursement	High degree of risk	No risk
Fee-for-service	High degree of risk	Low degree of risk
Per diem fees	High degree of risk	Low degree of risk
Per case reimbursement	Low to moderate degree of risk	Moderage to high degree of risk
Per case reimbursement plus outlier adjustment	Moderate degree of risk	Moderate degree of risk

11. Taking the fee per weighted case as $3,951 (the national Medicare payment rate for urban hospitals), the hospital would receive $12,236 per craniotomy.
13. Nursing homes can be funded on a per diem basis.
15. Members can be recruited on the basis of age.
17. (a) They have an incentive to increase membership. (b) They have an incentive to reduce services per member.

CHAPTER 8

1. (a) Price and quantity increase (demand curve shifts to right). (b) Price falls and quantity increases (demand curve shifts to right). (c) Price increases and quantity increases (demand curve shifts to right). (d) Price and quantity increase

(demand curve shifts to left). (e) Price and quantity decrease (demand curve shifts to left).

3. (a) Price increases and quantity falls (supply curve shifts to left). (b) Price decreases and quantity increases (supply curve shifts to right). (c) Price decreases and quantity increases (supply curve shifts to right). (d) Price decreases and quantity increases (supply curve shifts to right).

5. The FPL made $2.8 million in profits with an $8 million investment. Its return on capital (35 percent) is greater than in other industries. Capital will be attracted to this industry. Supply will increase and price and profits will fall.

7. Quantity demanded will increase to 250. Quantity supplied will fall to 50. There will be a shortage of 200. Quantity utilized will be 50.

9. Three hundred days are demanded at all rates. At a rate of $450, 200 days are supplied. At a rate of $600, 300 days are supplied. At a rate of $450, funding is $90,000, and 200 days are utilized. At a rate of $600, funding is $180,000, and total utilization is 300.

CHAPTER 9

1. The answers are contained in the following table:

Price	Quantity	Total Revenue	Marginal Revenue
$10	0	$0	
9	1	9	$9
8	2	16	7
7	3	21	5
6	4	24	3
5	5	25	1
4	6	24	−1

At a marginal cost of $3.50, the monopolist will supply up to the point where *MC* is above *MR*. This is at a volume of 3 and a price of $7.

3. The statistics for Group A are as follows.

Price	Quantity	Total Revenue	Marginal Revenue
$10	1	$10	$10
9	2	18	8
8	3	24	6
4	4	28	4
6	5	30	2

The corresponding statistics for Group B are these:

Price	Quantity	Total Revenue	Marginal Revenue
$12	1	$12	$12
11	2	22	10
10	3	30	8
9	4	36	6
8	5	40	4
7	6	42	2

The price in each market should be set where *MR* = *MC*. This is $9 for Group A and $10 for Group B.

5. The marginal cost to the hospital is given in the following table:

Quantity	Price	Total Cost	Marginal Cost
1	$1	$1	$1
2	2	4	3
3	3	9	5
4	4	16	7
5	5	25	9
6	6	36	11

The monopsonist will hire up to four nurses, at which point the marginal value of a nurse equals the marginal cost.

7. The consumers in the market may be influenced by the physicians to purchase more health care. In other words, the physicians could increase the elasticity of the demand curve.

CHAPTER 10

1. (a) With no insurance, the expected utility = $(.2 \times 84.4) + (.8 \times 100) = 96.88$. With insurance, the expected utility is 98.8. The individual should purchase insurance.

(b) At a price of $60, expected utility is 95.8, which is the utility of $940, or $1,000 – 60. This is less than a utility of 96.88, which is the expected utility if no insurance were bought. She would not buy insurance.

(c) If she got sick, and had no insurance, her wealth level would be $800 and utility would be 57.0. The expected utility with no insurance would be 91.4 ($-0.2 \times 57 + 0.8 \times 100$). This is less than the utility of 95.8 which is the utility if she buys insurance. She would therefore buy insurance. (d) Mrs. Smith is risk averse.

3. The price is $500 × (1 – .3), or $350.

5. The elasticity is $(\Delta Q/Q)/(\Delta P/P) = (400/1800)/(-40/100) = -5/9$.

7. (a) For healthy persons, the expected utility with no insurance is .2(87) + .8(100) = 97.8. The expected utility with insurance is U($975), which is greater than 98.8 (the utility of $970). A healthy person should buy insurance. For unhealthy persons, the expected utility with no insurance is .2(76) + .8(100) = 95.2. An unhealthy person should buy insurance.

(b) For healthy persons, the utility with no insurance = .2(89) + .8(100) = 97.8. The utility with insurance = U($980) = 99.4. A healthy person should buy insurance. For unhealthy persons, the utility with no insurance = .2(76) + .8(100) = 95.2. The utility with insurance =.8(utility at $950) + .2(utility at $980) = 98.4. An unhealthy person should buy insurance.

9. Administrative costs increase and payouts fall. Indeed, despite the improvement in utilization management, the added administrative costs could be enough to push the total costs higher than they were.

11. Information asymmetry occurs when the insurer and the consumer possess different information about risks. If the insurer had no information that it could use to distinguish risks between persons, it would charge a single premium rate.

CHAPTER 11

1. The relevant data for this exercise are contained in the following table:

Nursing Hours	Visits	Marginal Product	Value of the Marginal Product
1	12	12	$120
2	22	10	100
3	30	8	80
4	36	6	60
5	40	4	40

Midwest will hire additional nurses up to the point where the wage equals the value of the marginal product. In this case the quantity hired will be four.

3. (a) There is no effect on the curve but there is a movement down the curve. (b) The demand curve shifts outward. (c) The demand curve shifts outward. (d) There is no effect on the curve. (e) The demand curve shifts outward. (f) The demand curve shifts inwards.

5. The supply curve (relating wage rates and labor supplied) will shift downwards; if insurance is valued equally with wages, the curve will shift by the amount of the premium paid.

7. The supply of labor is lower for persons with poor health. At any given wage rate, persons with poor health will offer less labor, and their incomes will be lower.

CHAPTER 12

1. In the Paretean system, everyone's preferences count and in the delegatory system a person or group chooses for the society.

3. No further reallocation of resources can increase the net value of resources (i.e., $MV - MC$).

5. No, because if the MC is positive, eventually persons will receive so much care that the MV of this additional care will be low or zero and below the marginal cost of the care.

7. No, because the private market only ensures that each person obtains health care in relation to his or her own valuations and associated costs. If there are consumption externalities, there may be room for increases in social valuations through the philanthropic transfer of funds.

9. No, because the marginal cost of insurance may exceed gains (marginal value of insurance coverage) when the degree of coverage is already high.

11. With the extra-welfarist approach, judgments about social benefits are delegated to an authority. In health care, the delegated authority makes judgments on the valuations of the health states of the population. In the Paretean system, each person evaluates his or her own use of care.

CHAPTER 13

1. Out-of-pocket expenditures account for 17 percent, government for 31 percent, and private insurance for 32 percent of total health care expenses.

3. The subsidy will increase the demand for insurance. The amount of insurance purchased will increase.

5. A payroll tax is a tax on employment income. Payroll taxes lead to a reduction in employment and wages.

7. The income tax burden increases with income. The sales tax burden falls with income. The payroll tax burden falls with income. The insurance premium burden falls with income.

CHAPTER 14

1. Older persons (over 65) and persons with renal disease.
3. Part A is funded by payroll taxes levied by the federal government. Part B is funded by general government revenues and payroll taxes.
5. Hospital care, physician services, long-term care, and pharmaceuticals.
7. Medigap is private insurance that can be purchased to cover gaps in coverage due to Medicare premiums, deductibles, and copayments.
9. One quarter of the persons in this group are children, roughly half are employed, and many have poor health.
11. The stated goals are affordability, equity of payment, adequacy of care, feasibility of policies, and acceptance by concerned groups (providers, intermediaries, and consumers).
13. Medicaid faces the challenge of ensuring that there is adequate coverage (i.e., that persons who are eligible actually enroll) and acceptance by providers. Ensuring coverage can be achieved by extending the program's scope, and gaining acceptance can be achieved by setting adequate reimbursement rates.

CHAPTER 15

1. If insurers cannot determine consumer risk, then they will set prices at the group average. Low-risk persons may drop out of the market, leaving higher risk persons. Rates will spiral upwards and the market may disappear, even though persons would be willing to buy insurance and there are potential suppliers who would provide it at rates acceptable to the consumers (if the risks could be adequately determined).
3. The risk for small groups is higher than for large ones because there is a large variance in outcomes in small groups, which imposes a higher degree of risk on suppliers of insurance.
5. If there was community rating and the premiums exceeded the risk experience of some (more healthy) consumers, these consumers would not buy insurance, even though they could have at a rate that would cover their medical risks. In the second case, a person may simply choose not to insure, and be willing to retain the risks.
7. Salary provides a weak incentive to increase the volume of services. Fee-for-service provides a strong incentive to increase the volume of services. Capitation provides a weak incentive to decrease services per person but a strong incentive to enroll more members.
9. Non-managed-care insurers might lower their premiums, increase the monitoring of providers, or try to attract less costly consumers.

CHAPTER 16

1. The physician acts as an agent for two principals, the insurer and the patient.

3. If physicians can organize at a lower cost, they will tend to control the legislative process.
5. Patent rights allow drug companies sufficient time to recover their investment in the development of drugs (the development of a single drug can take many years and millions of dollars in investment).
7. It is called a combination in restraint of trade, and it is prohibited by Section 1 of the Sherman Act.
9. If the networks keep other physicians from practicing in a region (e.g., by denying them the right to admit patients to hospitals), then they would be illegal. However, if the networks result in greater efficiencies and enable physicians to lower costs, then this would be a justification for them to continue.

CHAPTER 17

1. He should use the concept of cost-utility, because survival and quality of life are both relevant outcomes. Also, two competing interventions are being compared.
3. She should use the concept of cost-benefit, as the question is whether the intervention should be used.
5. Nine hundred and sixty people lived the entire year. The 40 who died lived on average half a year, making a total of 20 extra life years. Therefore, the grand total is 980 life years.
7. Efficacy is the difference in outcomes under ideal conditions. Since 60 deaths per 100 would occur without the drug and 40 deaths per 100 would occur if everyone used the drug, the difference (efficacy) is 20 deaths less per 100 persons. Effectiveness = $60 - [(60/100) \times 25 + (40/100) \times 75] = 60 - 45 = 15$; that is, the effectiveness equals 15 deaths less per 100 persons.
9. The result for the case where she doesn't take the medicine is 1/2 year $\times$ .8 = .4 QALYs. The result if she does take the medicine is 7/12 years $\times$ 0.9 = .525 QALYs. The difference is 0.125 QALYs.

Index

A

Access, defined, 395
Acute care, defined, 395
Adjusted average per capita cost (AAPCC), defined, 395
Administrator as agent model, 140–142
Admission, 20
Adverse selection, 239
  defined, 395
  health insurance, 242–244
  insurance market reform, 333, 334
Agency, defined, 395
Agency theory, 86–92
  hospital reimbursement, 154–156
    per case payment, 155–156
      with adjustment for outliers, 156
    per diem fee, 155
    prospective fee-for-service system, 155
    retrospective payments, 154–155
  incentive
    health maintenance organization, 163–165
    managed care, 163–165
  physician reimbursement, 151
Agent, defined, 395
Aid to Families with Dependent Children, Medicaid, 310
All-payer system, defined, 395
Alternative level of care, defined, 395
Altruism
  resource allocation, 275–278
  valuation, 275–278
Ambulatory care, defined, 395
Ambulatory care group, defined, 395
Ambulatory visit group, defined, 395
American Medical Association, 216–217
Antitrust policy, 357–370
  competition, 368
  conceptual framework, 357–359
  federal guidelines, 369–370

health care market structure, 359–361
health insurer, 360–361
history, 361–362
hospital, 359–360
institutions, 361–362
managed care, 360–361, 368–369
merger, 363–366
monopolization, 366–368
nonprice competition, 368
pharmaceutical industry, 361
physician services, 360
quality, 368
The Statements of Enforcement Policy and Analytical Principles Relating to Health Care and Antitrust, 369–370
Appropriateness of care, defined, 396
Arc elasticity of demand, 66
Asymmetric information, defined, 396
Atypical patient, defined, 396
Availability, defined, 396
Average adjusted per capita cost, health maintenance organization, 161–162
Average cost, 104
  defined, 396
  marginal cost, relation, 106–108
  production, 106–108
Average fixed cost, 106
  defined, 396
Average total cost, 106
  fixed cost component, 108
  variable cost component, 108
Average variable cost, 106
  defined, 396

B

Basis of payment, defined, 396
Bed days, defined, 396
Benefit, defined, 396
Benefits, 250–251

labor supply, 255–256
on-the-job benefits, 141
Biased selection, 237–238
  defined, 396
  insurance market reform, 335–336
Blue Shield, monopolistic market, 208–210
Board of trustees, nonprofit agency, 136, 140
Burden, defined, 396

C

Capacity
  defined, 396
  measures, 30
Capital, defined, 396
Capital equipment, 108
Capital input, 30
Capitation, 41, 42, 150, 151
  defined, 396
  health maintenance organization, 161
Case management, defined, 397
Case mix, defined, 397
Case-mix group, defined, 397
Catastrophic insurance, 22
Charges, defined, 397
Clayton Act, 361–362, 363, 364, 367
Coinsurance, defined, 397
Community care, defined, 397
Community demand, 82–83
Community rating, 238, 241
  defined, 397
  efficiency, 336
  equity, 336
  insurance market reform, 335–336
Comorbidity, defined, 397
Competition
  antitrust policy, 368
  defined, 397
  Medicare, 320–322
Competitive bidding
  competitive market model, 188–190
  model, 189–190
Competitive equilibrium, defined, 400
Competitive labor market, 256–259
  assumptions, 256
  demand, 256–257
  predictions, 256–257
  supply, 256–257
  wage rate, 256–257
Competitive market model, 174–198
  assumptions, 175–176
  behavioral relationships, 175
  competitive bidding, 188–190
  consumer ignorance, 187–188
  demand shift
    price movement, 178–179
    quantity movement, 178–179
    stable supply, 178

evidence for and against, 185–188
fee differences among patients, 187
individual demand, 175
individual supply, 176, 177
long-run analysis, 180–181
market demand, 176, 177
market price, 176–178
market supply, 176, 177
phenomena to be explained, 175
predictions, 176–185
profit, excessive, 186
quality, 187
restricting competitive behavior, 187
shortage, 177, 182–183
supplier-induced demand, 187–188
supply shift
  price movements, 179–181
  quantity movements, 179–181
surplus, 177, 184
utilization, 179
Competitive price, defined, 397
Complement, defined, 397
Complementary commodity, demand, 59
Complication, defined, 397
Concurrent review, defined, 397
Conditions of entry, provider, 181
Conspiracy in restraint of trade, 362–363
Consumer choice, health care reform, 344–346
Consumer demand model, 60, 61–62, 253
  income, 253–254
  leisure time, 253–254
Consumer equilibrium, defined, 400
Consumer information, demand relationship, 62
Consumer taste, 88–89
  defined, 411
  demand, 60, 61–62
Consumerism, defined, 398
Consumer's surplus, defined, 397
Consumption, 30
  defined, 398
Contingent valuation
  cost-benefit analysis, techniques of valuation, 388–389
  defined, 398
Continuing care, defined, 398
Contract cost, 87
Cooperative pool, insurance market reform, 335
Copayment, 37, 82
  defined, 398
  Medicaid, 323
  Medicare, 40, 319
Core service, defined, 398
Cost, 44–49
  categorized, 45
  cost-effectiveness analysis, 382–383
  defined, 398
  health insurance, 118
  meanings, 44–45

monopolistic market, 204–205
output, relation, 99, 107, 128
profit, relation, 128
revenue
  relation, 128
  supply relation, 129–131
selected diseases, 48–49
Cost benefit, defined, 398
Cost curve
  defined, 398
  economy of scale, 117
  empirical estimation, 113–118
  group practice, 115–116
  hospital, 116–117
  marginal cost, 116–117
  nursing home, 117–118
  position, 108–110
Cost effectiveness, defined, 398
Cost function, defined, 398
Cost sharing, defined, 398
Cost shifting, defined, 398
Cost utility, defined, 398
Cost-benefit analysis, 376, 386–389
  contingent valuation, techniques of valuation,
    388–389
  cost-benefit ratio, 389
  human capital, 386–387
  risk preference, 387–388
  valuation of outcomes, 386
Cost-consequences analysis, 375
Cost-effectiveness analysis, 375
  cost, 382–383
  cost-effectiveness ratios, 383–384
  discounting future costs and benefits, 383
  effectiveness, 381
  efficacy, 381
  guidelines, 376–386
  interpreting results, 384–386
  outcomes, 378–380
  perspective, 377
  sensitivity analysis, 384
  time horizons, 378
Cost-minimization analysis, 376
Cost-of-illness study, 47–49
  incidence basis, 48
  prevalence basis, 48
Cost-output relation
  fixed cost, 103–104
  short-run, 103–108
  variable cost, 103–104
Cost-utility analysis, 375–376
Customary, prevailing, and reasonable, Medicare,
  151, 152

D

Day procedure group, defined, 399
Deductible, 71–73

defined, 399
Medicare, 319
Demand, 55–76. *See also* Specific type
  changes in, 58–60
  commodity, 56
  competitive labor market, 256–257
  complementary commodity, 59
  concept, 55–56
  consumer taste, 60
  defined, 399
  demand curve
    downward-sloping, 57
    labor, 250–251
  demand hypothesis, 56–57
  demand relationship, 57
  health, 85–86
  health insurance, 229–239
    assumptions of model, 229–230
    basic theory of demand, 229
    demand responsiveness to price, 236–237
    financial vulnerability factor, 232
    individual demand for insurance, 229–232
    limitations of theory, 232–233
    market demand for insurance, 233–234
    moral hazard, 234–236
    quantity demanded, 69–73
    risk aversion, 232
    risk perception factor, 232
  income, 58–59
  individual, 56–64
  labor, 249–252
    demand curve, 250–251
    effect of fringe benefits, 251–252
    firm's objectives, 250
    by individual firm, 249–252
    labor cost, 250
    marginal value product, 249–250
    market demand for labor, 252
    production function, 249, 250
    revenue derived from worker production,
      249–250
  measuring quantity responsiveness to price
    changes, 64–69
  medical care
    agency theory, 86–92
    demand for health promotion, 88–92
    discounting future values, 90–92
    external demand, 82–83
    influence of quality on, 83–84
    internal demand, 82
    private demand, 82
    social demand, 82–83
    supplier-induced demand, 86–92
    under uncertainty, 88–92
  monopolistic market, 203–204
  nursing home, 75–76
  out-of-pocket price, quantity demanded, 69–73
  price of related commodities, 59–60

price-quantity relation, 56–60
quantity demanded, 56–57, 58
simple model, 56–60
   behavioral assumption, 63
   shortcomings, 60–64
substitute commodity, 59–60
unit of measurement, 56
unitary elastic, 67
vertical demand curve, 57
Demand barrier, 285–286
Demand for health promotion, 88–92
Demand relationship, 57
   consumer information, 62
   consumer taste, 61–62
   deriving, 60–64
   health status, 61
   income, 62
   marginal utility, 61
   predictions, 63
   prices of other commodities, 62
   productivity of medical care, 62
   quality, 62
   utility maximization, 63
Demand shift
   competitive market model
      price movement, 178–179
      quantity movement, 178–179
      stable supply, 178
   simultaneous demand and supply shifts, 181, 182
Derived demand, 249
   defined, 399
Descriptive economics, 2
Diagnosis, defined, 399
Diagnosis-related group, 20, 38, 313
   breast disorder, 158
   case mix-adjusted admissions measure, 157–158
   defined, 399
   grouping diagnoses, 157–159
   hospital, 157–159
   medical education, 159
   Medicare, 157–159, 320
   outlier-related cost, 159
   Principal Inpatient Diagnostic Cost Group, 162
   reimbursement rate (standardized amount), 158–159
   relative weights, 157, 159
   setting rates, 157–159
   teaching hospital, 159
Diminishing marginal utility, 61
Direct cost, 45, 47
   defined, 399
Direct regulation, 350
Direct tax, 298
Direct teaching cost, defined, 399
Disability adjusted life expectancy, 26–27
Discharge planning, defined, 399
Discount, defined, 399
Disequilibrium, defined, 399

Distributional equity, 283–284
Downward-sloping demand curve, 57

E

Earned revenue, 127
Economic efficiency, 357
Economic evaluation, 374–389
   measures, 378
   purposes, 375
   study method selection, 375
   tools, 3–10
   types of comparative studies, 375
Economic profit, 104
Economic propositions, nature of, 8–10
Economic regulation, concept, 350–351
Economic Stabilization Program, monopolistic market, 208–210
Economic unit, 36–44
   employer, 38–39
   flows between units, 36–44
   flows in generic health care market, 37–38
   health maintenance organization, 41–42
   Medicaid, 40–41
   Medicare, 39–40
   preferred provider organization, 42–44
Economic variable, 3–8
   relations between economic variables, 4–8
      causal or noncausal, 4
      direction of relations, 5, 6
      graphic representation of relations, 5
      position of relations, 6–7, 8
      shape of relations, 7–8, 9
      slope of relations, 5–6, 7
Economics, 1–2
   descriptive economics, 2
   evaluative economics, 3
   explanatory economics, 2–3
   major tasks, 2–3
Economy of scale
   cost curve, 117
   defined, 400
   group practice, 115
   hospital, 117
   market, 213, 214
Economy of scope, 110–111
   complementary services, 111
   defined, 400
   diseconomies of scope, 111
Effectiveness
   cost-effectiveness analysis, 381
   defined, 400
Efficacy
   cost-effectiveness analysis, 381
   defined, 400
Efficiency
   community rating, 336
   efficient output levels, 271–280

Efficiency criterion, 270
    defined, 400
Elasticity of demand, defined, 400
Emergency care, defined, 400
Employee Retirement Income Security Act, 357
Employer coalition, 39
Encounter, defined, 400
Enforcement cost, 87
Episode of care, defined, 400
Episode of illness, defined, 400
Equality, 270, 271
Equilibrium, defined, 400
Equity
    community rating, 336
    concepts, 283–284
    defined, 400
    health policy
        of finance, 286–287
        of utilization, 286
Euroquol 5D, 25
Evaluative economics, 3
    value judgment, 269–287
Experience rating, 241
    defined, 401
Explanatory economics, 2–3
    purpose, 55
External benefits, 276
External demand, 82–83
External values, 276
Extra billing, defined, 401
Extra-welfarism, 270, 281–283

F

Federal Trade Commission Act, 362
Fee-for-service reimbursement, 148–150
    defined, 401
    fee schedule, 149–150
    Medicare, 312–313
    profit-maximizing model, 149
    relative value scale, 148–149
    supplier-induced demand, 87–88
    usual, customary, and reasonable reimbursement,
        149
15-D, 24–25
Firm, defined, 401
Fixed cost, 129, 131
    cost-output relation, 103–104
    defined, 401
Fixed input, 97–98
    defined, 401
Flat-of-the-curve medicine, 28
    defined, 401
Flow, 30
Food and Drug Administration, drug regulation,
    356
Free services, 45

Full cost, defined, 401
Funding, defined, 401

G

Global budget, defined, 401
Gross domestic product, defined, 401
Group model health maintenance organization,
    defined, 401
Group practice
    cost curve, 115–116
    defined, 401
    economy of scale, 115
Group rating, insurance market reform, 334

H

Health
    characteristics, 281
    defined, 401
    demand, 85–86
    labor market outcomes, 257–258
    medical care, relationship, 28–29
    valuation, 281–282
Health care
    defined, 402
    output, 17–30
    resources distributed according to need, 282–283
    too much, 1
    uncovered care, 313–314
Health care expenditure, 45–46
    growth, 1, 45, 46
    per capita, 46–47
    percent of gross domestic product, 46–47, 48
    by type of service, 46
    U.S. *vs.* other countries, 47, 48
Health care financing, 291–304
    alternative types
        administrative cost, 304
        incidence, 301–304
    burdens, 292–293
    economic analysis of alternative payment
        sources, 293–300
    means, 292–293
Health care reform, 330–346
    consumer choice, 344–346
    information, 344–346
    managed care, 338–344
Health insurance, 228–245. *See also* Insurance
    market reform
    adverse selection, 239, 242–244
    choice of health plan, 237–239
        biased selection, 237–238
    community rating, 238
    cost, 118
    defined, 402
    demand, 229–239
        assumptions of model, 229–230

basic theory of demand, 229
demand responsiveness to price, 236–237
financial vulnerability factor, 232
individual demand for insurance, 229–232
limitations of theory, 232–233
market demand for insurance, 233–234
moral hazard, 234–236
quantity demanded, 69–73
risk aversion, 232
risk perception factor, 232
distribution issues, 22
employer-provided, 38–39
income tax, 38–39
indemnity insurer regulatory controls, 44, 45
labor supply, 255–256
mandated benefit, 296–297
moral hazard, 281
optimal, 280–281
premium, 294
private, 293, 294–297
public, 307–324
trends, 314–317
regulation, 356–357
risk shifting, 21–23
cost sharing, 22
methods, 22
supply, 239–242
community rating, 241
experience rating, 241
insurer costs, 240–241
insurer revenues, 241
law of large numbers, 240
risk and insured population size, 240
supplier behavior, 239–240
supply predictions, 241–242
triple option package, 44
utility, 280
Health Insurance Experiment, 74–75
Health insurance purchasing coalition, 39
Health insurance purchasing cooperative,
defined, 402
Health insurer, antitrust policy, 360–361
Health maintenance organization, 339. See also
Managed care
average adjusted per capita cost, 161–162
capitation, 161
defined, 402
economic unit, 41–42
group model, 339
growth, 343–344
indemnity insurer regulatory controls, 44, 45
information asymmetry, 163
Medicare, 161–162
network model, 339
physician profiling, 44
provider optimal compensation, 164–165
services, 163–164
staff model, 339

supply incentives, 161
Health plan, defined, 402
Health policy
adequacy of supply, 286
demand barrier, 285–286
efficiency, 285–287
environmental conditions, 285
equity
of finance, 286–287
of utilization, 286
goals, 285–287
population health status, 287
public financial constraints, 287
quality, 286
technical efficiency, 286
Health promotion, defined, 402
Health promotion behavior, 88–92
discounting future values, 90–92
model limitations, 90
Health status, 23–30
concepts, 23
demand relationship, 61
individual health measures, 23–25
outcome, 27–29
population health measures, 25–27
Health technology, defined, 402
Health technology assessment, defined, 402
Health United States, output measurement
sources, 19
Health Utilities Index, 25
Health-related quality of life, 25
defined, 402
Herfindahl Index, defined, 402
Home care, defined, 402
Home support, defined, 402
Horizontal equity, 284
defined, 402
Horizontal integration, 36
defined, 403
Hospice, defined, 403
Hospital, 20
antitrust policy, 359–360
case mix-adjusted admissions measure, 157–158
cost curve, 116–117
diagnosis-related group, 157–159
economy of scale, 117
Hospital Intensity Index, 20–21
hospitalization rate, 25–26
marginal cost, 116–117
nonprofit *vs.* for-profit hospital, 142
output, 19
components, 21
measures, 20
Hospital Insurance Trust Fund, Medicare, 39
disbursements, 314–315, 316
Hospital Intensity Index, 20–21
Hospital reimbursement, 153–157
agency theory, 154–156

per case payment, 155–156
per case reimbursement with adjustment for
  outliers, 156
per diem fee, 155
prospective fee-for-service system, 155
retrospective payments, 154–155
all-payer system *vs.* multipayer system, 156
alternative bases of reimbursement, 153–154
  prospective, 154
  retrospective, 153–154
per admission reimbursement, 154
per diem reimbursement, 154
per service reimbursement, 154
prospective reimbursement experiments, 156–157
regulation, 353
  demand side regulation, 354
  hospital quality, 353
  supply side regulation, 353–354
Human capital, 30
Human capital approach, defined, 403

I

Incentive
  agency theory
    health maintenance organization, 163–165
    managed care, 163–165
  input-output relation, 101
Incidence, defined, 403
Income
  consumer demand model, 253–254
  demand, 58–59
  demand relationship, 62
Income tax, 38–39, 303
Incremental cost, defined, 403
Indemnity, defined, 403
Independent practice association, 42, 339
  defined, 403
Indigent, defined, 403
Indirect cost, 45, 47–48
  defined, 403
Indirect regulation, 350
Indirect tax, 298
Indirect teaching cost, defined, 403
Individual supply, competitive market model,
  176, 177
Individual supply curve, market supply curve,
  derivation of market supply curve, 134–135
Indivisibility, 108
Information, health care reform, 344–346
Information asymmetry
  health maintenance organization, 163
  insurance market reform, 333
Information symmetry, 332
Input-output relation
  basic relationship, 97–100
  incentive system, 101
  production, 97–103

quality, 100
relationship shifts, 100–101
substitution among inputs, 101–102
volume-outcome relationship, 102–103
Insurance market reform, 331–338
  adverse selection, 333, 334
  basic model, 331–333
  biased selection, 335–336
  community rating, 335–336
  cooperative pool, 335
  group rating, 334
  information asymmetry, 333
  mandate, 337
  need for, 331
  preferred risk selection, 334
  risk adjustment, 337–338
  risk selection limitation, 337–338
  subsidies, 334–335
  underwriting, 334
Intensity of care, defined, 403
Intensive care, defined, 403
Intergenerational equity, 284
Intermediate care facility, defined, 403
International Classification of Diseases, Ninth
  Revision, Clinical Modification (ICD-9-CM),
  defined, 403
Interpersonal comparison, 89
Intervention, defined, 404
Investment, 30
  defined, 404

J

Joint Commission on Accreditation of Healthcare
  Organizations, 353

L

Labor
  demand, 249–252
    demand curve, 250–251
    effect of fringe benefits, 251–252
    firm's objectives, 250
    by individual firm, 249–252
    labor cost, 250
    marginal value product, 249–250
    market demand for labor, 252
    monopolistic seller, 261, 262
    production function, 249, 250
    revenue derived from worker production,
      249–250
  supply, 252–256
    alternative labor supply curves, 254–255
    consumer demand model, 253
    health insurance benefits, 255–256
    impact of health, 257–258
    individual labor supply, 252–255
    market supply of labor, 256

wages, substitution effect of income for leisure, 254–255
Labor market, 248–262
  effect of mandated insurance coverage, 296–297
  market power, 259–262
    buyer's market power, 259–261
    revenues, 259–260
    supplier cost, 259, 260
    unions as monopoly sellers, 261–262
  occupational risk, 258–259
Law of large numbers, 240
Leisure time, consumer demand model, 253–254
Life expectancy, 26–27
Loading charge, defined, 404
Long run, defined, 404
Long-run analysis, 112
  competitive market model, 180–181
Long-run average cost curve, short-run average cost curve, 112–113
  relation, 112
Long-run cost curve, 112–113
  defined, 404
Long-term care, defined, 404
Long-term care facility, regulation, 353, 355
Long-term care facility reimbursement, 160–161
  per diem basis, 160
  Resource Utilization Group, 160–161
Lost-productivity cost, 45

M

Managed care, 338–344. *See also* health maintenance organization
  antitrust policy, 360–361, 368–369
  characterized, 44
  control of resource use, 340–341
  defined, 404
  health care reform, 338–344
  managed care organization types, 339–344
  market experience, 343–344
  Medicaid, 323–324
  Medicare, 309–310, 313, 320–322
  provider, 163–166
    agency theory and incentive contracts, 163–165
    compensation forms compared, 164–165
    management of provider behavior, 165–166
  quality, 341–343
  regulation, 356–357
  resource use, 341–343
  satisfaction, 341–343
  services, 163–164
Managed competition, defined, 404
Mandate
  defined, 404
  insurance market reform, 337
Mandated benefit
  economic analysis, 296–297

health insurance, 296–297
Marginal cost, 104
  average cost, relation, 106–108
  cost curve, 116–117
    shifts, 133–134
  defined, 404
  hospital, 116–117
  production, 105–106, 107
Marginal factor cost, monopsony, 212
Marginal out-of-pocket price, 71–73
Marginal product, 98–100
Marginal productivity, defined, 404
Marginal revenue, 127–129
  defined, 404
Marginal utility
  demand relationship, 61
  per dollar of expenditure, 63
Marginal valuation, 272
Marginal value product, 249–250
  defined, 404
Market. *See also* Specific type
  characterized, 174–175
  defined, 404
  economy of scale, 213, 214
  input prices and taxes, 215
  pricing, 213–215
  regulation, 215
  structure, 212–217
    defined, 404
    determinants, 213
Market concentration, 212–213
  defined, 397
  Herfindahl-Hirschman Index, 364–365
Market demand, 64, 65
  competitive market model, 176, 177
Market equilibrium, defined, 400
Market power, 202–222
  characterized, 202
  importance, 202–203
  increased concentration, 221–222
  labor market, 259–262
    buyer's market power, 259–261
    revenues, 259–260
    supplier cost, 259, 260
    unions as monopoly sellers, 261–262
  monopolistic competition, 218–222
  nonprice competition, 217–222
  physician services market, 216–217
  teaching hospital, 216–217
Market price, competitive market model, 176–178
Market supply, 134–135
  competitive market model, 176, 177
Market supply analysis, nonprofit agency, 137–138
Market supply curve, individual supply curve, derivation of market supply curve, 134–135
Medicaid, 40–41, 310–311
  Aid to Families with Dependent Children, 310
  competitive bidding by suppliers, 323

copayment, 323
defined, 405
managed care, 323–324
medically needy, 310
monopolistic market, 208–210
policy alternatives, 322–324
program scope, 322–323
provider payment, 323
services covered, 311
Supplemental Security Income, 310
who is covered, 310
Medical association, 216–217
Medical care, 18–21
  ability to improve health, 81
  defined, 405
  demand
    agency theory, 86–92
    demand for health promotion, 88–92
    discounting future values, 90–92
    external demand, 82–83
    influence of quality on, 83–84
    internal demand, 82
    private demand, 82
    social demand, 82–83
    supplier-induced demand, 86–92
    under uncertainty, 88–92
  health, relationship, 28–29
  multiperiod analysis, 81–82
  output measurement sources, 19
Medical education, 30
  diagnosis-related group, 159
  Medicare, 159
Medical profession
  competitive practices, 216–217
  control mechanism, 216
Medically needy, Medicaid, 310
Medicare, 39–40, 293, 308–310
  competition, 320–322
  copayment, 40, 319
  customary, prevailing, and reasonable, 151, 152
  deductible, 319
  defined, 405
  diagnosis-related group, 157–159, 320
  economic analysis, 318–319
  fee-for-service, 312–313
  financing, 308–309
  gaps in coverage, 314
  goals, 317–318
  health maintenance organization, 161–162
  Hospital Insurance Trust Fund, 39
    disbursements, 314–315, 316
  managed care, 309–310, 313, 320–322
  medical education, 159
  monopolistic market, 208–210
  outlier-related cost, 159
  out-of-pocket expenditures, 316–317
  Part A, 39–40
  Part B, 40

policy alternatives, 318–322
premium, 319
Principal Inpatient-Diagnostic Cost Group, 162
program scope, 319
prospective payment system, 313
provider payment, 312–313, 320
services covered, 308, 309
supplementary medical insurance, 308, 310
who is covered, 308
Medicare + Choice, 162, 320–321
defined, 405
Medigap insurance, 22–23, 40, 293, 311–312
defined, 405
Merger
  antitrust policy, 363–366
  pharmaceutical industry, 366
  state government, 366
Money cost, 84–85
  defined, 405
Monitoring cost, 87
Monopoly, 203–210, 358
  antitrust policy, 366–368
  Blue Shield, 208–210
  cost, 204–205
  deadweight loss due to monopoly, 358
  defined, 405
  demand, 203–204
  Economic Stabilization Program, 208–210
  market power, 218–222
  Medicaid, 208–210
  Medicare, 208–210
  nursing home, 210
  preferred provider organization, 219–221
  price discrimination, 206–208
  public program, 208–210
    physician pricing and supply, 208–210
  simple monopoly, 203
Monopsony, 210–212
  basic model, 210–212
  defined, 405
  marginal factor cost, 212
Moral hazard, 86–87, 234–236, 281
  defined, 405
Morbidity, 23
  defined, 405
Morbidity rate, 25–26
Mortality, 23
  defined, 405
Mortality rate, 25–26
Most responsible diagnosis, defined, 405
Multimarket analysis, competitive market model, 184–185
Multiproduct firm, defined, 405
Mundt Resolution, 217

N

National Health Interview Survey, 19

National Practitioner Data Base, 355
Need, defined, 405
Network, defined, 405
Nonpatient revenue, 133
Nonprice competition
  antitrust policy, 368
  market power, 217–222
  quality, 222
Nonprofit agency
  board of trustees, 136, 140
  market supply analysis, 137–138
  supply behavior
    administrator as agent model, 140–142
    output maximization hypothesis, 135–138
Nonprofit (not-for-profit), defined, 406
Normal profit, 104
Nursing home
  cost curve, 117–118
  defined, 406
  demand, 75–76
  monopolistic market, 210

O

Occupational risk, labor market, 258–259
Oligopolistic market, 221, 358–359
Opportunity cost, 45, 84–85
  defined, 406
Outcome, 18, 83
  confounding factors, 27
  measurement problems, 27–28
Outlier, defined, 406
Outlier-related cost
  diagnosis-related group, 159
  Medicare, 159
Outlying day, 159
Out-of-pocket payment, 37
Out-of-pocket price
  defined, 406
  demand, quantity demanded, 69–73
Outpatient care, defined, 406
Output
  case mix dimension, 111
  classes, 30
  cost, relation, 99, 107, 128
  cross-sectional comparisons, 19
  defined, 406
  efficient output level, 271–280
    alternative delivery arrangements, 278–280
    individual valuations of commodities or
      activities, 271–272
  measurements, 18–19
  output maximization hypothesis, 135–138
  product line dimension, 111
  profit, relation, 128
  revenue, relation, 128
  technical efficiency assumption, 274
  time series comparisons, 19

P

Paretean system, 271, 281–282
Patient, volume, 98
Patient day, defined, 406
Patient revenue, 127
Payroll tax, 298–300, 302
Peer review organization, 355
Per admission reimbursement, hospital, 154
Per capita payment, 150
  defined, 406
Per case payment, 150, 155–156
  with adjustment for outliers, 156
Per diem payment, 155
  defined, 406
  hospital, 154
Per service payment, hospital, 154
Perspective, defined, 406
Pharmaceutical industry
  antitrust policy, 361
  merger, 366
Pharmacist, state regulation, 356
Philanthropy, 275, 278, 279–280
Physical capital, 30
Physician
  antitrust policy, 360
  market power, 216–217
  monopoly, 208–210
  price formation, 193–195
  procedures or services, 20
  profiling by health maintenance organization, 44
  regulation, 355
    pricing, 355
    quality, 355
    services, 355
    utilization, 355
Physician reimbursement, 148–153
  agency theory, 151
Physician visit, 18–19
Plant, defined, 406
Point elasticity formula, 66
Point-of-service plan, defined, 406
Potential years of life lost, 25–26
Preadmission certification, defined, 406
Preferred provider organization, 339
  defined, 406
  economic unit, 42–44
  monopolistic competition, 219–221
Preferred risk selection, insurance market
  reform, 334
Premium, 21–22, 37, 293, 302
  defined, 407
  health insurance, 294
  Medicare, 319
  taxation, 294–296
Prepaid group practice, defined, 407
Prescription drug, 317
Prevention, defined, 407

Preventive medicine, defined, 407
Price
  competitive market model, 178–181
  defined, 407
  demand shift, 178–179
  insurance demand, 236–237
  of other commodities, demand relationship, 62
  physician services, 193–195
  price change effect on demand, 64–69
  profit-maximizing supply points at alternative
    prices, 132
  supply shift, 179–181
Price collusion, 221
Price discrimination
  defined, 407
  monopolistic market, 206–208
Price elasticity of demand, 66
  controlled experiment, 73–75
  estimates, 73–76
  natural experiments, 73, 74
Price fixing, 362–363
Price taker, defined, 407
Price-quality competition, 217–222
Pricing
  market, 213–215
  nonprofit *vs.* for-profit hospital, 142
Primary care, defined, 407
Principal, defined, 407
Principal diagnosis, defined, 407
Principal Inpatient Diagnostic Cost Group,
  313, 321
  diagnosis-related group, 162
  Medicare, 162
Principal-agent relationship, 86
  among payers and providers, 148
  reimbursement, 148
Procedure, defined, 407
Process, 18, 83
Producer equilibrium, defined, 400
Product differentiation, 187
Production
  average cost, 106–108
  defined, 407
  input-output relation, 97–103
  marginal cost, 105–106, 107
  process, 98
  total cost, 104–105
  volume-outcome relationship, 102–103
Production function, defined, 407
Productivity, defined, 407
Productivity of medical care, demand
  relationship, 62
Products of ambulatory care, defined, 408
Products of ambulatory surgery, defined, 408
Profit
  competitive market model, excessive profits, 186
  cost, relation, 128
  defined, 408

  normal, 104
  output, relation, 128
  profit-maximizing supply points at alternative
    prices, 132
Profit-maximizing model, fee-for-service
  reimbursement, 149
Prospective fee-for-service system, 155
Prospective payment
  defined, 408
  Medicare, 313
Provider
  conditions of entry, 181
  defined, 408
  managed care, 163–166
    agency theory and incentive contracts,
      163–165
    compensation forms compared, 164–165
    management of provider behavior, 165–166
Provider equilibrium, defined, 400
Provider payment, 147–167
  Medicaid, 323
  Medicare, 312–313, 320
Public health, defined, 408
Public ownership, 350
Public program, monopolistic market, 208–210
  physician pricing and supply, 208–210

Q

Quality of care, 18, 286, 352, 353, 355
  antitrust policy, 368
  aspects, 18
  competitive market model, 187
  defined, 408
  demand relationship, 62
  hospital, 20
    Hospital Intensity Index, 20–21
  influence on demand, 83–84
  input-output relation, 100
  managed care, 341–343
  meaning, 18
  measuring, 18–19
  nonprice competition, 222
  quantity, trade-off, 138, 140
  supply, 138–140
    supply model, 138–140
Quality of life, 24
  defined, 408
Quality-adjusted life year, 25
  defined, 408
Quantity, quality, trade-off, 138, 140
Quantity demanded, defined, 408
Quantity supplied, defined, 408

R

Rand Health Insurance Experiment, 82
Rate, defined, 408

Rate setting, defined, 408
Ratio of marginal utility to price, 63
Referral, 217
Refined diagnosis-related group, defined, 408
Regulation, 350–357
    to correct market failure, 351–352
    defined, 408
    economic regulation, 350–351
    Food and Drug Administration, 356
    forms, 350
    health insurance, 44, 45, 356–357
    health maintenance organization, 44, 45
    hospital, 353
        demand side regulation, 354
        hospital quality, 353
        supply side regulation, 353–354
    long-term care facility, 353, 355
    managed care, 356–357
    market, 215
    pharmaceutical industry, 355–356
    pharmacist, state regulation, 356
    physician, 355
        pricing, 355
        quality, 355
        services, 355
        utilization, 355
    as political good, 352
Reimbursement, 37–38. See also Specific type
    defined, 409
    principal-agent relationship, 148
    system impact on physician practices, 150
Relative value, defined, 409
Relative value scale, fee-for-service reimbursement,
    148–149
Resource, defined, 409
Resource allocation
    altruism, 275–278
    socially optimum quantity of medical care,
        274–275
Resource intensive weight, defined, 409
Resource use, managed care, 341–343
Resource utilization group
    defined, 409
    long-term care facility reimbursement, 160–161
Resource-based relative value system, 150,
    151–153, 313
    defined, 409
    development, 151
    supply analysis, 152–153
Retrospective payment, 154–155
    defined, 409
Retrospective review, defined, 409
Returns to scale, defined, 409
Revenue
    cost
        relation, 128
        supply relation, 129–131
    defined, 409

output, relation, 128
Right to health care, 271
Risk, defined, 409
Risk adjustment, insurance market reform, 337–338
Risk averse, 89
    defined, 409
Risk factor, defined, 410
Risk neutral, defined, 410
Risk pooling, 22
    defined, 410
Risk selection limitation, insurance market reform,
    337–338
Risk shifting, health insurance, 21–23
    cost sharing, 22
    methods, 22
Risk taker, defined, 410

S

Salary reimbursement, 150
Sales tax, 300, 301, 302–303
Satisfaction, managed care, 341–343
Scarcity, 1
Schedule demand curve, defined, 399
Search cost, 87
Second surgical opinion, defined, 410
Secondary care, defined, 410
Selective contracting, defined, 410
Sensitivity analysis
    cost-effectiveness analysis, 384
    defined, 410
Sherman Act, 361, 366, 367
Short run, defined, 410
Shortage
    competitive market model, 177, 182–183
    defined, 410
Short-run average cost curve, long-run average cost
    curve, 112–113
    relation, 112
Short-run cost curve, defined, 410
Signout case, defined, 410
Single-payer system, defined, 410
Single-product firm, defined, 410
Skilled nursing facility, defined, 410
Social cost, 47
    defined, 410
Solo practice, defined, 410
Staff model health maintenance organization,
    defined, 410
Standardized mortality rate, defined, 411
Stock, 30
Structure, 18, 83
Substitute, defined, 411
Substitute commodity, demand, 59–60
Substitution effect
    defined, 411
    of income for leisure, 254–255
Supplemental medical insurance, 40

expenditures, 315
revenues, 315
Supplemental Security Income, Medicaid, 310
Supplier-induced demand, 30, 86–92
  competitive market model, 187–188
  defined, 411
  fee-for-service, 87–88
  objectives, 191–193
  pedagogic model, 190–191
  supply, 191
Supply
  competitive labor market, 256–257
  defined, 411
  health insurance, 239–242
    community rating, 241
    experience rating, 241
    insurer costs, 240–241
    insurer revenues, 241
    law of large numbers, 240
    risk and insured population size, 240
    supplier behavior, 239–240
    supply predictions, 241–242
  labor, 252–256
    alternative labor supply curves, 254–255
    consumer demand model, 253
    health insurance benefits, 255–256
    impact of health, 257–258
    individual labor supply, 252–255
    market supply of labor, 256
  quality, 138–140
    supply model, 138–140
Supply analysis, resource-based relative value scale, 152–153
Supply behavior model
  basic model, 127–133
  individual for-profit company, 127
  nonpatient revenue, 133
  nonprofit agency
    administrator as agent model, 140–142
    output maximization hypothesis, 135–138
  supply curve shifts, 133–134
Supply curve
  defined, 411
  physician services, 152–153
Supply function, defined, 411
Supply shift
  competitive market model
    price movements, 179–181
    quantity movements, 179–181
  simultaneous demand and supply shifts, 181, 182
Surplus
  competitive market model, 177, 184
  defined, 411
Survival time, 25

T

Taxation, 251–252, 293

direct tax, 298
health care funding, 298–300, 301
income tax, 38–39, 303
indirect tax, 298
payroll tax, 298–300, 302
premium, 294–296
Teaching hospital, 30. *See also* Medical education
  diagnosis-related group, 159
  market power, 216–217
Technical efficiency, 357
Technical efficiency assumption, 274
Tertiary care, defined, 411
Third-party payment, defined, 411
Time cost, 84–85
  defined, 411
Time discount, defined, 399
Total cost
  behavior, 104
  components, 154
  defined, 412
  production, 104–105
  total cost curve, 104
  total fixed cost, defined, 412
  total variable cost, defined, 412
Total product, defined, 412
Transaction cost, defined, 412
Transfer case, defined, 412
Transfer payment, defined, 412
Trim point, defined, 412
Typical patient, defined, 412

U

Underwriting, insurance market reform, 334
Uninsured population, 1, 313–314
Union
  labor market effects, 261–262
  as monopoly sellers of labor, 261–262
Unitary elastic, 67
Usual, customary, and reasonable reimbursement, 149
Utility, 61
  defined, 412
  health insurance, 280
  wealth, 230–232
    financial vulnerability factor, 232
    limitations of theory, 232–233
    relationship, 89
    risk aversion, 232
    risk perception factor, 232
Utilization
  competitive market model, 179
  defined, 412
Utilization management, defined, 412

V

Valuation

alternative delivery arrangements, 278–280
altruism, 275–278
competitive market with no philanthropy, 278
competitive market with philanthropy, 278–280
contingent, 388
free and unlimited care, 278
health, 281–282
individual valuations of commodities or
    activities, 271–272
marginal valuation, 272
private (or internal) valuation, 272
socially optimum quantity of medical care,
    274–275
techniques, 388–389
values in selfish market, 272–274
Value judgment
defined, 412
evaluative economics, 269–287
Value system
alternative, 270–271
ranking schemes, 271
Values, ways of deriving
delegatory or top-down, 270
participatory or bottom-up, 270
Variable cost, 129, 131
cost-output relation, 103–104

defined, 413
Variable input, 97–98, 129
defined, 413
Vertical demand curve, 57
Vertical equity, 284
defined, 413
Vertical integration, defined, 413
Volume, defined, 413
Volume-outcome relationship
input-output relation, 102–103
production, 102–103

W

Wage rate, competitive labor market, 256–257
Wages, substitution effect of income for leisure,
    254–255
Wants, 60
defined, 413
Wealth, utility, 230–232
financial vulnerability factor, 232
limitations of theory, 232–233
relationship, 89
risk aversion, 232
risk perception factor, 232
Willingness-to-pay approach, defined, 413